Nutra-Cosmeceuticals from Algae for Health and Wellness

Nutra-Cosmeceuticals from Algae for Health and Wellness

Editors

**María Lourdes Mourelle
Herminia Domínguez
Jose Luis Legido**

MDPI • Basel • Beijing • Wuhan • Barcelona • Belgrade • Manchester • Tokyo • Cluj • Tianjin

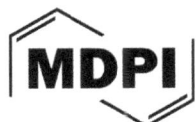

Editors
María Lourdes Mourelle
Department of Applied Physics,
Universidad de Vigo
Spain

Herminia Domínguez
CINBIO, Departamento de
Enxeñería Química,
Facultade de Ciencias,
Universidade de Vigo
(Campus Ourense)
Spain

Jose Luis Legido
Department of Applied Physics,
Universidad de Vigo
Spain

Editorial Office
MDPI
St. Alban-Anlage 66
4052 Basel, Switzerland

This is a reprint of articles from the Special Issue published online in the open access journal *Marine Drugs* (ISSN 1660-3397) (available at: http://www.mdpi.com).

For citation purposes, cite each article independently as indicated on the article page online and as indicated below:

LastName, A.A.; LastName, B.B.; LastName, C.C. Article Title. *Journal Name* **Year**, *Volume Number*, Page Range.

ISBN 978-3-0365-3204-2 (Hbk)
ISBN 978-3-0365-3205-9 (PDF)

© 2022 by the authors. Articles in this book are Open Access and distributed under the Creative Commons Attribution (CC BY) license, which allows users to download, copy and build upon published articles, as long as the author and publisher are properly credited, which ensures maximum dissemination and a wider impact of our publications.

The book as a whole is distributed by MDPI under the terms and conditions of the Creative Commons license CC BY-NC-ND.

Contents

About the Editors vii

Preface to "Nutra-Cosmeceuticals from Algae for Health and Wellness" ix

Ana Regueiras, Álvaro Huguet, Tiago Conde, Daniela Couto, Pedro Domingues,
Maria Rosário Domingues, Ana Margarida Costa, Joana Laranjeira da Silva,
Vitor Vasconcelos and Ralph Urbatzka
Potential Anti-Obesity, Anti-Steatosis, and Anti-Inflammatory Properties of Extracts from the
Microalgae *Chlorella vulgaris* and *Chlorococcum amblystomatis* under Different Growth Conditions
Reprinted from: *Mar. Drugs* 2022, 20, 9, doi:10.3390/md20010009 1

Ratih Pangestuti, Monjurul Haq, Puji Rahmadi and Byung-Soo Chun
Nutritional Value and Biofunctionalities of Two Edible Green Seaweeds (*Ulva lactuca* and
Caulerpa racemosa) from Indonesia by Subcritical Water Hydrolysis
Reprinted from: *Mar. Drugs* 2021, 19, 578, doi:10.3390/md19100578 17

Marta Salvador Ferreira, Diana I. S. P. Resende, José M. Sousa Lobo, Emília Sousa and
Isabel F. Almeida
Marine Ingredients for Sensitive Skin: Market Overview
Reprinted from: *Mar. Drugs* 2021, 19, 464, doi:10.3390/md19080464 35

Yerin Jin, Sora Yu, Dong Hyun Kim, Eun Ju Yun and Kyoung Heon Kim
Characterization of Neoagarooligosaccharide Hydrolase BpGH117 from a Human Gut
Bacterium *Bacteroides plebeius*
Reprinted from: *Mar. Drugs* 2021, 19, 271, doi:10.3390/md19050271 51

Eun Ju Yun, Sora Yu, Young-Ah Kim, Jing-Jing Liu, Nam Joo Kang, Yong-Su Jin and
Kyoung Heon Kim
In Vitro Prebiotic and Anti-Colon Cancer Activities of Agar-Derived Sugars from Red Seaweeds
Reprinted from: *Mar. Drugs* 2021, 19, 213, doi:10.3390/md19040213 65

João Cotas, Diana Pacheco, Glacio Souza Araujo, Ana Valado, Alan T. Critchley and
Leonel Pereira
On the Health Benefits vs. Risks of Seaweeds and Their Constituents: The Curious Case of the
Polymer Paradigm
Reprinted from: *Mar. Drugs* 2021, 19, 164, doi:10.3390/md19030164 79

M. Lourdes Mourelle, Carmen P. Gómez and José L. Legido
Microalgal Peloids for Cosmetic and Wellness Uses
Reprinted from: *Mar. Drugs* 2021, 19, 666, doi:10.3390/md19120666 99

Lucía López-Hortas, Noelia Flórez-Fernández, Maria D. Torres, Tania Ferreira-Anta,
María P. Casas, Elena M. Balboa, Elena Falqué and Herminia Domínguez
Applying Seaweed Compounds in Cosmetics, Cosmeceuticals and Nutricosmetics
Reprinted from: *Mar. Drugs* 2021, 19, 552, doi:10.3390/md19100552 115

Javier Echave, Maria Fraga-Corral, Pascual Garcia-Perez, Jelena Popović-Djordjević,
Edina H. Avdović, Milanka Radulović, Jianbo Xiao, Miguel A. Prieto and
Jesus Simal-Gandara
Seaweed Protein Hydrolysates and Bioactive Peptides: Extraction, Purification, and
Applications
Reprinted from: *Mar. Drugs* 2021, 19, 500, doi:10.3390/md19090500 145

About the Editors

María Lourdes Mourelle received her Degree in Pharmacy from the University of Santiago de Compostela and received her PhD in Applied Physics from the University of Vigo. She belongs to the research group FA2 of Applied Physics (University of Vigo), where she works in the field of thermalism, peloids, thalassotherapy, and wellness, as well as researching algae and microalgae for wellness and cosmetic uses.

Herminia Domínguez received her PhD in Chemistry from the University of Santiago de Compostela. She is professor of Chemical Engineering at University of Vigo, Campus Ourense (Spain), where she has been working on the extraction of bioactive compounds from underutilized and residual sources using green technologies; she has a particular interest in pressurized solvent extraction and membrane technology.

José Luis Legido received his Degree in Chemistry and PhD in Physics from the University of Santiago de Compostela. He is a professor of Applied Physics at University of Vigo, where he has been working on the thermophysical characterization of complex materials, such as thermal peloids, for therapeutic and cosmetic applications.

Preface to "Nutra-Cosmeceuticals from Algae for Health and Wellness"

The increase in the life expectancy of the population has led to growing interest, that of both consumers and public administrations, in health and well-being through physical activity, a balanced diet, and the use of functional foods and nutraceuticals. Well-being activities also include care in thermal centers and wellness centers in general.

The Global Wellness Institute (GWS) defines wellness as "the active search of activities, options and lifestyles that lead to a holistic state of health". Accordingly, wellness is not a passive state, but instead, an "active exercise", associated with intentions, options encountered, and actions taken as people work towards an optimum state of health and wellness. Wellness is related to holistic health, which has many different dimensions (physical, mental, environmental, spiritual, emotional, and social) that should work together in harmony. Within the context of an integrative and holistic wellness, nutrition is one of the pillars of well-being, and algae and microalgae contribute to this objective; although, this should not only be seen from the point of view of food consumed, but also should also encompass preventive treatments through water and its derivatives, such as peloids and marine muds (thermal spa centers and thalassotherapy centers), and the activities that take place around them.

Algae and microalgae have been consumed for centuries by different cultures and along coasts and lakes worldwide. Their nutritional importance lies not only in the macronutrients (proteins, soluble and insoluble carbohydrates, polyunsaturated fatty acids) and micronutrients (vitamins, minerals) they contain, but also in a variety of different compounds, such as fucoidans, carotenoids, polyphenols, and phlorotannins—some of which are exclusively found in these organisms. Edible algae are included in the diet in different forms (salads, soups, stews, as condiments, etc.), but are also increasingly included—the algae as a whole or some of its phytochemicals—in nutritional supplements and nutraceuticals with different purposes; these include the prevention of cardiovascular disorders, the regulation of glucose levels, as modulators of the immune response, and as antioxidants, among other purposes. Likewise, algae and microalgae have become an important source of active ingredients for cosmetics and dermocosmetics because they are an abundant resource and, in the case of microalgae, they are easy to cultivate.

Within this abundant context, this Special Issue presents the nutritional and bio-functional contributions of microalgal and macroalgal compounds to human health and wellness.

María Lourdes Mourelle, Herminia Domínguez, Jose Luis Legido
Editors

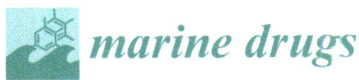

Article

Potential Anti-Obesity, Anti-Steatosis, and Anti-Inflammatory Properties of Extracts from the Microalgae *Chlorella vulgaris* and *Chlorococcum amblystomatis* under Different Growth Conditions

Ana Regueiras [1,2], Álvaro Huguet [1], Tiago Conde [3], Daniela Couto [3,4], Pedro Domingues [3,4], Maria Rosário Domingues [3,4], Ana Margarida Costa [5], Joana Laranjeira da Silva [5], Vitor Vasconcelos [1,2] and Ralph Urbatzka [1,*]

[1] Blue Biotechnology and Ecotoxicology Group, CIIMAR/CIMAR, Interdisciplinary Centre of Marine and Environmental Research, Terminal de Cruzeiros do Porto de Leixões, University of Porto, 4450-208 Matosinhos, Portugal; aregueiras@ciimar.up.pt (A.R.); alvarohl96@gmail.com (Á.H.); vmvascon@fc.up.pt (V.V.)

[2] Departamento de Biologia, Faculdade de Ciências, Universidade do Porto, Rua do Campo Alegre, Edifício FC4, 4169-007 Porto, Portugal

[3] Mass Spectrometry Centre, LAQV-REQUIMTE, Department of Chemistry, University of Aveiro, Santiago University Campus, 3810-193 Aveiro, Portugal; tiagoalexandreconde@ua.pt (T.C.); danielacouto@ua.pt (D.C.); p.domingues@ua.pt (P.D.); mrd@ua.pt (M.R.D.)

[4] CESAM—Centre for Environmental and Marine Studies, Department of Chemistry, University of Aveiro, Santiago University Campus, 3810-193 Aveiro, Portugal

[5] Allmicroalgae, R&D Department, Rua 25 de Abril, 2445-287 Pataias, Portugal; margarida.costa@niva.no (A.M.C.); joana.g.silva@allmicroalgae.com (J.L.d.S.)

* Correspondence: rurbatzka@ciimar.up.pt

Citation: Regueiras, A.; Huguet Á.; Conde, T.; Couto, D.; Domingues, P.; Domingues, M.R.; Costa, A.M.; Silva, J.L.d.; Vasconcelos, V.; Urbatzka, R. Potential Anti-Obesity, Anti-Steatosis, and Anti-Inflammatory Properties of Extracts from the Microalgae *Chlorella vulgaris* and *Chlorococcum amblystomatis* under Different Growth Conditions. *Mar. Drugs* **2022**, *20*, 9. https://doi.org/10.3390/md20010009

Academic Editors: María Lourdes Mourelle, Herminia Domínguez and Jose Luis Legido

Received: 16 November 2021
Accepted: 20 December 2021
Published: 22 December 2021

Publisher's Note: MDPI stays neutral with regard to jurisdictional claims in published maps and institutional affiliations.

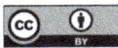

Copyright: © 2021 by the authors. Licensee MDPI, Basel, Switzerland. This article is an open access article distributed under the terms and conditions of the Creative Commons Attribution (CC BY) license (https:// creativecommons.org/licenses/by/ 4.0/).

Abstract: Microalgae are known as a producer of proteins and lipids, but also of valuable compounds for human health benefits (e.g., polyunsaturated fatty acids (PUFAs); minerals, vitamins, or other compounds). The overall objective of this research was to prospect novel products, such as nutraceuticals from microalgae, for application in human health, particularly for metabolic diseases. *Chlorella vulgaris* and *Chlorococcum amblystomatis* were grown autotrophically, and *C. vulgaris* was additionally grown heterotrophically. Microalgae biomass was extracted using organic solvents (dichloromethane, ethanol, ethanol with ultrasound-assisted extraction). Those extracts were evaluated for their bioactivities, toxicity, and metabolite profile. Some of the extracts reduced the neutral lipid content using the zebrafish larvae fat metabolism assay, reduced lipid accumulation in fatty-acid-overloaded HepG2 liver cells, or decreased the LPS-induced inflammation reaction in RAW264.7 macrophages. Toxicity was not observed in the MTT assay in vitro or by the appearance of lethality or malformations in zebrafish larvae in vivo. Differences in metabolite profiles of microalgae extracts obtained by UPLC-LC-MS/MS and GNPS analyses revealed unique compounds in the active extracts, whose majority did not have a match in mass spectrometry databases and could be potentially novel compounds. In conclusion, microalgae extracts demonstrated anti-obesity, anti-steatosis, and anti-inflammatory activities and could be valuable resources for developing future nutraceuticals. In particular, the ultrasound-assisted ethanolic extract of the heterotrophic *C. vulgaris* significantly enhanced the anti-obesity activity and demonstrated that the alteration of culture conditions is a valuable approach to increase the production of high-value compounds.

Keywords: microalgae; anti-obesity; anti-inflammation; anti-steatosis; molecular networking

1. Introduction

Obesity, according to the World Health Organization (WHO), is defined as an abnormal or excessive fat accumulation that may impair health, reduce well-being, and increase morbidity and mortality. Nowadays, it is considered a global epidemic, leading to more than 2.8 million deaths per year. Obesity prevalence almost tripled in 40 years (1975–2016), and in 2016, the WHO estimated that 380 million children under 19 were overweight or obese, and up to 1.9 billion adults were overweight [1]. The excessive accumulation of fat tissue accompanied by mild chronic inflammation of the tissue defines obese individuals [2]. Obesity is correlated with an exponential increase of metabolic syndrome (MetS) [3], leading to type 2 diabetes, nonalcoholic fatty liver disease (NAFLD), cardiovascular diseases, cancer, musculoskeletal diseases (e.g., arthritis), sleep apnea, respiratory conditions (such as asthma), and others. MetS is characterized by specific pathologic conditions, including obesity, insulin resistance, hypertension, and hyperlipidemia [4]. NAFLD presents liver steatosis in the absence of alcohol abuse and is closely linked to metabolic syndrome [5]. Currently, NAFLD is the most important cause of chronic liver disease, ranging from simple steatosis to severe tissue inflammation (steatohepatitis), fibrosis, cirrhosis, and hepatocellular carcinoma [6].

Treatment options for obesity are based on lifestyle changes (healthy diet, physical exercise, and behavioral therapies), pharmacotherapy, and bariatric surgery. Pharmacotherapy, allied with exercise and diet, is a standard support for obesity treatment, although some drugs have been considered non-efficacious, unsafe, and showed dangerous side effects [7,8]. Due to the exposed facts, the development of more specific, effective, and directed treatments and drugs against obesity and obesity-related pathologies is still in need. Natural products are known as a source of novel molecules for treating human diseases, and a significant portion of the approved drugs (> 60%) has origin in nature or inspired the synthesis of pharmacophores. One of the FDA-approved drugs for the treatment of obesity is derived from the bacterium *Streptomyces* (orlistat), which targets the inhibition of gastric and pancreatic lipases [3].

Researchers have been focusing on terrestrial environments for new natural compounds discovery for centuries, while research has only started looking at aquatic environments in the last few decades. Despite the apparent difficulties of isolating novel compounds from marine organisms in a sustainable way, currently, 14 FDA-approved drugs from marine environments exist for the treatment of cancer, pain, or hypertriglyceridemia (https://www.midwestern.edu/departments/marinepharmacology/clinical-pipeline, accessed on 6 December 2021). Oceans comprise more than 71% of the Earth's surface and represent a huge potential reservoir for discovering new natural compounds [9]. Microalgae are known to be a source of lipids, proteins, and carbohydrates [10,11], as well as being rich in exploitable molecules, vitamins, polyunsaturated fatty acids (PUFAs), pigments, carotenoids, other antioxidant compounds, peptides, and toxins [12,13]. The macronutrients produced vary depending on the microalgae species and its cultivation mode (autotrophic, heterotrophic, and mixotrophic) [13]. As a source of high-value products and molecules, microalgae became interesting for commercial purposes, such as biotechnological and pharmaceutical exploitation, biodiesel production, and food and dietary supplements, among others.

The microalgae *Chlorella vulgaris*, the first algae isolated and grown in pure culture is often used for bioremediation and treatment of wastewater [14,15], and is approved for production and commercialization as a health/food supplement. The regular dietary supplementation of *C. vulgaris* can protect against specific types of cancer, oxidative stress and help in the reduction of hyperlipidemia [16]. Recent studies have demonstrated *C. vulgaris's* ability to produce carotenoids, chlorophyll pigments, a range of fatty acids and complex lipids (glycerophospholipids, glycolipids) [17], and vitamins (B3 and B5), among other interesting compounds [18]. In contrast to the commonly cultivated green algae *C. vulgaris*, *Chlorococcum* sp. is a green microalga from the family Chlorococcaceae, which is still poorly explored in terms of its biotechnological potential. *Chlorococcum* sp. is known for accumulating large amounts of lipids [19] and producing high amounts of carotenoids [20]. Furthermore, *Chlorococcum* sp. has anticholinesterase and antioxidant activity, and the presence of phenolic compounds, polysaccharides, and omega 3 polar lipids [21] was shown by Olasehinde et al. [22], making this microalga a possible interesting nutraceutical producer.

The present work aimed to search for novel bioactivities from microalgae with human health applications, particularly for metabolic diseases. This work focussed on two microalgae, *Chlorococcum amblystomatis* grown autotrophically and *Chlorella vulgaris* grown auto- and heterotrophically, and their biomass was extracted using organic solvents. Those extracts were evaluated in various in vivo and in vitro bioassays for their activities towards obesity, steatosis, and inflammation. Additionally, potential toxicity was assessed, and the first characterization of their metabolite profile by untargeted LC-MS/MS was performed to identify putative compounds involved in the observed bioactivities. The identification of bioactive extracts for metabolic diseases from microalgae and their responsible metabolites will be an important step for the future development of novel nutraceuticals or functional food.

2. Results

2.1. Lipid-Reducing Activity

Microalgae extracts were subjected to a bioactivity screening to identify their potential lipid-reducing activities using zebrafish larvae in vivo, namely the Nile Red fat metabolism assay. Results are represented in Figure 1. Dimethyl sulfoxide (0.1% DMSO) was used as solvent control and resveratrol (50 µM REV) as a positive control. Figure 1a–b shows a visualization of Nile Red staining of neutral lipid reservoirs for the solvent control and the positive control, respectively. Results from bioactivity screening are presented in Figure 1c and expressed as a percentage of fluorescence intensity relative to the solvent control (DMSO). Seven of the analyzed samples reduced significant Nile Red fluorescence. In particular, heterotrophic *C. vulgaris* (CH), extracted with ethanol and ultrasounds (UAE), revealed very promising results, similar to the ones obtained from the positive control, REV. Even though most of the results showed an elevated variability, with large standard deviations (SD) for most samples, CH-UAE extract showed very small SD. No toxicity or visible malformation was detected during the assays, assuming the absence of toxicity in zebrafish larvae at the tested concentration.

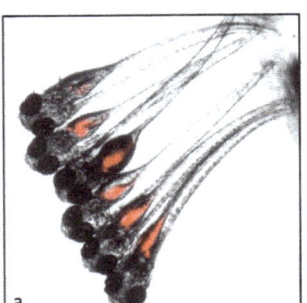
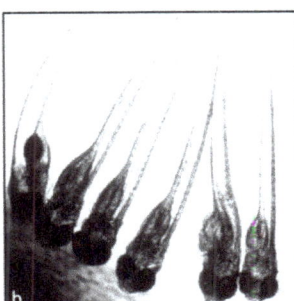
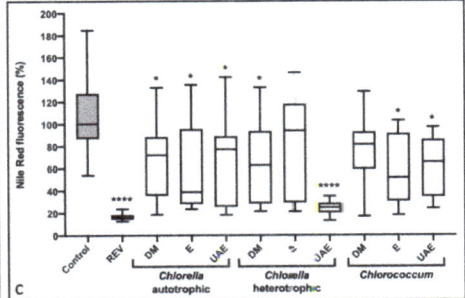

Figure 1. Lipid-reducing activity of the extracts (10 µg/mL) in the Nile Red fat metabolism assay using zebrafish larvae. a–b: images of zebrafish larvae, with overlay of bright field picture and red fluorescence channel; (**a**): solvent control with 0.1% of DMSO; (**b**): positive control with 50 µM of REV. (**c**): Results of the screening for lipid-reducing activity. Data are shown relative to DMSO (100%) as box-and-whisker plots (5–95 percentiles) and were obtained from three independent assays with 6–7 individual larvae each (n = 18–21). Statistically significant different results from control (DMSO) were marked with asterisk (* $p < 0.05$; **** $p < 0.0001$). Solvents used for preparation of the extracts: DM: dichloromethane-methanol (2:1); E: ethanol; UAE: ultrasound-assisted extraction with ethanol.

Comparing the heterotrophic, most active extract (CH-UAE, 75% lipid reduction) with the equivalent autotrophic extract (CA-UAE, 20% lipid reduction), it is possible to infer that the cultivation mode plays an essential role in the production of bioactive compounds present in the extracts.

2.2. Anti-Inflammatory Activity

The anti-inflammatory activity was assessed using the RAW264.7 cell line exposed to 10 and 25 µg/mL extracts. Results from 10 µg/mL are presented in the Supplementary Materials (Figure S1). Figure 2 shows the results from the extracts at 25 µg/mL. Eight of the nine samples resulted in statistically significant nitric oxide (NO) reduction, ranging from approximately 25% to more than a 40% reduction in NO content (Figure 2a). Analyzing Figure 2b, which represents viability, no cytotoxicity was observed for extracts at 25 µg/mL extracts. In contrast, one extract significantly increased viability (CA-DM; 42% average viability increase).

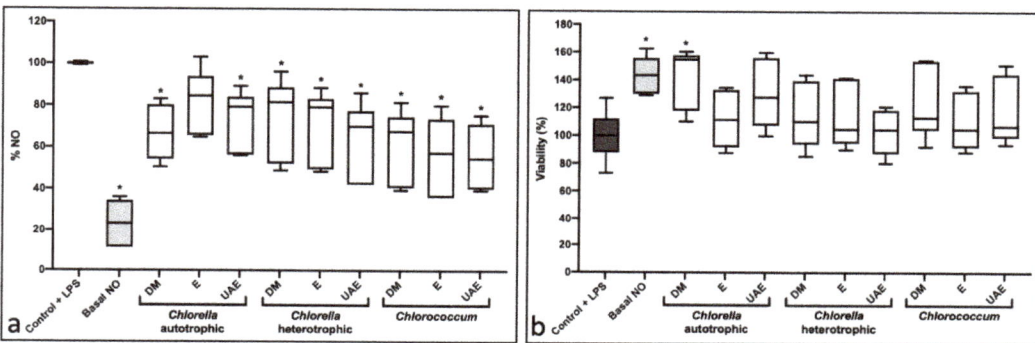

Figure 2. Anti-inflammatory and viability assays in RAW264.7 cell line exposed to 25 µg/mL of extracts. Dark grey represents inflammation control (induced by LPS and containing the same DMSO content as extracts); light grey represents basal NO without induction of inflammation by LPS. (**a**) Results for the anti-inflammatory assay; (**b**) results for cell viability. Solvents used for preparation of the extracts: DM: dichloromethane-methanol (2:1); E: ethanol; UAE: ultrasound-assisted extraction with ethanol. The data for both assays are derived from three independent experiments in duplicates and shown as box-and-whisker plots (5–95 percentiles). Statistical differences compared to DMSO control are indicated by asterisks (* $p < 0.05$).

2.3. Anti-Steatosis Assay

The steatosis assay quantifies the lipid content through the fluorescence emitted by the Nile Red dye, which stains neutral lipid droplets, and cell viability through the intensity of fluorescence emitted by HO-33342 that stains the nucleus (Figure 3a). Results presented in Figure 3b consists of a ratio between the intensity emitted by the Nile Red per cytoplasm and the intensity emitted by the HO-33342, giving the results as the lipid content normalized for cell density for each well. At 10 µg/mL, no significant results were obtained (Figure S2). At 25 µg/mL, six of the nine extracts showed slight, but significant anti-steatosis activity, when compared to the fat-overloaded control (control + SO). Like the results obtained from the zebrafish Nile Red assay, ultrasound-assisted extraction with ethanol in heterotrophic *C. vulgaris* (CH-UAE) showed a 20% reduction in lipid content in HepG2 cells, reinforcing this as the most promising extract. Results observed in the SrB assay (Figure 3c) discarded significant cytotoxicity for all samples.

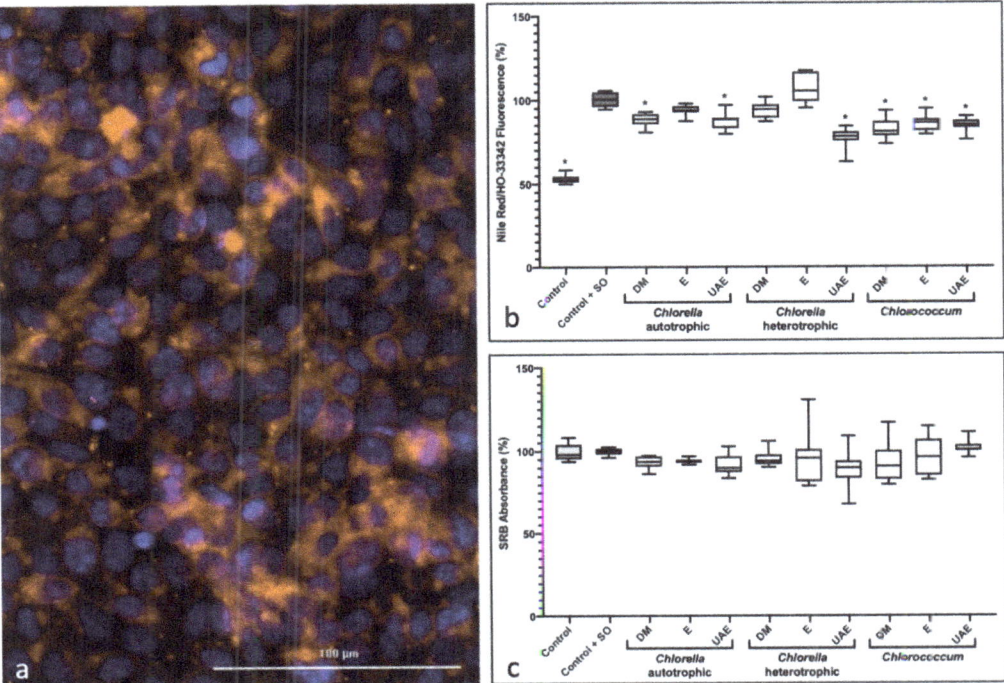

Figure 3. Anti-steatosis activity assay in fatty-acid-overloaded HepG2 cells and cell viability by SrB method, at 25 μg/mL extract. (**a**) HepG2 cells stained under fluorescent light; in orange, lipidic content stained by NileRed; in blue, cell nucleus stained by HO-33342 (DAPI). (**b**) Nile Red and HO-33342 fluorescence quantification ratio expressed as percentage compared to fat-overloaded control (Control + SO); (**c**) HepG2 cell viability using SrB method. Light grey represents DMSO control; dark grey represents control + SO. Solvents used for preparation of the extracts: DM: dichloromethane-methanol (2:1); E: ethanol; UAE: ultrasound-assisted extraction with ethanol. Data were derived from two independent experiments in triplicates and shown as box-and-whisker plots (5–95 percentiles). Statistical differences compared to DMSO + SO control is indicated by asterisks (* $p < 0.05$).

2.4. Metabolite Profiling

For the untargeted metabolite profiling, the extracts were chosen and compared, forming three groups: autotrophic *Chlorella vulgaris* (CA-DM; CA-E; CA-UAE), heterotrophic *Chlorella vulgaris* (CH-DM; CH-E; CH-UAE), and *Chlorococcum amblystomatis* (C-DM; C-E; C-UAE). The molecular network (Figure 4) allowed the visualization of the metabolites present in each group or shared between groups, their precursor mass, and putative identifications (http://gnps.ucsd.edu/ProteoSAFe/status.jsp?task=9f0f25a1f005406eab16a5e5711a19ea, accessed on 25th of October 2021). The original Cytoscape file is provided in Supplementary Materials (Figure S3).

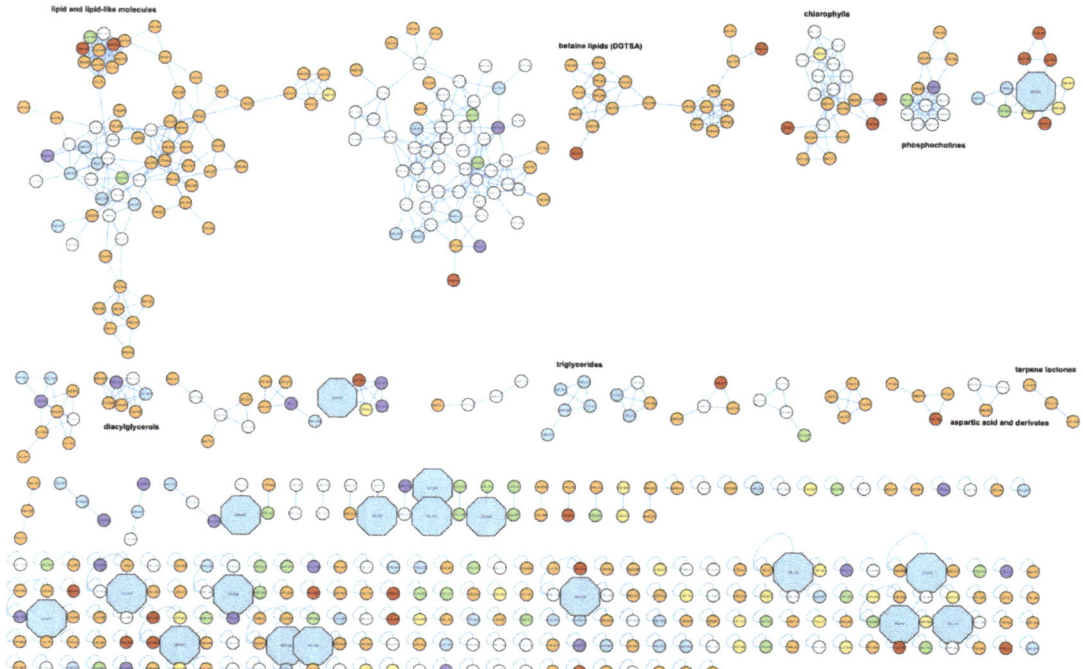

Figure 4. Metabolite profiling using LC-MS/MS and GNPS. Unique mass peaks, exclusively present in the most bioactive extract CH-UAE, are presented as octagonal nodes and highlighted by size. The color of the nodes corresponds to their presence in the analyzed extracts: yellow: only in autotrophic *C. vulgaris*; blue: only in heterotrophic *C. vulgaris*; red: only in *C. amblystomatis*; green: shared between auto- and heterotrophic *C. vulgaris*; orange: shared between autotrophic *C. vulgaris* and *C. amblystomatis*; purple: shared between heterotrophic *C. vulgaris* and *C. amblystomatis*; white: shared by all.

Most molecules are shared between all three groups (white nodes) or between both autotrophically grown microalgae (orange nodes). For example, although chlorophylls are shared by all three groups, some chlorophyll metabolites are exclusive to *C. amblystomatis* extracts (red nodes) or autotrophic growth (orange nodes). Betaine lipids and terpene lactones metabolites were only detected in autotrophic growing conditions. On the other hand, we were able to identify a cluster of triglycerides only identified in heterotrophically grown *C. vulgaris*. These results suggest that culture conditions may play an important role for the production of the metabolites present in the extracts, even more than the species itself. Metabolites shared with both *C. vulgaris* groups and colored in green are scarce in the molecular network.

Metabolites only present in CH-UAE extract, identified in the previous assays as the most promising ones, were highlighted in Figure 4 in blue and octagonal nodes. From this extract, 18 unique nodes in clusters were identified. Table 1 shows the results obtained for those 18 nodes, with their putative identifications.

Table 1. Putative identification of unique compounds in the active extract CH-UAE derived from the molecular network at Figure 4, by GNPS tools, DNP, and NPA. Identifications were based on the MS2 fragmentation on GNPS and on m/z values +/− 0.002 against the databases DNP and NPA. Possible matches were only considered if the calculated mass error was lower than 5ppm. From the original 18 compounds, 8 putative identifications were found. M + H$^+$: mass + hydrogen; RT: retention time; ppm: parts per million; DNP: Dictionary of natural products; NPA: natural products atlas.

M + H$^+$	RT	Putative Identification	ppm	Formula	Source
358.202	519.548	Benzanoid			GNPS
409.162	549.5865	2,6-Diamino-2,6-dideoxyidose; L-form, Dibenzyl dithioacetal or 3-(4-Hydroxybenzyl)-3,6-bis(methylthio)-2,5-piperazinedione; (3R,6R)-form, O-(3-Methyl-2-butenyl), 1,4-N-di-Me	0.1	$C_{20}H_{28}N_2O_3S_2$	DNP
		Urauchimycin C	2.2	$C_{19}H_{24}N_2O_8$	DNP
333.136	749.917	Anhydrocehydrotylophorinidine; 3-O-De-Me	−1.5	$C_{21}H_{18}NO_3$	DNP
		Pandangolide 2; Me ester	−3.6	$C_{15}H_{24}O_6S$	DNP
		Xanthine; 7H-form, 1,7-Dibenzyl	2.5	$C_{19}H_{16}N_4O_2$	DNP
393.167	652.9033	7,8-Dihydroxy-1-methyl-β-carboline; 3,4-Dihydro, O^7-Me, 8-O-β-D-Glucopyranoside	2.1	$C_{19}H_{24}N_2O_7$	DNP
749.391	550.2385	Biscarpamontamine A or Conodiparine A; 19′-Ketone or Conodiparine B; 19′-Ketone or Conodiririne A or Conodiririne B or Coryzeylamine or Tabercorymine A or Tabernaricatine B; 19R,20S-Epoxide or Tabernaricatine B; 19S,20R-Epoxide or Tabernaricatine D; $\Delta^{1',2'}$-Isomer, 7′β-hydroxy	−0.6	$C_{44}H_{52}N_4O_7$	DNP
451.119	735.559	Aspergillazine B or Aspergillazine B; 2-Epimer	3.3	$C_{20}H_{22}N_2O_8S$	DNP
		2,2′,3,3′,7,7′-Hexahydroxy-1,1′-biphenanthrene or 2,2′,4,4′,7,7′-Hexahydroxy-1,1′-biphenanthrene or 2,2′,4,4′,7,7′-Hexahydroxy-1,3′-biphenanthrene or 2,4,4′,5,5′,7′-Hexahydroxy-1,1′-biphenanthrene or 3,3′,4,4′,7,7′-Hexahydroxy-1,1′-biphenanthrene or 2,4,4′,7,7′-Pentahydroxy-1,2′-biphenanthrene ether or 2,4,5′,7,7′-Pentahydroxy-1,2′-biphenanthrene ether	1.8	$C_{28}H_{18}O_6$	DNP
		Rhizoferrin; (R,R)-form, 2-Oxo	−2.3	$C_{16}H_{22}N_2O_{13}$	DNP
		Aspergillazine C or Penispirozine C ou Perispirozine D	−3.3	$C_{20}H_{22}N_2O_8S$	NPA
729.368	732.944500	2,15-Dihydroxy-18-nor-16-kauren-19-oic acid; (ent-2α,15β)-form, 2-O-[β-D-Glucopyranosyl-(1→3)-2-O-(3-methylbutanoyl)-β-D-glucopyranoside] or 3,5,11,14-Tetrahydroxycard-20(22)-enolide; (3β,5β,11α,14β)-form, 3-O-[3-O-Methyl-β-D-glucopyranosyl-(1→4)-6-deoxy-α-L-glucopyranoside]	−2.4	$C_{36}H_{56}O_{15}$	DNP
227.075	648.9525	3-Buten-1-ol; 4-Methylbenzenesulfonyl or 3-Buten-1-ol; 4-Methylbenzenesulfonyl or 2,4-Dihydroxy-3,5,6-trimethylthiobenzoic acid; S-Me ester or 4-Phenyl-3-buten-1-ol; (Z)-form, Methanesulfonyl	3.6	$C_{11}H_{14}O_3S$	DNP
		1-(2′,4′-dihydroxy-5′-methyl-3′-methylsulfanyl-lmethylphenyl)ethanone or Mortivinacin A	3.4	$C_{11}H_{14}O_3S$	NPA

Table 1. Cont.

M + H⁺	RT	Putative Identification	ppm	Formula	Source
666.062	979.23				
543.447	887.89275				
415.142	734.2515				
743.346	590.652499				
402.176	711.7333				
160.841	387.5715				
761.357	554.2535				
763.178	827.886				
715.388	650.252				
713.373	775.4403				

3. Discussion

The use of cell lines for bioactivity screening in metabolic diseases, as obesity and associated co-morbidities, have proved to be an essential tool; however, they do not represent the complexity of whole organisms. Zebrafish (*Danio rerio*) surged as an attractive model organism. It has high physiological and genetic homology with mammals, relatively low-cost maintenance, larvae with optical transparency, and fast development. Similarities between zebrafish and mammalian lipid metabolism have been recorded [23], allowing the development of specific screening assays. The zebrafish Nile Red fat metabolism assay [23] allows the quantification of the neutral lipidic content (in the intestine and yolk sac region) in zebrafish larvae, enabling us to understand if certain compounds have lipid-reducing activity. The zebrafish Nile Red assay has been successfully used for screening of new secondary metabolites from cyanobacterial fractions [24] and for the isolation of known and novel chlorophyll derivatives (13^2-hydroxypheophytine a, 13^2-hydroxy-farnesyle a) from the cyanobacteria *Nodosilinea* sp. and *Cyanobium* sp. [25].

To the best of our knowledge, this assay was not yet employed in microalgae extracts, and we report, for the first time, strong bioactivity for heterotrophic *Chlorella vulgaris* extracted with ethanol and ultrasound-assisted extraction, which reduced 70% of neutral lipids in the zebrafish larvae. In comparison, autotrophic *C. vulgaris* only reduced 20% of neutral lipid levels. In concordance with these results, *C. vulgaris* anti-obesity activity has long been identified and studied [26–28]. In high-fat-diet fed rats, supplementation with *C. vulgaris* effectively reduced total serum lipids, liver triglycerides, and cholesterol [28].

Various authors revealed differences between autotrophic and heterotrophic cultivation. Chen et al. [29] had demonstrated that the lipid content and microalgae composition are species- and cultivation-dependent. Heterotrophic growth is more profitable in terms of lipid content when compared to traditional autotrophic growth conditions [30,31]. Although both culture conditions were closed systems with a more controlled environment, the heterotrophic conditions are axenic, allowing an easier manipulation and production of more constant biomass while decreasing the probability of culture contamination [32]. Autotrophic cultivation is described to lead to a higher content of glycolipids and omega-3 polyunsaturated fatty acids, whereas heterotrophic growth increased phospholipids, saturated fatty acids, and omega-6 polyunsaturated fatty acid levels [17]. Autotrophic cells were shown to have a higher concentration of pigments (chlorophyll and carotenoid), while heterotrophic cells have lower pigment content [33].

Molecular networking allowed further investigation of putative compounds associated with the bioactivity previously identified in the heterotrophic extract from *C. vulgaris* (CH-UAE). The comparison between microalgae and growth conditions revealed unique metabolites in this bioactive extract. Of those presented in Table 1, none was yet described in the scientific literature for their lipid-reducing activity. Additionally, such compounds' production is not associated with microalgae but with bacteria, plants, or fungi, in accordance with the information in the databases. The other 12 peaks with no match in the searched databases may represent novel compounds. In accordance, many studies using similar untargeted metabolite profiling approaches demonstrated a large percentage of not-known compounds, which still remain to be isolated and identified [24,34–36]. In the future, CH-UAE extract should be fractionated to reduce the complexity of the material and identify the responsible compounds for the observed anti-obesity activity.

As obesity is characterized by chronic inflammation, it is essential to assess the anti-inflammatory activity of the extracts. Our results showed a reduction in the production of NO of about 30–40% for *C. vulgaris* and *C. amblystomatis*. Couto et al. [17], when comparing both autotrophic and heterotrophic *C. vulgaris*, were able to conclude that both growing conditions had high anti-inflammatory and antioxidant properties. However, results in that study were obtained using 500 μg/ml extracts, which is 20x higher than those used in the present study (25 μg/mL). The production of bioactive compounds with anti-inflammatory activity has already been reported in *C. vulgaris* [37] and *Chlorococcum* sp. [22]. A study from Kwak et al. [38] showed anti-inflammatory and immunostimulatory effects through an increase in natural killer cells activity and the production of cytokines in healthy people after *C. vulgaris* biomass consumption for an eight-week period. The carotenoid violaxanthin from *Chlorella ellipsoidea* had been associated with anti-inflammatory activity [39], capable of inhibiting NO production in a dose-dependent way [39].

Steatosis, one of the NAFLD states, is common in obese patients [40]. The assay employed here to determine anti-steatosis activity relies on the importance of the liver in fatty assay metabolism and used HepG2 cell lines exposed to sodium oleate, known to induce steatosis in cells, as described by Costa et al. [24]. Although both microalgae under different growth conditions demonstrated significant results, there are differences in these activities. Extraction with dichloromethane–methanol 2:1 (DM) and ultrasound-assisted extraction with ethanol (UAE) resulted in higher anti-steatosis activity compared with ethanol (E) extracts. The effect of ultrasound-assisted extraction, when compared to extraction just with ethanol, was also observed at the anti-inflammatory assay. Ethanol extracts from *Coffea arabica* L. leaves have been characterized to be more efficient for extracting chlorophylls, carotenoids, and higher antioxidant activity when compared to dichloromethane or hexane extracts [41]. Solvent mixtures, compared to single solvents, were found to be more efficient, with higher yields in extracts of *Annona muricata* L. leaves [42]. Ultrasound extraction presents a variety of advantages, such as lower time consumption, as well as improved extraction yield for organic compounds, compared to conventional methods [43–45].

Regarding *C. amblystomatis* extracts, not much research has been reported on lipid-reducing activity in in vitro or in vivo models of obesity or steatosis. This microalga is not accepted for human consumption, and therefore cannot be subjected to human trials, which may explain the lack of further studies. Our results for *C. amblystomatis* extracts are promising, as it shows a significant reduction in neutral lipids in fatty-acid-overloaded liver cells compared with the ones obtained for heterotrophic *Chlorella*. In accordance with the zebrafish Nile Red fat metabolism assay results, ultrasound-assisted ethanolic extract of heterotrophic *C. vulgaris* demonstrated the highest bioactivity in preventing the formation of lipid droplets in HepG2 cells. Our study allows inferring that both microalgae species have a lipid-lowering effect that may be useful for the treatment of NAFLD.

4. Materials and Methods

4.1. Microalgae Biomass Production

Chlorella vulgaris and *Chlorococcum amblystomatis* are deposited at Allmicroalgae industrial collection under the internal codes 0002CA and 0066CA, respectively. These microalgae were cultivated as previously described [17,46]. Briefly, autotrophic cultivation was carried using Guillard f/2-based medium. The scale-up started in 5 L flask reactors under laboratory-controlled conditions, which were sequentially scaled up, at an approximate proportion of 1:5 until reaching an outdoor 10 m^3 photobioreactor (PBR) at Allmicroalgae production plant facilities. The pH was kept constant by pulse injections of CO_2. For heterotrophic cultivation, a C:N ratio of 6.7:1 and glucose (Sapecquimica, Vila Nova de Gaia, Portugal) was used as the source of organic carbon. The heterotrophic culture was carried step-wise from 50 mL Erlenmeyer's until reaching the industrial 5000 L fermenter. All fermenters were operated in fed-batch under controlled temperature, pH, and dissolved oxygen.

4.2. Microalgae Extraction

Microalgae biomass extraction was performed using 25 mg of *Chlorella vulgaris* (grown autotrophically and heterotrophically) and *Chlorococcum amblystomatis* using ethanol 96% (E), dichloromethane:methanol 2:1 (DM), and ultrasound-assisted extraction (UAE) with ethanol 96%. The UAE was performed using a Sonics VCX 130 sonifier (Sonics & Materials INC., Newtown, CT., USA, output power 130 W, output frequency 20 kHz, power density 3.56 W/cm^3), with a microtip probe set to six 20 second pulses of 70% of amplitude, each followed by one minute cool down in ice, as described in Figueiredo et al. [47]. Samples were vortexed for 2 min and centrifuged at 2000 rpm for 10 min. The organic phases were collected and dried under a N_2 stream.

Crude microalgae extracts were weighed in pre-weighed amber vials. For bioactivity assays, dry crude extracts were diluted in DMSO at a concentration of 10 mg/mL.

4.3. Zebrafish Larvae Nile Red Fat Metabolism Assay

The lipid-reducing activity of compounds was analyzed using the zebrafish Nile Red assay as previously described [8]. According to the EC Directive 86/609/EEC for animal experiments, the chosen procedures are not considered animal experiments using non-autonomous feeding stages, and no permission was necessary. Zebrafish embryos were raised from one DPF (days post-fertilization) in egg water (60 µg/mL marine sea salt dissolved in distilled H_2O) with 200 µM PTU (1-phenyl-2-thiourea) to inhibit pigmentation. From three DPF to five DPF, zebrafish larvae were exposed to the samples at a final concentration of 10 µg/mL with daily renewal of water and extracts in a 48-well plate with a density of 6–8 larvae/well (n = 6–8). A solvent control (0.1% DMSO) and positive control (REV, resveratrol, final concentration 50 µM) were included in the assay. Neutral lipids were stained with Nile Red overnight at the final concentration of 10 ng/mL. For imaging, the larvae were anesthetized with tricaine (MS-222, 0.03%) for 5 min and fluorescence analyzed with a fluorescence microscope (Olympus, BX-41, Hamburg, Germany). Fluorescence intensity was quantified in individual zebrafish larvae by ImageJ (http://rsb.info.nih.gov/ij/index.html, accessed on 1 July 2021).

4.4. Cell Assays

The murine macrophage cell line RAW 264.7 (American Type Culture Collection, ATCC) was selected to determine the anti-inflammatory potential. RAW 264.7 were cultured in Dulbecco's Modified Eagle Medium (DMEM, Roti-CELL) with glutamine, without pyruvate, supplemented with 10% (v/v) of inactivated fetal bovine serum (FBS) and 1% (v/v) penicillin-streptomycin (penicillin 100 IU/L, streptomycin 100 µL/mL). Human-hepatoma-derived cell line HepG2 cells (ATCC) were used for the anti-steatosis assay. Cells were cultured in Dulbecco Modified Eagle's Medium (DMEM) and grown in DMEM supplemented with 10% (v/v) fetal bovine serum, 1% penicillin/streptomycin (100 IU mL^{-1} and 10 mg mL^{-1}, respectively), and 0.1% amphotericin. Both cell lines were incubated in a humidified atmosphere with 5% CO_2 at 37 °C. The culture medium was renewed twice a week, and cell passages (scraping for RAW 264.7 and trypsinization for HepG2) were made at about 80% confluence. All samples were tested at a final concentration of 10 µg/mL.

4.4.1. Anti-Inflammatory Assay

The anti-inflammatory assay was performed as described by Lopes et al. [48]. RAW 264.7 cells were stimulated with LPS (1 µg/mL) and incubated for 22 h. After the incubation period, NO was measured in the culture medium through a Griess reaction. A total of 75 µL of Griess reagent (sulfanilamide 10 mg/mL and ethylenediamine 1 mg/mL, prepared in 2% H_3PO_4) was mixed with 75 µL cell supernatant and incubated in the dark for 10 min. The absorbance of the reaction product was measured at 562 nm. Results were expressed as the percentage of NO from the LPS control. Three independent assays were performed, each assay in duplicate for each sample. To assess the direct effect of the extracts on basal NO production, the assay was also performed in RAW 264.7 cells in the absence of LPS (pro-inflammatory activity).

Cytotoxicity of the extracts was monitored through the 3-(4,5-dimethylthiazole-2-yl)-2,5-diphenyltetrazolium bromide (MTT) assay, as described by Lopes et al. [18]. The assay consisted of the reduction in the yellow MTT to insoluble purple formazan crystals by dehydrogenizing metabolically active cells. After the incubation period of 24 h, 100 µL of MTT solution (0.5 mg/mL), freshly prepared in DMEM at 37 °C, was added to each well and incubated at 37 °C for 45 min. The supernatant was removed after the incubation period, and the resulting formazan crystals were dissolved in 100 µL DMSO. The absorbance of the colored product was determined at 515 nm. Cytotoxicity was expressed as the percentage of cell viability vs. the solvent control. Three independent assays were performed in duplicate for each sample.

4.4.2. Steatosis Assay

The anti-steatosis assay was performed as described by Costa et al. [24]. Cells were seeded at 10^5 cells/mL in 96-well plates and adhered overnight (24 h). The cells were washed in PBS and changed to incomplete DMEM supplemented with 62 µM sodium oleate. DMSO and 0.5% MeOH were used as solvent control. Cells were incubated at 37 °C for 6 h. After, cells were changed to Hank's Buffered Salt Solution (HBSS) (0.137 M NaCl, 5.4 mM KCl, 0.25 mM Na_2HPO_4, 0.44 mM KH_2PO_4, 1.3 mM $CaCl_2$, 1.0 mM $MgSO_4$, 4.2 mM $NaHCO_3$, glucose-free) with HO-333424 (1:100) and Nile Red5 (1:400), and incubated for 15 min at 37 °C in the dark. Cells were then washed twice with HBSS. Fluorescence was read at 485/572 nm excitation/emission for Nile Red and 360/460 nm for HO-33342.

Cytotoxicity of the fractions was also tested on HepG2 cell line using the SRB colorimetric assay. Following the anti-steatosis assay, cells were fixed for 1 h at 4 °C, in the dark, adding 50% (w/v) ice-cold trichloroacetic acid (TCA) to the culture medium. Cells were washed four times with deionized water and the plates air-dried. Then, 0.4% (w/v) SRB in 1% acetic acid was added to each well for 15 min, followed by five washes with 1% acetic acid. The plates were air-dried, and 10 mmol L−1, pH 10.5 Tris–HCl was added to each well. Absorbance was read at 492 nm with reference at 650 nm on a Synergy HT Multi-detection microplate reader.

4.5. Metabolite Profiling

A total of 40 µl of each sample replica (DMSO, 10 mg/mL) was dried and then resuspended to a concentration of 1 mg/mL in acetonitrile for LC-MS. Experimental conditions are described in Ribeiro et al. [49]. The chromatographic step was carried out in an ACE UltraCore 2.5 Super C18 column (75 mm × 2.1 mm, Advanced Chromatography Technologies, Aberdeen, United Kingdom). Briefly, mobile phase A was a mixture of water (H_2O; 95%), methanol (MeOH; 5%), and formic acid (0.1%); while mobile phase B consisted of a mixture of isopropanol (95%), MeOH (5%) and formic acid (0.1%). The gradient flux was 0.35 mL/min, and the program ran for 20 min. The separation temperature was kept at 40 °C for the entire analysis. Q Exactive™ Focus Hybrid Quadrupole carried out the LC/MS analysis—Orbitrap™ Mass Spectrometer (Thermo Scientific™, Waltham, MA, USA) coupled to an Electrospray Ionization (ESI) source, operating in positive mode.

As described by Bellver et al. [34], molecular networking analysis was conducted with some modifications. Raw data were converted using the software program MSConvert to mzXML format for molecular networking and metabolomic analysis. Converted data were uploaded to GNPS (Global Natural Products Social Molecular Networking) [50] (https://gnps.ucsd.edu/, accessed on 25 October 2021). A molecular network was created using the online workflow (https://ccms-ucsd.github.io/GNPSDocumentation/, accessed on 29 October 2021) on the GNPS website (http://gnps.ucsd.edu, accessed on 25 October 2016) [50]. The data were filtered by removing all MS/MS fragment ions within +/− 17 Da of the precursor m/z. MS/MS spectra were window filtered by choosing only the top 6 fragment ions in the +/- 50Da window throughout the spectrum. The precursor ion mass tolerance was set to 0.02 Da and an MS/MS fragment ion tolerance of 0.02 Da. A network was then created where edges were filtered to have a cosine score above 0.7 and more than 6 matched peaks. Further, edges between two nodes were kept in the network if and only if each of the nodes appeared in each other's respective top 10 most similar nodes. Finally, the maximum size of a molecular family was set to 100, and the lowest-scoring edges were removed from molecular families until the molecular family size was below this threshold. The spectra in the network were then searched against GNPS' spectral libraries. The library spectra were filtered in the same manner as the input data. All matches kept between network spectra and library spectra were required to have a score above 0.7 and at least 6 matched peaks. Bioinformatic tools of GNPS were also used, including the Dereplicator [51], Dereplicator+ [52]. To enhance chemical structural information within the molecular network, information from in silico structure annotations from GNPS Library Search, Dereplicator, were incorporated into the network using the GNPS MolNetEnhancer workflow (https://ccms-ucsd.github.io/GNPSDocumentation/molnetenhancer/, accessed on 29 October 2021) on the GNPS website (http://gnps.ucsd.edu, accessed on 29 Octoner 2021) [50,51]. Chemical class annotations were performed using the ClassyFire chemical ontology [53]. Precursor mass was searched in GNPS as well as in other databases, such as the "Dictionary of Marine Natural Compounds" [54] (https://dnp.chemnetbase.com/, accessed on 29 October 2021) and the "Natural Products Atlas" [55] (https://www.npatlas.org/, accessed on 28 October 2021), applying a search filter of 0.002 m/z and a deviation of <5 ppm. Bioactive peaks were manually checked in the Xcalibur software (version 4.1, Thermo Scientific Exactive Series 2.9) for peak intensity, H-isotopes, and Na$^+$ adducts. The MS-error was calculated in parts per million (ppm) and restricted to <5 ppm.

The obtained results from the GNPS platform were then visualized and analyzed using the software program Cytoscape 3.4.0 [56]. Nodes were grouped with different colors, and the ones with significant bioactivity were highlighted in octagonal shape and bigger size.

4.6. Statistical Analysis

Data were first analyzed using normality, Shapiro–Wilk, and Kolmogorov–Smirnov tests to check for Gaussian distribution of samples and a Bartlett's test ($p < 0.05$) to determine equal variance of the samples. If the normal distribution was confirmed, a one-way analysis of variance (ANOVA) was used to find differences among means, followed by a multi-comparisons Dunnett test ($p < 0.05$) as post hoc test. If there were no normal distribution, Kruskal–Wallis test for nonparametric distribution of values would be used, using Dunn's post hoc test. Analyses were performed using GraphPad Prism 9.0.1.

5. Conclusions

In conclusion, the present study shows that microalgae species, namely, *Chlorella vulgaris* and *Chlorococcum amblystomatis*, have significant anti-obesity, anti-steatosis, and anti-inflammatory activities and could be valuable resources for the development of future nutraceuticals. In particular, heterotrophic cultivation of *C. vulgaris* strongly increased the lipid-reducing activity in the zebrafish assay, confirming that alteration of culture conditions can be a valuable approach to increase the production of high-value compounds in microalgae.

Supplementary Materials: The following are available online at https://www.mdpi.com/article/10.3390/md20010009/s1, Figure S1. Anti-inflammatory and viability assays in RAW264.7 cell line exposed to 10 µg/mL of extracts. Figure S2. Anti-steatosis activity assay in fatty-acid-overloaded HepG2 cells and cell viability by SrB method, at 10 µg/mL extract. Figure S3. Cytoscape file from metabolite profiling, network created by GNPS.

Author Contributions: A.R. and Á.H. bioactivity screening, metabolite networking, data analysis, writing; T.C. and D.C. extraction of biomass; M.R.D. and P.D. funding, supervision, methodology. A.M.C. and J.L.d.S. culture and collection of microalgae, funding, methodology; R.U. supervision, conceptualization, funding, methodology, writing; V.V. supervision, funding. All authors have read and agreed to the published version of the manuscript.

Funding: This work was supported by the AlgaValor project (POCI-01-0247-FEDER-035234), financed by the European Regional Development Fund (ERDF) through the COMPETE2020-Operational Programme for Competitiveness and Internationalisation (POCI) and PORTUGAL2020, and national funds through FCT UIDB/04423/2020 and UIDP/04423/2020. Thanks are due to the University of Aveiro and FCT/MCT for the financial support to LAQV/REQUIMTE (UIDB/50006/2020), CESAM (UIDB/50017/2020+UIDP/50017/2020), CICECO—Aveiro Institute of Materials, (UIDB/50011/2020 and UIDP/50011/2020) and to RNEM—Portuguese Mass Spectrometry Network (LISBOA-01-0145-FEDER-402-022125) through national funds and, where applicable, co-financed by the FEDER, within the PT2020 Partnership Agreement.

Institutional Review Board Statement: According to the EC Directive 86/609/EEC for animal experiments, zebrafish larvae in non-independent feeding stages of development are not considered animal experimentation. Hence, ethical review and approval were not necessary

Data Availability Statement: All data are contained within the article and Supplementary Materials.

Conflicts of Interest: The authors declare no conflict of interest.

References

1. UNICEF, United Nations Children's Fund; WHO, World Health Organization; WB, World Bank (WB) Joint Child Malnutrition Estimates—Levels and Trends; WHO: Geneva, Switzerland, 2017.
2. González-Muniesa, P.; Mártinez-González, M.-A.; Hu, F.B.; Després, J.-P.; Matsuzawa, Y.; Loos, R.J.F.; Moreno, L.A.; Bray, G.A.; Martinez, J.A. Obesity. *Nat. Rev. Dis. Primers* **2017**, *3*, 17034. [CrossRef]
3. Castro, M.; Preto, M.; Vasconcelos, V.; Urbatzka, R. Obesity: The Metabolic Disease, Advances on Drug Discovery and Natural Product Research. *Curr. Top. Med. Chem.* **2016**, *16*, 2577–2604. [CrossRef]
4. Rochlani, Y.; Pothineni, N.V.; Kovelamudi, S.; Mehta, J.L. Metabolic Syndrome: Pathophysiology, Management, and Modulation by Natural Compounds. *Ther. Adv. Cardiovasc. Dis.* **2017**, *11*, 215–225. [CrossRef]
5. Marchisello, S.; Di Pino, A.; Scicali, R.; Urbano, F.; Piro, S.; Purrello, F.; Rabuazzo, A.M. Pathophysiological, Molecular and Therapeutic Issues of Nonalcoholic Fatty Liver Disease: An Overview. *Int. J. Mol. Sci.* **2019**, *20*, 1948. [CrossRef] [PubMed]
6. Pettinelli, P.; Obregon, A.M.; Videla, L.A. Molecular Mechanisms of Steatosis in Nonalcoholic Fatty Liver Disease. *Nutr. Hosp.* **2011**, *26*, 441–450. [CrossRef] [PubMed]
7. Bessesen, D.H.; Van Gaal, L.F. Progress and challenges in anti-obesity pharmacotherapy. *Lancet Diabetes Endocrinol.* **2018**, *6*, 237–248. [CrossRef]
8. Urbatzka, R.; Freitas, S.; Palmeira, A.; Almeida, T.; Moreira, J.; Azevedo, C.; Afonso, C.; Correia-da-Silva, M.; Sousa, E.; Pinto, M.; et al. Lipid Reducing Activity and Toxicity Profiles of a Library of Polyphenol Derivatives. *Eur. J. Med. Chem.* **2018**, *151*, 272–284. [CrossRef]
9. Cragg, G.M.; Newman, D.J. Biodiversity: A Continuing Source of Novel Drug Leads. *Pure Appl. Chem.* **2005**, *77*, 7–24. [CrossRef]
10. Becker, E.W. Micro-Algae as a Source of Protein. *Biotechnol. Adv.* **2007**, *25*, 207–210. [CrossRef]
11. Elser, J.J.; Fagan, W.F.; Denno, R.F.; Dobberfuhl, D.R.; Folarin, A.; Huberty, A.; Interlandi, S.; Kilham, S.S.; McCauley, E.; Schulz, K.L.; et al. Nutritional Constraints in Terrestrial and Freshwater Food Webs. *Nature* **2000**, *408*, 578–580. [CrossRef]
12. Koyande, A.K.; Chew, K.W.; Rambabu, K.; Tao, Y.; Chu, D.-T.; Show, P.-L. Microalgae: A Potential Alternative to Health Supplementation for Humans. *Food Sci. Hum.* **2019**, *8*, 16–24. [CrossRef]
13. Rizwan, M.; Mujtaba, G.; Memon, S.A.; Lee, K.; Rashid, N. Exploring the Potential of Microalgae for New Biotechnology Applications and Beyond: A Review. *Renew. Sustain. Energy Rev.* **2018**, *92*, 394–404. [CrossRef]
14. Ge, S.; Qiu, S.; Tremblay, D.; Viner, K.; Champagne, P.; Jessop, P.G. Centrate Wastewater Treatment With Chlorella vulgaris: Simultaneous Enhancement of Nutrient Removal, Biomass and Lipid Production. *Chem. Eng. J.* **2018**, *342*, 310–320. [CrossRef]
15. Sydney, E.B.; Sycney, A.C.N.; de Carvalho, J.C.; Soccol, C.R. Chapter 4—Potential Carbon Fixation of Industrially Important Microalgae. In *Biofuels from Algae (Second Edition)*; Pandey, A., Chang, J.-S., Soccol, C.R., Lee, D.-J., Chisti, Y., Eds.; Elsevier: Amsterdam, The Netherlands, 2019; pp. 67–88.

16. Panahi, Y.; Darvishi, B.; Jowzi, N.; Beiraghdar, F.; Sahebkar, A. Chlorella vulgaris: A Multifunctional Dietary Supplement with Diverse Medicinal Properties. *Curr. Pharm. Des.* **2016**, *22*, 164–173. [CrossRef] [PubMed]
17. Couto, D.; Melo, T.; Conde, T.A.; Costa, M.; Silva, J.; Domingues, M.R.M.; Domingues, P. Chemoplasticity of the Polar Lipid Profile of the Microalgae Chlorella vulgaris Grown Under Heterotrophic and Autotrophic Conditions. *Algal Res.* **2021**, *53*, 102128. [CrossRef]
18. Pantami, H.A.; Ahamad Bustamam, M.S.; Lee, S.Y.; Ismail, I.S.; Mohd Faudzi, S.M.; Nakakuni, M.; Shaari, K. Comprehensive GCMS and LC-MS/MS Metabolite Profiling of Chlorella vulgaris. *Mar. Drugs* **2020**, *18*, 367. [CrossRef] [PubMed]
19. Lv, J.; Wang, X.; Liu, W.; Feng, J.; Liu, Q.; Nan, F.; Jiao, X.; Xie, S. The Performance of a Self-Flocculating Microalga Chlorococcum sp. *GD in Wastewater with Different Ammonia Concentrations. Int. J. Environ. Res.* **2018**, *15*, 434. [CrossRef]
20. Laje, K.; Seger, M.; Dungan, B.; Cooke, P.; Polle, J.; Holguin, F.O. Phytoene Accumulation in the Novel Microalga Chlorococcum sp. *Using the Pigment Synthesis Inhibitor Fluridone. Mar. Drugs* **2019**, *17*, 187. [CrossRef]
21. Conde, T.A.; Couto, D.; Melo, T.; Costa, M.; Silva, J.; Domingues, M.R.; Domingues, P. Polar Lipidomic Profile Shows Chlorococcum amblystomatis as a Promising Source of Value-Added Lipids. *Sci. Rep.-UK* **2021**, *11*, 4355. [CrossRef]
22. Olasehinde, T.A.; Olaniran, A.O.; Okoh, A.I. Cholinesterase Inhibitory Activity, Antioxidant Properties, and Phytochemical Composition of Chlorococcum sp. Extracts. *J. Food Biochem.* **2021**, *45*, e13395. [CrossRef]
23. Jones, K.S.; Alimov, A.P.; Rilo, H.L.; Jandacek, R.J.; Woollett, L.A.; Penberthy, W.T. A High Throughput Live Transparent Animal Bioassay to Identify Non-Toxic Small Molecules or Genes That Regulate Vertebrate Fat Metabolism for Obesity Drug Development. *Nutr. Metab. (Lond)* **2008**, *5*, 23. [CrossRef] [PubMed]
24. Costa, M.; Rosa, F.; Ribeiro, T.; Hernandez-Bautista, R.; Bonaldo, M.; Gonçalves Silva, N.; Eiríksson, F.; Thorsteinsdóttir, M.; Ussar, S.; Urbatzka, R. Identification of Cyanobacterial Strains With Potential for the Treatment of Obesity-Related Co-Morbidities by Bioactivity, Toxicity Evaluation and Metabolite Profiling. *Mar. Drugs* **2019**, *17*, 280. [CrossRef]
25. Freitas, S.; Silva, N.G.; Sousa, M.L.; Ribeiro, T.; Rosa, F.; Leão, P.N.; Vasconcelos, V.; Reis, M.A.; Urbatzka, R. Chlorophyll Derivatives from Marine Cyanobacteria with Lipid-Reducing Activities. *Mar. Drugs* **2019**, *17*, 229. [CrossRef]
26. Sano, T.; Tanaka, Y. Effect of Dried, Powdered Chlorella vulgaris on Experimental Atherosclerosis and Alimentary Hypercholesterolemia in Cholesterol-Fed Rabbits. *Artery* **1987**, *14*, 76–84. [CrossRef]
27. Shibata, S.; Oda, K.; Onodera-Masuoka, N.; Matsubara, S.; Kikuchi-Hayakawa, H.; Ishikawa, F.; Iwabuchi, A.; Sansawa, H. Hypocholesterolemic Effect of Indigestible Fraction of Chlorella regularis in Cholesterol-Fed Rats. *J. Nutr. Sci. Vitaminol.* **2001**, *47*, 373–377. [CrossRef] [PubMed]
28. Lee, H.S.; Park, H.J.; Kim, M.K. Effect of Chlorella vulgaris on Lipid Metabolism in Wistar Rats Fed High Fat Diet. *Nutr. Res. Pract.* **2008**, *2*, 204–210. [CrossRef]
29. Chen, B.; Wan, C.; Mehmood, M.A.; Chang, J.-S.; Bai, F.; Zhao, X. Manipulating Environmental Stresses and Stress Tolerance of Microalgae for Enhanced Production of Lipids and Value-Added Products–A Review. *Bioresour. Technol.* **2017**, *244*, 1198–1206. [CrossRef]
30. Xie, T.; Xia, Y.; Zeng, Y.; Li, X.; Zhang, Y. Nitrate Concentration-Shift Cultivation to Enhance Protein Content of Heterotrophic Microalga Chlorella vulgaris: Over-Compensation Strategy. *Bioresour. Technol.* **2017**, *233*, 247–255. [CrossRef] [PubMed]
31. Barros, A.; Pereira, H.; Campos, J.; Marques, A.; Varela, J.; Silva, J. Heterotrophy as a Tool to Overcome the Long and Costly Autotrophic Scale-Up Process for Large Scale Production of Microalgae. *Sci. Rep.-UK* **2019**, *9*, 13935. [CrossRef]
32. Liu, J.; Sun, Z.; Gerken, H. *Recent Advances in Microalgal Biotechnology*; OMICS Group eBooks: Foster City, CA, USA, 2016.
33. Xu, H.; Miao, X.; Wu, Q. High Quality Biodiesel Production From a Microalga Chlorella prototheocoides by Heterotrophic Growth in Fermenters. *J. Biotechnol.* **2006**, *126*, 499–507. [CrossRef]
34. Bellver, M.; Costa, S.L.D.; Sanchez, B.A.; Vasconcelos, V.; Urbatzka, R. Inhibition of Intestinal Lipid Absorption by Cyanobacterial Strains in Zebrafish Larvae. *Mar. Drugs* **2021**, *19*, 161. [CrossRef] [PubMed]
35. Santos, J.D.; Vitorino, I.; De la Cruz, M.; Díaz, C.; Cautain, B.; Annang, F.; Pérez-Moreno, G.; Gonzalez Martinez, I.; Tormo, J.R.; Martín, J.M.; et al. Bioactivities and Extract Dereplication of Actinomycetales Isolated From Marine Sponges. *Front. Microbiol.* **2019**, *10*, 727. [CrossRef] [PubMed]
36. Bel Mabrouk, S.; Reis, M.; Sousa, M.L.; Ribeiro, T.; Almeida, J.R.; Pereira, S.; Antunes, J.; Rosa, F.; Vasconcelos, V.; Achour, L.; et al. The Marine Seagrass Halophila stipulacea as a Source of Bioactive Metabolites Against Obesity and Biofouling. *Mar. Drugs* **2020**, *18*, 88. [CrossRef]
37. Sibi, G.; Rabina, S. Inhibition of Pro-Inflammatory Mediators and Cytokines by Chlorella vulgaris Extracts. *Pharmacogn. Res.* **2016**, *8*, 118–122. [CrossRef]
38. Kwak, J.H.; Baek, S.H.; Woo, Y.; Han, J.K.; Kim, B.G.; Kim, O.Y.; Lee, J.H. Beneficial Immunostimulatory Effect of Short-Term Chlorella Supplementation: Enhancement of Natural Killercell Activity and Early Inflammatory Response (Randomized, Double-Blinded, Placebo-Controlled Trial). *Nutr. J.* **2012**, *11*, 53. [CrossRef]
39. Soontornchaiboon, W.; Joo, S.S.; Kim, S.M. Anti-Inflammatory Effects of Violaxanthin Isolated From Microalga Chlorella ellipsoidea in Raw 264. *7 Macrophages. Biol. Pharm. Bull.* **2012**, *35*, 1137–1144. [CrossRef] [PubMed]
40. Polyzos, S.A.; Kountouras, J.; Mantzoros, C.S. Obesity and Nonalcoholic Fatty Liver Disease: From Pathophysiology to Therapeutics. *Metabolism* **2019**, *92*, 82–97. [CrossRef] [PubMed]
41. Marcheafave, G.G.; Tormena, C.D.; Pauli, E.D.; Rakocevic, M.; Bruns, R.E.; Scarminio, I.S. Experimental Mixture Design Solvent Effects on Pigment Extraction and Antioxidant Activity from Coffea arabica L. Leaves. *Microchem. J.* **2019**, *146*, 713–721. [CrossRef]

42. Ribeiro de Souza, E.B.; da Silva, R.R.; Afonso, S.; Scarminio, I.S. Enhanced Extraction Yields and Mobile Phase Separations by Solvent Mixtures for the Analysis of Metabolites in Annona muricata L. Leaves. *J. Sep. Sci.* **2009**, *32*, 4176–4185. [CrossRef]
43. Cai, Z.; Qu, Z.; Lan, Y.; Zhao, S.; Ma, X.; Wan, Q.; Jing, P.; Li, P. Conventional, Ultrasound-Assisted, and Accelerated-Solvent Extractions of Anthocyanins From Purple Sweet Potatoes. *Food Chem.* **2016**, *197*, 266–272. [CrossRef]
44. Medina-Torres, N.; Ayora-Talavera, T.; Espinosa-Andrews, H.; Sánchez-Contreras, A.; Pacheco, N. Ultrasound Assisted Extraction for the Recovery of Phenolic Compounds from Vegetable Sources. *Agronomy* **2017**, *7*, 47. [CrossRef]
45. Rodríguez-Pérez, C.; Quirantes-Piné, R.; Fernández-Gutiérrez, A.; Segura-Carretero, A. Optimization of Extraction Method to Obtain a Phenolic Compounds-Rich Extract from Moringa oleifera Lam Leaves. *Ind. Crops Prod.* **2015**, *66*, 246–254. [CrossRef]
46. Correia, N.; Pereira H.; Silva, J.T.; Santos, T.; Soares, M.; Sousa, C.B.; Schüler, L.M.; Costa, M.; Varela, J.; Pereira, L.; et al. Isolation, Identification and Biotechnological Applications of a Novel, Robust, Free-living Chlorococcum (Oophila) ambystomatis Strain Isolated from a Local Pond. *Appl. Sci.* **2020**, *10*, 3040. [CrossRef]
47. Figueiredo, A.R.P.; da Costa, E.; Silva, J.; Domingues, M.R.; Domingues, P. The Effects of Different Extraction Methods of Lipids from Nannochloropsis oceanica on the Contents of Omega-3 Fatty Acids. *Algal Res.* **2019**, *41*, 101556. [CrossRef]
48. Lopes, G.; Clarinha, D.; Vasconcelos, V. Carotenoids from Cyanobacteria: A Biotechnological Approach for the Topical Treatment of Psoriasis. *Microorganisms* **2020**, *8*, 302. [CrossRef] [PubMed]
49. Ribeiro, I.; Girão, M.; Alexandrino, D.A.M.; Ribeiro, T.; Santos, C.; Pereira, F.; Mucha, A.P.; Urbatzka, R.; Leão, P.N.; Carvalho, M.F. Diversity and Bioactive Potential of Actinobacteria Isolated from a Coastal Marine Sediment in Northern Portugal. *Microorganisms* **2020**, *8*, 1691. [CrossRef]
50. Wang, M.; Carver, J.J.; Phelan, V.V.; Sanchez, L.M.; Garg, N.; Peng, Y.; Nguyen, D.D.; Watrous, J.; Kapono, C.A.; Luzzatto-Knaan, T.; et al. Sharing and community curation of mass spectrometry data with Global Natural Products Social Molecular Networking. *Nat. Biotechnol.* **2016**, *34*, 828–837. [CrossRef]
51. Mohimani, H.; Gurevich, A.; Mikheenko, A.; Garg, N.; Nothias, L.-F.; Ninomiya, A.; Takada, K.; Dorrestein, P.C.; Pevzner, P.A. Dereplication of Peptidic Natural Products Through Database Search of Mass Spectra. *Nat. Chem. Biol.* **2017**, *13*, 30–37. [CrossRef]
52. Mohimani, H.; Gurevich, A.; Shlemov, A.; Mikheenko, A.; Korobeynikov, A.; Cao, L.; Shcherbin, E.; Nothias, L.-F.; Dorrestein, P.C.; Pevzner, P.A. Dereplication of Microbial Metabolites Through Database Search of Mass Spectra. *Nat. Commun.* **2018**, *9*, 4035. [CrossRef]
53. Feunang, Y.D.; Eisner, R.; Knox, C.; Chepelev, L.; Hastings, J.; Owen, G.; Fahy, E.; Steinbeck, C.; Subramanian, S.; Bolton, E.; et al. ClassyFire: Automated Chemical Classification with a Comprehensive, Computable Taxonomy. *J. Cheminform.* **2016**, *8*, 61. [CrossRef] [PubMed]
54. Dictionary of Natural Products 30.1. Available online: https://dnp.chemnetbase.com/faces/chemical/ChemicalSearch.xhtml (accessed on 30 November 2021).
55. Van Santen, J.A.; Jacob, G.; Singh, A.L.; Aniebok, V.; Balunas, M.J.; Bunsko, D.; Neto, F.C.; Castaño-Espriu L., Chang, C.; Clark, T.N.; et al. The Natural Products Atlas: An Open Access Knowledge Base for Microbial Natural Products Discovery. *ACS Cent. Sci.* **2019**, *5*, 1824–1833. [CrossRef] [PubMed]
56. Shannon, P.; Markiel, A.; Ozier, O.; Baliga, N.S.; Wang, J.T.; Ramage, D.; Amin, N.; Schwikowski, B.; Ideker, T. Cytoscape: A Software Environment for Integrated Models of Biomolecular Interaction Networks. *Genome Res.* **2003**, *13*, 2498–2504. [CrossRef] [PubMed]

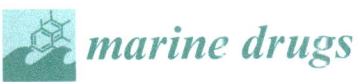

Article

Nutritional Value and Biofunctionalities of Two Edible Green Seaweeds (*Ulva lactuca* and *Caulerpa racemosa*) from Indonesia by Subcritical Water Hydrolysis

Ratih Pangestuti [1,*], Monjurul Haq [2], Puji Rahmadi [3] and Byung-Soo Chun [4,*]

1. Research & Development Divisions for Marine Bio Industry (BBIL), National Research and Innovation Agency (BRIN), North Lombok 83352, Indonesia
2. Department of Fisheries & Marine Bioscience, Jashore University of Science & Technology, Jashore 7408, Bangladesh; mr.haq@just.edu.bd
3. Research Center for Oceanography, National Research and Innovation Agency (BRIN), Jakarta 14430, Indonesia; puji.rahmad@lipi.go.id
4. Department of Food Science & Technology, Pukyong National University, 45 Yongso-ro, Nam-gu, Busan 48513, Korea
* Correspondence: ratih.pangestuti@lipi.go.id (R.P.); bschun@pknu.ac.kr (B.-S.C.); Tel.: +82-51-629-5830 (B.-S.C.)

Citation: Pangestuti, R.; Haq, M.; Rahmadi, P.; Chun, B.-S. Nutritional Value and Biofunctionalities of Two Edible Green Seaweeds (*Ulva lactuca* and *Caulerpa racemosa*) from Indonesia by Subcritical Water Hydrolysis. *Mar. Drugs* 2021, 19, 578. https://doi.org/10.3390/md19100578

Academic Editors: Bill J. Baker, María Lourdes Mourelle, Herminia Domínguez and Jose Luis Legido

Received: 30 August 2021
Accepted: 13 October 2021
Published: 15 October 2021

Publisher's Note: MDPI stays neutral with regard to jurisdictional claims in published maps and institutional affiliations.

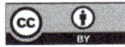

Copyright: © 2021 by the authors. Licensee MDPI, Basel, Switzerland. This article is an open access article distributed under the terms and conditions of the Creative Commons Attribution (CC BY) license (https://creativecommons.org/licenses/by/4.0/).

Abstract: *Caulerpa racemosa* (sea grapes) and *Ulva lactuca* (sea lettuces) are edible green seaweeds and good sources of bioactive compounds for future foods, nutraceuticals and cosmeceutical industries. In the present study, we determined nutritional values and investigated the recovery of bioactive compounds from *C. racemosa* and *U. lactuca* using hot water extraction (HWE) and subcritical water extraction (SWE) at different extraction temperatures (110 to 230 °C). Besides significantly higher extraction yield, SWE processes also give higher protein, sugar, total phenolic (TPC), saponin (TSC), flavonoid contents (TFC) and antioxidant activities as compared to the conventional HWE process. When SWE process was applied, the highest TPC, TSC and TFC values were obtained from *U. lactuca* hydrolyzed at reaction temperature 230 °C with the value of 39.32 ± 0.32 GAE mg/g, 13.22 ± 0.33 DE mg/g and 6.5 ± 0.47 QE mg/g, respectively. In addition, it also showed the highest antioxidant activity with values of 5.45 ± 0.11 ascorbic acid equivalents (AAE) mg/g and 8.03 ± 0.06 trolox equivalents (TE) mg/g for ABTS and total antioxidant, respectively. The highest phenolic acids in *U. lactuca* were gallic acid and vanillic acid. Cytotoxic assays demonstrated that *C. racemosa* and *U. lactuca* hydrolysates obtained by HWE and SWE did not show any toxic effect on RAW 264.7 cells at tested concentrations after 24 h and 48 h of treatment ($p < 0.05$), suggesting that both hydrolysates were safe and non-toxic for application in foods, cosmeceuticals and nutraceuticals products. In addition, the results of this study demonstrated the potential of SWE for the production of high-quality seaweed hydrolysates. Collectively, this study shows the potential of under-exploited tropical green seaweed resources as potential antioxidants in nutraceutical and cosmeceutical products.

Keywords: *Caulerpa racemosa*; *Ulva lactuca*; nutritional; potential; SWE

1. Introduction

Seaweed, also known as marine macroalgae, comprises photosynthetic organisms and includes more than 12,000 species [1,2]. Based on photosynthetic pigment, they can be categorized into: Rhodophyceae (red seaweeds), Phaeophyceae (brown seaweeds) and Chlorophyceae (green seaweeds) [3]. Seaweeds play an important ecological, socio-economic role for coastal communities and are also used for many purposes such as food, medicinal, building materials, feed and many others. Seaweeds are rich in bioactive materials such as polysaccharides, proteins, peptides, amino acids and secondary metabolites including polyphenolic compounds and natural pigments. These bioactive materials have been demonstrated to possess various biological activities and medicinal and health beneficial effects. In addition, many studies have found that countries where seaweeds are consumed on a daily basis have significantly fewer diet-related diseases and longer life expectancy [1]. Seaweeds' bioactive compounds have become a driving factor for their increased demand in food, nutraceutical and cosmeceutical products [4].

Seaweeds are widely distributed and can be found in all zones on the Earth from polar, temperate to tropical regions. Indonesia is an archipelagic country with a long coastline and lies within the heart of the Coral Triangle, the center of the highest marine biodiversity on Earth [5]. The earliest documentation of seaweeds diversity in Indonesia is reported by Rumphius (1750), who established the botanical foundations of the flora of Indonesia. Further, in 1912, van Bosse documented 782 seaweed species in Indonesia, which consisted of 196 species of green seaweeds, 452 species of red seaweeds and 134 species of brown seaweeds. Recently, it was reported that around 1000 seaweeds species can be found in Indonesia [4,6]. Despite the great diversity of seaweed species in Indonesia, only a few species have been used for foods, supplements, nutraceutical and cosmeceutical industries. Among tropical seaweeds species, *Caulerpa racemosa* (known as sea grapes or green caviar) and *Ulva lactuca* (known as sea lettuces) belong to the green algae (Chlorophyta) represent under-exploited seaweed resources in Indonesia. Sulfated polysaccharides from *Ulva* spp. have beneficial effects for cancer chemoprevention, anti-hypertensive and immune-modulating activities [7–9]. In addition, the aqueous extract of *Caulerpa* spp. showed anti-photoaging activity in UVB-irradiated mice [10]. Unfortunately, bioactive compounds, as well as biofunctionalities of *C. racemosa* and *U. lactuca* from Indonesia, are not well characterized. In addition, fewer studies were conducted concerning the bioactive compounds from green seaweeds and their biological activities compared to other seaweed classes [11].

Generally, hot water extraction (HWE), organic solvents' extraction and acid/base extraction were used to extract bioactive compounds from seaweeds [4]. However, exposure to organic solvents and strong acids/bases can lead to deleterious effects on human health and environmental concerns. Therefore, environmentally friendly technologies such as microwave-assisted extraction (MAE), ultrasound-assisted extraction (UAE), enzymatic hydrolysis (EAE), ultrasound-assisted extraction (UAE) and subcritical water hydrolysis (SWE) are gaining more attention for development in many sectors. Bioactive compounds such as polysaccharides, carotenoids and phenolic compounds have been extracted from seaweeds by SWE [12,13]. During the SWE process, solvents were maintained in a subcritical state, between boiling point (100 °C; 0.10 MPa) and critical point (374 °C; 22 MPa), where they remain as a liquid due to the high pressure [4]. Temperature is one of the crucial factors that affect the efficiency and selectivity in the SWE process [5]. Previous studies have demonstrated that the seaweed hydrolysates obtained from SWE have better biological activities as compared to hydrolysates obtained by the conventional HWE process [14]. Considering its high productivity, effectiveness, extraction time, low cost and environmental friendliness, the SWE process has shown many benefits over conventional HWE and other extraction methods.

The main objective of this work was to characterize bioactive compounds in two edible under-exploited tropical seaweeds. First, proximate compositions and fatty acid profiles of *U. lactuca* and *C. racemosa* were analyzed. These two green seaweeds species were further hydrolyzed by conventional HWE at 100 °C and SWE at four different temperature conditions (110 °C, 150 °C, 190 °C and 230 °C). The hydrolysates from HWE and SWE were further analyzed for biochemical compositions, including total protein, sugar, phenolic, flavonoid and saponin contents. Biological activities of *C. racemosa* and *U. lactuca* were tested using radical scavenging assays, and cytotoxic potentials were studied to gain insight into the potential toxicity of seaweeds hydrolysates. The data obtained and presented in this research on the chemical composition of two edible seaweeds can provide the foundations for the explorations of under-exploited seaweeds in Indonesia and fill the gaps for future

research in the development of functional foods, nutraceuticals and cosmeceuticals from
U. lactuca and *C. racemosa*.

2. Results and Discussion

2.1. Proximate and Fatty Acid Composition of C. racemosa and U. lactuca

Carbohydrates were the major component of *C. racemosa* and *U. lactuca*, accounting for 38.62 ± 0.01 and $61.83 \pm 0.01\%$ of the proximate content, respectively (Table 1). Both green seaweeds also contained protein (7.60 ± 0.01 and $10.0 \pm 0.01\%$), ash (38.41 ± 1.90 and $17.36 \pm 0.87\%$), lipids (0.71 ± 0.01 and $0.13 \pm 0.01\%$) and moisture contents (14.66 ± 0.43 and $10.18 \pm 0.04\%$). When *C. racemosa* and *U.lactuca* were compared directly, the protein and carbohydrates contents of *U. lactuca* were higher than those of *C. racemosa*. The carbohydrate contents of *U. lactuca* found in this study were slightly higher than reported in other studies [15–17]. For example, Rasyid et al. (2017) reported that carbohydrate contents of *U. lactuca* from Pamengpeu, and West Java–Indonesia were 58.1% [15]. The carbohydrates contents in seaweeds are likely to be dependent on geographic location, the season of harvest and algal maturity [18]. Many studies have reported that seaweeds contain high carbohydrates and/or protein but low lipid contents. High carbohydrate contents in *U. lactuca* suggest that these green seaweeds could be an important source of polysaccharides for industrial uses. One of the major sulfated polysaccharides found in the genera *Ulva* spp. is ulvan, which may constitute 8 to 40% of the seaweed biomass [19]. Although the industrial applications based on ulvans are still limited, these sulfated polysaccharides have been demonstrated to possess a broad range of bioactivities such as immunomodulating, antiviral, antioxidant, antihyperlipidemic and anticancer activities [20]. Ulvan has been demonstrated to promote gastrointestinal health and has been linked to a reduction in the incidence of non-communicable diseases (NCD) [21,22]. Ulvan has the potential to be applied as bioactive compounds in foods, nutraceuticals and cosmeceuticals; however, the structural and biological properties of ulvan from *U. lactuca* require thorough investigation.

Table 1. Proximate composition of seaweeds.

	Moisture	Ash	Lipid	Protein	Carbohydrate
Caulerpa racemosa	14.66 ± 0.43	38.41 ± 1.90	0.71 ± 0.01	7.60 ± 0.01	38.62 ± 0.01
Ulva lactuca	10.18 ± 0.04	17.86 ± 0.87	0.13 ± 0.01	10.0 ± 0.01	61.83 ± 0.01

In terms of lipid content, the values found in both species were relatively low, indicating that both *C. racemosa* and *U. lactuca* are an ideal choice for people who require a low-fat diet [23]. The differences in proximate contents of seaweeds could be attributed to the differences in species, biological conditions, postharvest treatment and preparative methods. The fatty acids composition (area%) of *C. racemosa* and *U. lactuca* are given in Table 2. The Table 2 shows that 11 of 37 types of authentic standard fatty acids were identified in *U. lactuca*, while 24 of 37 types of authentic standard fatty acids were identified in *C. racemosa*. In *C. racemosa* and *U. lactuca*, palmitic acid (C16:0) showed maximum quantities of 50.73 ± 1.41 and $46.64 \pm 1.12\%$, respectively. The proportion of PUFAs in *C. racemosa* found in this study was higher compared to *U. lactuca*, with linolenic acid (C18:3) found as the major omega-3 PUFAs in both species. Our results show that EPA (C20:5n3), DHA (C22:6n3) and AA(C20:4n6) were not detected in both seaweeds, but they contained essential fatty acids such as linoleic acid (C18:2n6) and linolenic acid (C18:3). In contrast, previous studies reported the presence of EPA and DHA in *C. racemosa* and *U. lactuca* [17,24]. It has been reported by Nelson et al. (2002) that variations in fatty acid compositions are attributable to environmental and genetic differences. Ratios of omega-6/omega-3 fatty acids found in this study were relatively low, at 2.71 and 1.18 for *C. racemosa* and *U. lactuca*, respectively. As regards international organizations, the World Health Organization recommends that the ratio of omega-6/omega-3 fatty acids should not exceed 10 in the daily diet [17], since high omega-6/omega-3 fatty acids ratios will increase risk of many diseases [25]. Hence, the low omega-6/omega-3 fatty acids ratios found in *C. racemosa* and *U. lactuca* suggest that both seaweeds are a good source of omega-3 fatty acids and also an important source of supply of omega-3 fatty acids for homeostasis and maintaining human health [26].

Table 2. Fatty acid compositions of two green seaweeds from Indonesia.

Fatty Acids	C. racemosa	U. lactuca
Caproic acid (C6:0)	0.40 ± 0.01	ND
Capric acid (C10:0)	ND	ND
Undecanoic acid (C11:0)	0.62 ± 0.02	ND
Lauric acid (C12:0)	0.61 ± 0.02	ND
Tridecanoic acid (C13:0)	0.51 ± 0.02	ND
Mystric acid (C14:0)	3.87 ± 0.07	4.05 ± 0.42
Myristoleic acid (C14:1n5)	0.73 ± 0.02	ND
Pentadaecanoic acid (C15:0)	0.71 ± 0.02	4.05 ± 0.42
Palmitic acid (C16:0)	50.73 ± 1.41	46.62 ± 1.12
cis-10-pentadecanoic acid (C15:1)	2.48 ± 0.07	1.92 ± 0.03
Palmitoleic acid (C16:1)	3.45 ± 0.09	2.83 ± 0.07
Cis-10-heptadecanoic acid (C17:0)	0.44 ± 0.01	ND
Stearic acid (C18:0)	3.51 ± 0.09	3.31 ± 0.30
Linolelaidic acid (C18:2n6)	2.50 ± 0.28	ND
Eleic acid	3.27 ± 0.09	5.41 ± 0.17
Elaidic acid	0.37 ± 0.01	17.46 ± 0.46
Arachidic acid (C20:0)	ND	ND
Linoleic acid (C18:2n6)	3.69 ± 0.10	2.59 ± 0.19
Linolenic acid (C18:3)	2.59 ± 0.09	2.20 ± 0.08
cis-11,14-eicosadienoic acid (C20:2)	0.47 ± 0.06	ND
cis-8,11,14-eicosatrienoic acid (C20:3n3)	ND	ND
cis-11,14,17-eicosatrienoic acid (C20:3n3)	ND	ND
cis-5,8,11,14,17-eicosapentanoic acid (20:5n3, EPA)	ND	ND
Behenic acid (C22:0)	1.83 ± 0.05	3.40 ± 0.10
Erucic acid (C22:1)	2.30 ± 0.40	ND
cis-13, 16-docosadienoic acid (C22:2)	0.37 ± 0.00	ND
cis-4,7,10-13,16,19-docosahexanoic acid (DHA) (C22:6n3)	ND	ND
Arachidonic acid (C20:4n6)	ND	ND
Tricosanoic acid (C23:0)	0.54 ± 0.01	ND
Lignoceric acid (C24:0)	11.65 ± 0.33	ND
Nervonic acid (C24:1)	2.19 ± 0.06	ND
Σω-3 PUFAs	2.59	2.20
Σω-6 PUFAs	7.03	2.59
ΣPUFAs	9.62	4.79
ΣSFAa	88.07	95.21
ΣMUFAs	2.30	-
Σω-3/ Σω-6	0.37	0.85
Σω-6/ Σω-3	2.71	1.18

alues are means±standard deviations (n = 3). Abbreviations: ND: not detected, ω-3: omega-3; ω-6: omega-6; PUFAs: polyunsaturated fatty acids; SFAs: saturated fatty acids; MUFAs: monounsaturated fatty acids.

2.2. Extraction Yield of C. racemosa and U. lactuca

During the hydrolysis process, HWE was maintained at 100 °C and SWE at temperatures of 110 °C, 150 °C, 190 °C and 230 °C. The reaction times taken were 2 h and 10 min for HWE and SWE, respectively. The pressure of the SWE process was monitored using the pressure gauge and maintained at 5–7 MPa. The extraction yields ranged from 16.37 to 36.38% and 41.49 to 52.08% (dry weight) for *C. racemosa* and *U. lactuca*, respectively (Figure 1A). Compared to the conventional HWE, the SWE process showed higher extraction yields. The temperature and SWE process directly affected the extraction yield of green seaweed and reached the highest yield at 190 °C. It has been reported that temperature is one of the important parameters during the SWE process. The increased extraction yield in SWE at higher temperatures can be correlated with the change in the dielectric constant of water. As the temperatures during SWE process increase, the dielectric constant will also increase; hence, bioactive materials would also increase significantly. Higher temperatures in SWE led to increases in mass transfer, rapid extraction, lower surface tension and higher solubility of bioactive materials [27]. However, some compounds will also be degraded at elevated temperatures. The change in pH value can be related to those processes (Figure 1B). The solvent pH prior to hydrolysis was 7.2, and following the SWE process, seaweed hydrolysate tended to be acidic. The pH reached the lowest value at hydrolysis temperatures of 230 °C, with the value of 4.32 ± 0.01 and 4.24 ± 0.01 for *C. racemosa* and *U. lactuca*, respectively. The low pH value might correlate with the degradation of sugar into organic acids, which further increased the acidity of green seaweed hydrolysates. In accordance with the findings of our study, Park et al. (2019) found that the pH value of red seaweeds *Porphyra yezoensis* hydrolysates following SWE process were decreased from 7.15 ± 0.01 to 4.16 ± 0.06 at hydrolysis temperatures of 210 °C [28].

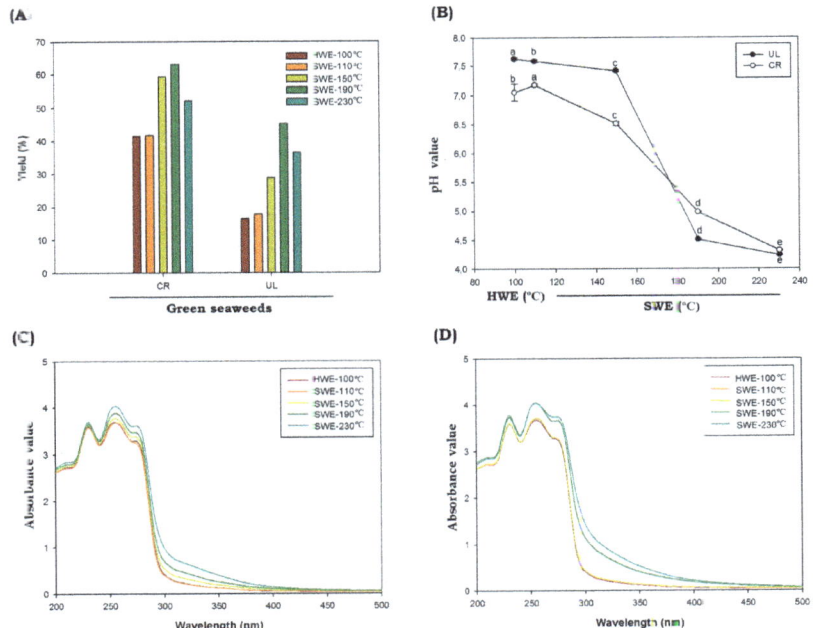

Figure 1. Chemical characteristics of *C. racemosa* and *U. lactuca*. Yield (**A**), pH (**B**), UV-absorbance spectra of *C. racemosa* (**C**) and *U. lactuca* (**D**) obtained by subcritical water hydrolysis. Abbreviations: HWE: hot water extractions; SWE: subcritical water extractions; UL: *Ulva lactuca*; CR: *caulerpa racemosa*. Different letters (a–e) denote a statistically significant difference ($p < 0.05$).

The UV absorption spectra of *C. racemosa* and *U. lactuca* hydrolysates are shown in Figure 1C,D. A peak observed at 235 nm was attributed to n–π* transition; the absorption peak near 275 nm was attributed to n→σ* transition for the amino groups; and the spectral absorption at 300 nm was assigned to n→π* transition for the carbonyl or carboxyl groups [29]. When *C. racemosa* and *U. lactuca* were hydrolyzed by SWE at temperatures of 190 °C and 230 °C, the intensities of the absorption peaks significantly increased, probably because the total protein and other bioactive compounds such as polyphenolic compounds were higher compared to HWE and SWE at lower temperatures. In addition, *C. racemosa* and *U. lactuca* showed strong absorption in the ultraviolet (UV)-B region around 280 to 320 nm (Figure 1C,D) indicating that both green species were rich in UVB-absorbing compounds. In marine environments, light variations occur on much shorter timescales, ranging from seconds to minutes, hours and even days. As a result, seaweeds including *C. racemosa* and *U. lactuca* must avoid the contradiction between effective light absorption on the one hand and a quick photoprotective response to photoinhibitory light intensities on the other [30]. In addition, Wiraguna et al. (2018) has reported UVB-protective activity of *Caulerpa* sp from Indonesia [31]. The presence of UVB-absorbing compounds in *C. racemosa* and *U. lactuca* will allow for future perspectives to understand the photoprotective mechanisms in these tropical green seaweeds. Further, these UVB-absorbing compounds can be used as UVB filters to absorb the entire spectrum of UVB radiation, and these potential compounds can be delivered for the development in the cosmeceutical applications [4].

Analysis of the seaweed hydrolysates' color is shown in Table 3, in which the HWE and SWE at low extraction temperature gave the highest lightness (L*) value. One possible reason for the lighter color observed in HWE and SWE at 110 °C is a shorter exposure to the heat treatment as compared to the higher reaction temperatures. The L* value then decreased when the reaction temperature increased [32]. The L* values of hydrolysates obtained in this study ranged from 32.43 to 54.47 and 23.64 to 56.18 for *C. racemosa* and *U. lactuca*, respectively. It can be seen that L* values were remarkably lower in hydrolysates obtained by SWE at higher temperatures ($p < 0.05$), which showed the significant effect of the temperature and hydrolysis process on L* values. Accordingly, redness (a*) and blueness (b*) values were higher as the temperature of SWE increased, and the lowest values were obtained from the HWE process. There was a significant difference due to the hydrolysis process ($p < 0.05$). The chroma (C*) value indicates the degree of saturation of color and is proportional to the strength of the color. In this study, we found changes in variations in C* values between HWE and SWE. In addition, the C* values also varied at different hydrolysis temperatures ($p < 0.05$). The highest C value was found for seaweed hydrolysates obtained by HWE. In addition, hue angle (H*) is another parameter often used to determine the color of hydrolysates. In our study, we found that H* values of seaweed hydrolysates obtained by SWE at higher temperatures (190 °C and 230 °C) were higher than those of HWE and SWE at lower temperatures ($p < 0.05$). Our results showed that the hydrolysis process especially by SWE at higher temperatures gives greater a*, b*, C* and H* to the seaweed hydrolysates. Pourali et al. (2010) reported that dark color following the SWE process might be correlated with the formation of 5-hydroxymethyl-2-furfural (HMF) and soluble polymers from the decomposition of the produced soluble sugars in a subcritical medium [33]. In addition, the dark color observed at higher temperatures is also attributed to the formation of undesired materials undergoing the Maillard reaction products (MRPs). The UV absorbance at 420 nm is often used to monitor the browning intensity caused by brown polymeric substances, such as melanoidins, which are formed at the final phase of MRPs [34]. Temperature is an important parameter of MRPs, as increasing the temperature could reduce the surface tension and viscosity of water, which resulted in an enhanced solubility of the analytes in the solvent, which further increased reaction rate. As demonstrated in Table 4, compared to the HWE, the MRPs levels were increased under the SWE process. The MRPs product level was the highest under SWE extraction conditions of 230 °C ($p < 0.05$). This subset of MRPs contributes to the coloration of many processed products. The intensity of brown color of these extracts increased with elevation in temperature, supporting the occurrence of MRPs during the SWE process. The MRPs provide a unique aroma and changes in food quality parameters. The process could be indicated from the appearance of the extract, as the color of extracts turned dark brown at temperatures above 150 °C. Interestingly, in our study, we noticed a burning odor in the seaweed hydrolysates obtained by SWE at an extraction temperature above 150 °C. Similar observations (in terms of solution color and odor) have been reported in several studies [34,35].

Table 3. Color characteristics of green seaweed hydrolysates.

Green Seaweed	Conditions	L*	a*	b*	C*	H*
C. racemosa	HWE	52.57 ± 0.57 [a]	−0.75 ± 0.01 [d]	10.15 ± 0.21 [e]	10.17 ± 0.21 [e]	−4.20 ± 0.04 [e]
	SWE 110 °C	54.57 ± 0.35 [b]	−0.87 ± 0.01 [d]	14.54 ± 0.14 [d]	14.57 ± 0.14 [d]	−3.40 ± 0.01 [d]
	SWE 150 °C	36.13 ± 0.37 [d]	11.13 ± 0.11 [c]	38.91 ± 0.19 [c]	40.46 ± 0.21 [c]	15.96 ± 0.07 [b]
	SWE 190 °C	32.43 ± 0.23 [e]	17.58 ± 0.01 [a]	45.60 ± 0.08 [b]	48.86 ± 0.06 [b]	21.08 ± 0.03 [a]
	SWE 230 °C	39.33 ± 0.40 [c]	14.49 ± 0.13 [b]	51.52 ± 0.27 [a]	53.52 ± 0.30 [a]	15.70 ± 0.06 [c]
U. lactuca	HWE	56.18 ± 0.61 [a]	−1.59 ± 0.04 [e]	19.84 ± 0.82 [e]	19.90 ± 0.82 [e]	−4.57 ± 0.09 [e]
	SWE 110 °C	55.81 ± 0.26 [a]	−1.07 ± 0.00 [d]	22.33 ± 0.52 [c]	22.35 ± 0.52 [c]	−2.74 ± 0.06 [d]
	SWE 150 °C	42.65 ± 0.53 [b]	0.72 ± 0.03 [c]	21.51 ± 0.35 [d]	21.52 ± 0.35 [d]	1.92 ± 0.04 [c]
	SWE 190 °C	25.07 ± 0.42 [c]	24.04 ± 0.08 [b]	36.73 ± 0.64 [a]	43.89 ± 0.58 [b]	33.21 ± 0.37 [b]
	SWE 230 °C	23.64 ± 0.05 [d]	27.58 ± 0.28 [a]	35.92 ± 0.34 [b]	45.29 ± 0.44 [a]	37.52 ± 0.02 [a]

Abbreviations: HWE: hot water extraction; SWE: subcritical water extraction; L*: lightness; a*: red/green coordinate b*: yellow/blue coordinate; C*: chroma; H*: hue. Values correspond to mean ± SD from three independent experiments. Different letters (a–d, a–d) denote a statistically significant difference ($p < 0.05$).

Table 4. Maillard Reaction Products (MRPs) of green seaweed hydrolysates

Green Seaweed	Conditions	294	420	294/420
C. racemosa	HWE	0.84 ± 0.02 [d]	0.05 ± 0.00 [d]	17.23 ± 0.48 [a]
	SWE 110 °C	0.84 ± 0.06 [d]	0.05 ± 0.00 [d]	16.41 ± 1.08 [b]
	SWE 150 °C	0.98 ± 0.01 [c]	0.07 ± 0.00 [c]	13.38 ± 0.12 [c,d]
	SWE 190 °C	1.17 ± 0.01 [b]	0.09 ± 0.00 [b]	12.77 ± 0.16 [d]
	SWE 230 °C	1.49 ± 0.01 [a]	0.11 ± 0.00 [a]	14.05 ± 0.27 [c]
U. lactuca	HWE	0.86 ± 0.01 [d]	0.05 ± 0.00 [d]	16.41 ± 0.34 [a]
	SWE 110 °C	0.86 ± 0.02 [d]	0.05 ± 0.00 [d]	16.43 ± 0.09 [a]
	SWE 150 °C	0.88 ± 0.01 [c]	0.06 ± 0.00 [c]	14.52 ± 0.35 [b]
	SWE 190 °C	1.62 ± 0.02 [b]	0.13 ± 0.00 [b]	12.46 ± 0.14 [d]
	SWE 230 °C	1.99 ± 0.01 [a]	0.15 ± 0.00 [a]	13.09 ± 0.08 [c]

Abbreviations: MRPs: Maillard Reaction Products; HWE: hot water extraction; SWE: subcritical water extraction. Values correspond to mean ± SD from three independent experiments. Values correspond to mean ± SD from three independent experiments. Different letters (a–d, a–d) denote a statistically significant difference ($p < 0.05$).

2.3. Total Protein, Sugars and Reducing Sugar Contents of C. racemosa and U. lactuca Hydrolysates

The total protein contents in C. racemosa and U. lactuca hydrolysates obtained by HWE and SWE at various temperatures are provided in Figure 2A. In this study, we found that the protein contents of green seaweeds were not significantly different in HWE and SWE processes at extraction temperatures of up to 150 °C ($p < 0.05$). Interestingly, at higher temperatures (above 150 °C), the protein contents were increased dramatically. The highest protein yield (330.37 mg/g ± 5.46) was obtained from the U. lactuca hydrolyzed at 230 °C. Protein has low solubility at low temperature, due to robust aggregation via hydrophobic interactions [36,37]. When the temperature rises, the water ionization constant rises, increasing the protein yield observed in C. racemosa and U. lactuca.

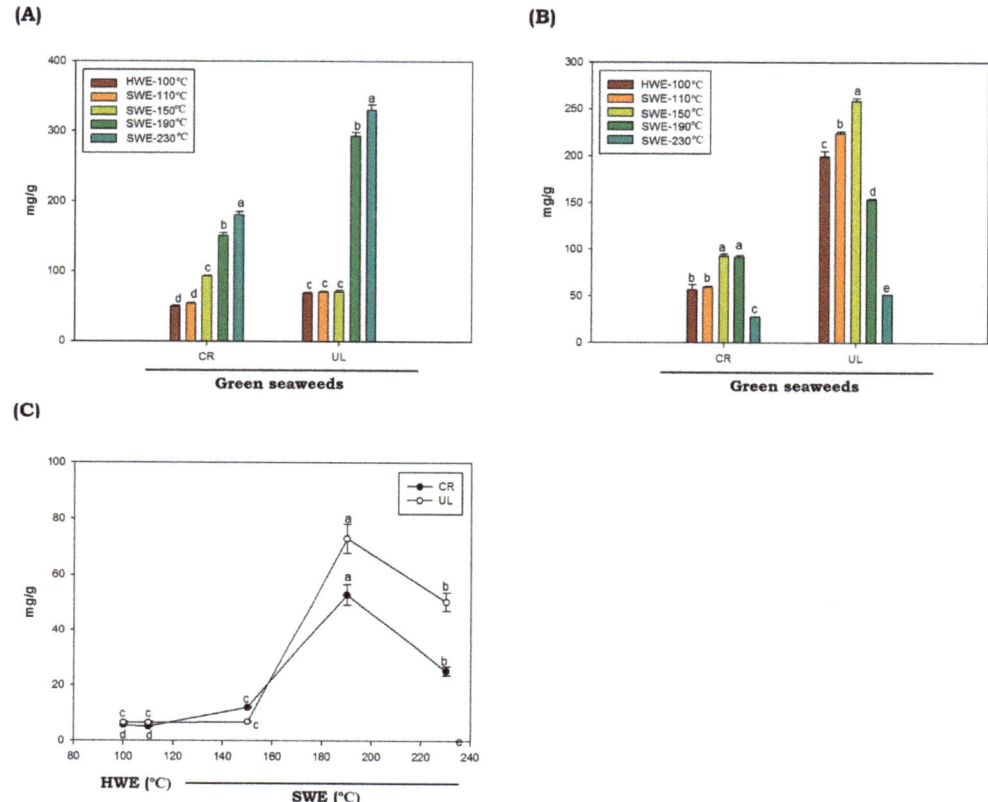

Figure 2. Total protein (**A**), sugar (**B**) and reducing sugar (**C**) of green seaweed hydrolysates obtained by HWE and SWE. CR: *C. racemosa*; UL: *U. lactuca*. Values correspond to mean ± SD from three independent experiments. Different letters (a–e) denote a statistically significant difference ($p < 0.05$).

The total sugar values of *C. racemosa* and *U. lactuca* hydrolysates are shown in Figure 2B. The proportions of total sugars of *C. racemosa* and *U. lactuca* ranged from 56.88 to 93.04 mg/g and 51.67 to 258.95 mg/g, respectively. Total sugar of *C. racemosa* and *U. lactuca* with the highest content was obtained by SWE at 150 °C, with values of 93.04 ± 2.13 mg/g and 258.93 ± 2.71 mg/g, respectively. Compared to *C. racemosa*, *U. lactuca* showed higher total sugar contents. The sugar contents of *U. lactuca* found in this study are comparable to the total sugar contents of *U. lactuca* from Tunisia and Israel, which were 272 mg/g and 68.10 to 159.29 mg/g, respectively [38,39]. However, compared to Arctic *U. lactuca*, the sugar contents found in this study were slightly lower [40]. It was reported that the variations in total sugar contents could be affected by temporal or spatial variations in sugar contents of particular seaweed species, and also by methodological differences. In addition, we found that the levels of total sugars in both green seaweeds were decreased at temperatures above 150 °C. The hydrolysis of poly- or oligosaccharides and the degradation of monosaccharides caused by the high ionic product of solvent at elevated temperature under SWE conditions were thought to be the cause of the decrease in total sugar content [41]. Both *C. racemosa* and *U. lactuca* produce low amounts of reduced sugars when hydrolyzed by HWE or SWE at temperatures of up to 150 °C. The highest reducing sugar levels of both *C. racemosa* and *U. lactuca* were obtained by SWE at temperatures of 190 °C with values of 53.06 ± 3.65 mg/g 73.00 ± 5.15 mg/g, respectively. It was demonstrated that reducing sugar content from the seaweeds polysaccharides by SWE increased up to certain reaction temperatures and then decreased [42]. The lower levels of reducing sugar may be correlated to the decomposition of sugar into other products, such as ketones and aldehydes, from which organic acids can be produced

2.4. Phenolics, Saponins and Flavonoid Contents of C. racemosa and U. lactuca Hydrolysates

Polyphenols are naturally present in plants such as seaweeds, which help them to eliminate free radicals. In this study, results for total phenolic (TPC), saponin (TSC) and flavonoid (TFC) *C. racemosa* and *U. lactuca* hydrolysates are shown in Figure 3. The values of TPC, TSC and TFC were represented as gallic acid equivalent (GAE), diosgenin equivalent (DE) and quercetin equivalent (QE), respectively. The values of TPC, TSC and TFC of *C. racemosa* and *U. lactuca* hydrolysates extracted by HWE and SWE at 110 up to 150 °C are low. However, as temperatures increased from 190 to 230 °C, the TPC, TSC and TFC of both *C. racemosa* and *U. lactuca* were significantly increased ($p < 0.05$). The highest TPC, TSC and TFC of both green seaweeds were obtained at reaction temperatures of 230 °C. The TPC, TSC and TFC values were obtained from *U. lactuca* hydrolyzed at 230 °C with the value of 39.82 ± 0.32 GAE mg/g, 13.22 ± 0.33 DE mg/g and 6.5 ± 0.47 QE mg/g, respectively. It has been reported that temperature is one of the most important factors affecting TPC, TSC and TSC in SWE process. In addition, it was reported that when the dielectric constant SWE decreases as the temperature rises, more nonpolar phenolics are being extracted [43].

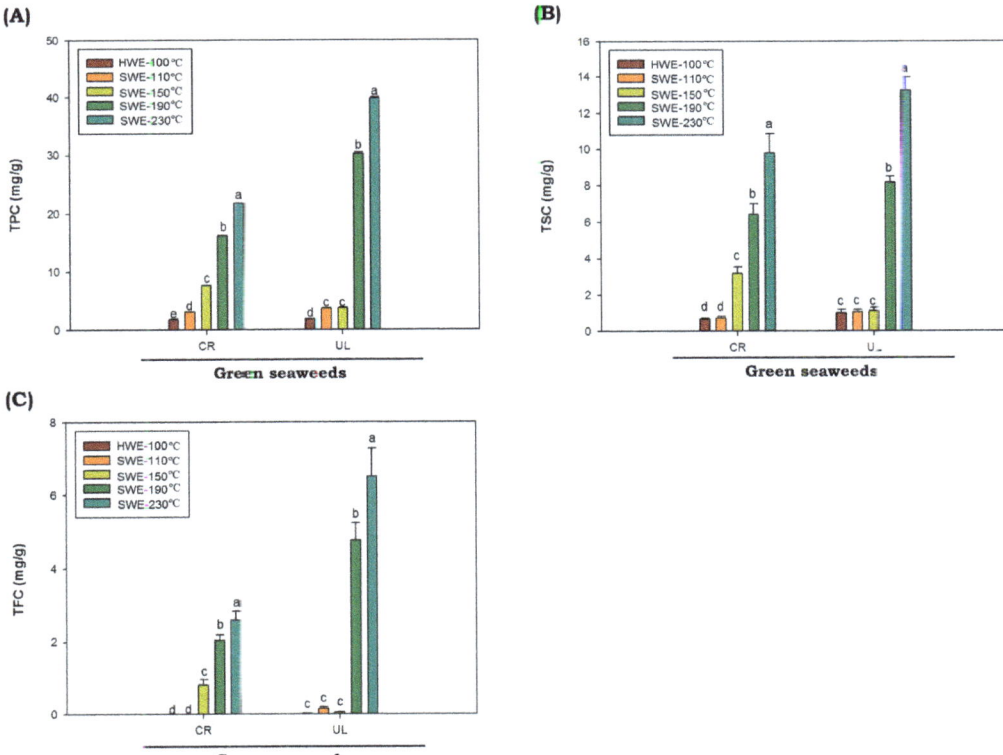

Figure 3. Total phenolic (**A**), flavonoid (**B**) and saponin (**C**) contents of green seaweed hydrolysates were obtained by HWE and SWE. CR: *C. racemosa*; UL: *U. lactuca*. Values correspond to mean ± SD from three independent experiments Different letters (a–e) denote a statistically significant difference ($p < 0.05$).

Total phenolic contents of *C. racemosa* and *U. lactuca* hydrolysates are higher as compared to the TSC and TFC. Therefore, phenolic acid constituents from both green seaweed hydrolysates were quantified by HPLC. The contents of phenolic compounds in *C. racemosa* and *U. lactuca* hydrolysates were estimated based on the reference phenolic acid standards calibration curves. The main constituents of the phenolic acids present in *C. racemosa* and *U. lactuca* are summarized in Table 5. The phenolic acids with the highest levels in *U. lactuca* were gallic acid and vanillic acid. Interestingly, phenolic acids in both green seaweeds hydrolysates obtained by SWE generally increased at elevated temperatures up to 230 °C. However, a previous study reported a loss of phenolic acids, which were hydrolyzed using SWE at high temperatures (above 200 °C). Decreased phenolic acid levels in the SWE hydrolysates at elevated temperatures may be related to the conversion of phenolic acid into decarboxylation products and other gaseous products [44]. At elevated temperatures, phenolic compounds degraded much faster. Khuwijitjaru et al., (2014) demonstrated that only the chlorogenic, p-hydroxybenzoic, protocatechuic and syringic acids were present at 200 °C after 1h of SWE treatments. Notably, in this study, we found an increment in chlorogenic, p-hydroxybenzoic and protocatechuic acid at temperatures of 190 and 230 °C. It was reported that substituent groups on the ring structure of phenolic acids, such as amino, hydroxyl and methoxyl, acted as an activating group in the SWE process, assisting the thermal decarboxylation of benzoic acid derivatives [45].

Table 5. Phenolic acid constituents of green seaweed hydrolysates obtained by HWE and SWE (mg/g dry material).

Green Seaweed	Conditions	Gallic Acid	Chlorogenic Acid	Gentisic Acid	Protocatechuic Acid	p-Hydroxybenzoic Acid	Vanillic Acid
C. racemosa	HWE	9.26 ± 0.06 [c]	ND	ND	ND	ND	ND
	SWE 110 °C	7.52 ± 0.17 [d]	ND	ND	ND	ND	ND
	SWE 150 °C	15.74 ± 0.38 [a]	0.22 ± 0.02 [c]	ND	ND	ND	ND
	SWE 190 °C	16.11 ± 0.07 [a]	1.32 ± 0.04 [b]	14.62 ± 0.32 [b]	ND	6.95 ± 0.08 [b]	ND
	SWE 230 °C	13.91 ± 0.11 [b]	1.41 ± 0.04 [a]	27.40 ± 0.51 [a]	ND	11.21 ± 0.21 [a]	ND
U. lactuca	HWE	9.25 ± 0.05 [e]	ND	ND	ND	ND	ND
	SWE 110 °C	14.47 ± 0.21 [d]	ND	ND	ND	ND	ND
	SWE 150 °C	26.84 ± 0.19 [b]	ND	ND	ND	ND	ND
	SWE 190 °C	31.27 ± 0.58 [a]	3.83 ± 0.07 [b]	11.69 ± 0.28 [b]	1.31 ± 0.04 [b]	5.03 ± 0.12 [a]	47.15 ± 0.56 [a]
	SWE 230 °C	19.74 ± 0.44 [c]	5.39 ± 0.15 [a]	20.63 ± 0.45 [a]	3.26 ± 0.27 [a]	4.05 ± 0.09 [b]	32.42 ± 0.52 [b]

Abbreviations: HWE: hot water extraction; SWE: subcritical water extraction; L: lightness; a: red/green coordinate; b: yellow/blue coordinate; C: chroma; H: hue. Values correspond to mean ± SD from three independent experiments. Different letters (a–d, a–e) denote a statistically significant difference ($p < 0.05$).

2.5. Potential of Cytotoxic and Antioxidant Activities of C. racemosa and U. lactuca Hydrolysates

Potential cytotoxic effects *C. racemosa* and *U. lactuca* hydrolysates were tested at 50 μg/mL using MTT cell viability assay in cultured macrophage (RAW 264.7 cells). As shown in Figure 4, all green seaweed hydrolysates obtained by HWE as well as SWE did not show any toxic effect on RAW 264.7 cells at tested concentrations after 24 h and 48 h of treatment ($p < 0.05$). These results showed that *C. racemosa* and *U. lactuca* hydrolysates were safe and non-toxic. Similar non-toxic properties of *C. racemosa* and *U. lactuca* aqueous extracts have been reported by previous studies [46,47]. These results showed the potential of *C. racemosa* and *U. lactuca* to be developed in nutraceutical and cosmeceutical products.

Seaweeds, including green seaweeds, have been continuously demonstrated to possess a wide range of bioactive materials as well as biological activities [10]. In this study, the antioxidant potential of green seaweed hydrolysates obtained by HWE and SWE was tested using ABTS radical scavenging and total antioxidant assays, which are represented as ascorbic acid equivalents (AAE) and trolox equivalents (TE), respectively. The antioxidant potentials of *C. racemosa* and *U. lactuca* hydrolysates are shown in Table 6. The antioxidant activity of both *C. racemosa* and *U. lactuca* reaches a maximum value with SWE at 230 °C. During the subcritical process at certain temperatures, solvents could extract more bioactive compounds that could not be extracted at lower temperatures and/or by conventional HWE. A temperature of 230 °C was found to be the most optimal condition to obtain bioactive materials from *C. racemosa* and *U. lactuca* using SWE. It was reported that the potential antioxidant activity of *U. lactuca* could be attributed to the higher content of polyphenols, flavonoids, saponins and sulfated polysaccharides compounds, with a known ability to scavenge synthetic radicals in in vitro tests (i.e ABTS) [48]. In addition, in our previous study, we found that the antioxidant activities of seaweeds are strongly correlated with their phenolic contents [5]. The results of the present study demonstrated that green seaweed hydrolysates obtained by SWE could be effective and safe alternatives to fight against radicals. In addition, green seaweed hydrolysates could be used as effective sources for antioxidative nutraceutical and cosmeceutical ingredients. Furthermore, more attention has been raised about the use of natural antioxidants as "natural" entities in nutraceutical and cosmeceutical products [49,50]. These will increase the potency of seaweeds extracts obtained by green extraction methods in various industries since it is of natural origin and environmental friendly.

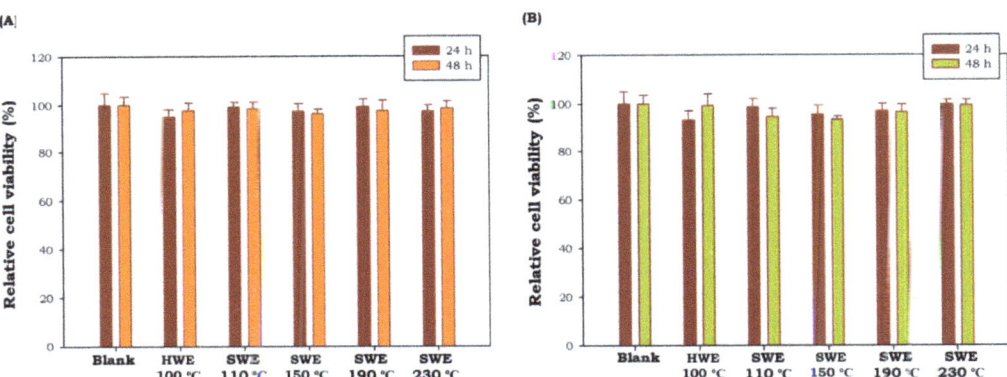

Figure 4. Effects of *C. racemosa* (**A**) and *U. lactuca* (**B**) on the viability of RAW 264.7 cells. HWE: hot water extraction; SWE: subcritical water extraction. Results are the percentage of three independent experiments and are shown as the percentage of viable cells compared with the viability of untreated cells. Values correspond to mean ± SD from three independent experiments.

Table 6. Antioxidant activity of green seaweed hydrolysates.

Green Seaweed	Conditions	ABTS (AAE mg/g)	Total Antioxidant (TE mg/g)
C. racemosa	HWE	0.09 ± 0.05 [d]	0.18 ± 0.03 [d]
	SWE 110 °C	0.11 ± 0.03 [d]	0.16 ± 0.04 [d]
	SWE 150 °C	1.12 ± 0.05 [c]	1.63 ± 0.07 [c]
	SWE 190 °C	3.48 ± 0.10 [b]	5.08 ± 0.09 [b]
	SWE 230 °C	5.45 ± 0.11 [a]	8.03 ± 0.06 [a]
U. lactuca	HWE	0.15 ± 0.05 [e]	0.22 ± 0.07 [d]
	SWE 110 °C	0.22 ± 0.03 [d]	0.32 ± 0.05 [d]
	SWE 150 °C	0.40 ± 0.05 [c]	3.37 ± 0.07 [c]
	SWE 190 °C	7.09 ± 0.00 [b]	10.30 ± 0.00 [b]
	SWE 230 °C	8.14 ± 0.02 [a]	11.82 ± 0.02 [a]

Abbreviations: HWE: hot water extraction; SWE: subcritical water extraction; AAE: ascorbic acids equivalents; TE: trolox equivalents. Values correspond to mean ± SD from three independent experiments. Different letters (a–d, c–e) denote a statistically significant difference ($p < 0.05$).

3. Materials and Methods

3.1. Materials

Two under-exploited green seaweed species (*C. racemosa* and *U. lactuca*) were collected from Tual, Southeast Maluku, in June 2018. A voucher specimen was deposited in Balai

Bioindustri Laut (BBIL), Lembaga Ilmu Pengetahuan Indonesia (LIPI) West Nusa Tenggara with the accession numbers of GSW-CR-180601 and GSW-UL-180602 for *Caulerpa racemosa* and *Ulva lactuca*, respectively. All the chemicals utilized in this study were obtained from Merck and Junsei Chemical Co., Ltd. (Tokyo, Japan) and were of analytical grade.

3.2. C. racemosa and U. lactuca Sample Preparation

Both *C. racemosa* and *U. lactuca* were washed with clean water; sand debris and other dirt were gently removed. The green seaweeds were further oven-dried at 45 °C for 120 h. In the next step, dried green seaweeds were further freeze-dried and then powderized into a very fine particle (passed through a 0.71 mm siever). The green seaweeds were further kept at −20 °C prior to analysis.

3.3. Proximate Analysis of C. racemosa and U. lactuca

The protein, ash, lipid, protein and moisture contents of *C. racemosa* and *U. lactuca* were measured according to the Association of Official Analytical Chemists methods [51]. Further, total carbohydrate content was estimated by subtracting the total mass of green seaweeds from the sum of other proximate contents.

3.4. Fatty Acid Composition Analysis of C. racemosa and U. lactuca

The fatty acid composition of *C. racemosa* and *U. lactuca* were determined using a Fatty Acid Composition Analysis (Agilent Technologies, Wilmington, NC, USA) gas chromatograph with a fused silica capillary column (Supelco, Bellefonte, PA, USA). Methylation of fatty acids (fatty acid methyl esters; FAMEs Supelco, Bellefonte, PA, USA) were prepared according to The American Oil Chemists' Society's protocols. The oven temperature was turned on at 130 °C and run for 180 s, and then the temperatures were increased up to 240 °C at a rate of 4 °C/min and then maintained at 240 °C for 600 s. Both the injector and the detector were set to 250 °C. The FAMEs were identified by comparison of retention time with a standard fatty acid methyl ester mixture (Supelco, Bellefonte, PA, USA).

3.5. Sample Extraction

3.5.1. Hot Water Extraction of Green Seaweeds

Fine powder of *C. racemosa* and *U. lactuca* was mixed with distilled water at normal pH (7.2) with the sample to solvent ratios of 1:40 (*w/v*). The mixtures were kept at 100 °C and agitated (200 rpm) for 2 h. The hydrolysate obtained after HWE processes was filtered and freeze-dried.

3.5.2. Subcritical Water Extraction (SWE) of Green Seaweeds

The SWE was operated in a continuous-type subcritical water system (Phosentech, South Korea). Fine powder of *C. racemosa* and *U. lactuca* was added into the reactor with distilled water at normal pH (7.2) at 1:40 ratios (*w/v*). The chamber was sealed tightly, purged with nitrogen gas and kept at the desired reaction temperature, pressure and speed (200 rpm) for 10 min. Hydrolyzed green seaweeds were immediately collected after the reaction was terminated and filtered with 0.45 μm membrane filter. The hydrolysate obtained after SWE processes was freeze-dried.

$$\text{Yield (\%)} = \frac{W_{hyd}}{W_0} \times 100\,\% \tag{1}$$

where W_{hyd} is the weight of freeze-dried hydrolysate and W_0 is the initial weight of green seaweeds.

3.6. Physical Properties of C. racemosa and U. lactuca (Color, pH and Maillard Reaction Products (MRPs))

Color properties of *C. racemosa* and *U. lactuca* hydrolysates were measured using a chromameter (Lovibond RT Series, Amesbury (Wiltshire), UK) [5]. The color characteristics of *C. racemosa* and *U. lactuca* were distinguished based on lightness value (L^*), redness value ($a*$) and yellowness value ($b*$). Chroma meter was standardized each time with black and white references prior to analysis. The hue angle ($h*ab$) and chroma ($C*ab$) of *C. racemosa* and *U. lactuca* hydrolysates were calculated based on the following equations:

$$H° = \tan^{-1}\left(\frac{b*}{a*}\right) \qquad (2)$$

$$C*ab = \sqrt{(a*)^2 + (b*)^2} \qquad (3)$$

Following the hydrolysis process, *C. racemosa* and *U. lactuca* were filtered and cooled down, and then pH was measured by using a pH meter (Mettler-Toledo, Greifensee, Switzerland). The MRPs were determined through the UV absorbance of samples, as described previously [52]. After the hydrolysis processes, 0.2 mL of filtered *C. racemosa* and *U. lactuca* (1 mg per mL) was measured at 294 and 420 nm.

3.7. Total Protein, Total Sugar and Reducing Sugar of C. racemosa and U. lactuca

The protein concentrations of *C. racemosa* and *U. lactuca* hydrolysates were determined following Lowry's method. The *C. racemosa* and *U. lactuca* hydrolysates (0.2 mL) were mixed with $CuSO_4$ reagent at 1:10 ratios (v/v) and vortexed. After incubation for 600 s at RT, 0.2 mL of 0.2 N Folin–Ciocalteu reagent (FCR) was loaded into the mixture and incubated for another 0.5 h. Total protein was determined through the UV absorbance of samples at 660 nm, and bovine serum albumin was used as the reference standard.

The total sugar value of *C. racemosa* and *U. lactuca* hydrolysates was measured based on the phenol sulfuric acid method. The *C. racemosa* and *U. lactuca* (0.2 mL) were mixed with 5% phenol (0.2 mL) and sulfuric acid (H_2SO_4; 1 mL) and 0.5 h at 100 °C. The total sugar was determined through the UV absorbance of samples at 490 nm, and $C_6H_{12}O_6$ was used as the reference standard.

Reducing sugar analyses of *C. racemosa* and *U. lactuca* hydrolysates were measured by using the 3,5-dinitrosalicylic (DNS) acid method with slight modifications. *C. racemosa* and *U. lactuca* hydrolysates (0.5 mL) were mixed with DNS reagent solution at 1:1 ratios. The mixtures were then incubated at 95 °C for 15 min. After incubation, 0.5 mL of $KNaC_4H_4O_6·4H_2O$ (40%) was added. Reducing sugar was determined through the UV absorbance of samples at 575 nm, and $C_6H_{12}O_6$ was used as the reference standard.

3.8 Total Flavonoid Content (TFC), Total Phenolic Content (TPC) and Total Saponin Content (TSC) of C. racemosa and U. lactuca

The TFC of *C. racemosa* and *U. lactuca* hydrolysates were measured according to previous methods [53]. Green seaweed hydrolysates (0.2 mL) were mixed with 0.4 mL of H_2O and 0.2 mL of 5% $NaNO_2$ and incubated at RT for 10 min. Following incubation periods, 10% $AlCl_3$ (0.03 mL) and 1 M NaOH (0.4 mL) were added. The mixtures were loaded onto 96-well plates, and the absorbance was measured at 510 nm using multimode microplate readers. Quercetin (Q) was used as the reference standard for flavonoids. The original reaction solution was used to convert the value of the diluted samples. The final results were given in mg Q equivalent/g dry weight (mg Q/g DW).

The TPC of *C. racemosa* and *U. lactuca* hydrolysates was measured using FCR methods [54]. The *C. racemosa* and *U. lactuca* (0.5 mL) were mixed with 0.2 N FCR solution (0.5 mL) and kept in the dark at RT for 10 min. A 7.5% mixture of Na_2CO_3 was added (0.5 mL) and kept in the dark at RT for 2 h. The TPC was determined through the UV absorbance of samples at 765 nm, and the final values were expressed as mg phloroglucinol equivalent/g dry weight (mg/g DW).

The TSC of *C. racemosa* and *U. lactuca* hydrolysates was measured using the methods described previously with slight modifications. *C. racemosa* and *U. lactuca* were placed into tubes, at volumes with MeOH at 80% and 0.25 mL; 0.25 mL of 8% vanillin reagent and 2.5 mL H_2O_4S (72%) were added. The mixtures were mixed properly and kept at 60 °C for 10 min. After 10 min, the mixtures were transferred into ice. The TSC was determined through the UV absorbance of samples at 544 nm, and the final values were expressed as mg diosgenin equivalent/g dry weight (mg/g DW).

3.9. High-Performance Liquid Chromatography (HPLC) Analysis of C. racemosa and U. lactuca Hydrolysates

The *C. racemosa* and *U. lactuca* hydrolysates were further analyzed for phenolic acid compositions using the HPLC system (Hitachi America Ltd., White Plains, NY, USA) on a Nucleosil C_8 column (Macherey-Nagel, Düren, Germany) with linear gradients of solvent A (H_2O with 0.1% CH_3COOH) and solvent B (C_2H_3N with 0.1% CH_3COOH) at a flow rate of 1 mL per min. The elution peaks were detected at 280 nm. The HPLC peak was confirmed with the reference phenolic acids and expressed as mg/g DW.

3.10. Antioxidant Activity

3.10.1. 2,2-Azino-bis(3-ethylbenzothiazoline-6-sulfonic acid) Scavenging Assay

The 2,2-azino-bis(3-ethylbenzothiazoline-6-sulfonic acid) (ABTS) (7 mmol/L) and $K_2S_2O_8$ (2.45 mmol/L) were prepared in a separate bottle, and both solutions were kept in the dark at RT. After 24 h, both solutions were mixed. The radical mixtures were diluted with MeOH to obtain absorbance values of 0.72. The *C. racemosa* and *U. lactuca* hydrolysates were mixed with ABTS radical mixture at 1:5 ratios (*v/v*). The ABTS scavenging activity was determined through the UV absorbance of samples at 734 nm, and MeOH was used as the negative control. In comparison, different concentrations of ascorbic acid were used as standard and evaluated. The results are expressed in terms of AAE.

3.10.2. Total Antioxidant Capacity (TAC)

The *C. racemosa* and *U. lactuca* hydrolysates (0.1 mL) were mixed with 3 mL of radical mixture consist of 0.6 M H_2SO_4, 28 mM Na_3PO_4 and 4 mM $(NH_4)_6Mo_7O_{24}$. The mixtures were maintained at 95 °C for 180 min. The total antioxidant activity was determined through the measurements of UV absorbance at 695 nm, and MeOH was used as negative control. In comparison, different concentrations of trolox were used as standard and evaluated. The results are expressed in terms of TE.

3.11. Effects of Seaweeds Hydrolysates on Cell Viability

Cytotoxic effects of *C. racemosa* and *U. lactuca* hydrolysates were determined by MTT reduction assay [55]. First, macrophage (RAW 264.7) cells were seeded into cell culture plates at a cell density of 2×10^4 cells/well in serum-free DMEM. The *C. racemosa* and *U. lactuca* hydrolysates (50 µg/mL) were then loaded in the cell culture and then incubated for 24 h. One hundred microliters of an MTT (0.5 mg/ml) solution was loaded into the cultures, and incubation was continued for another 240 min. MTT was used as an indicator of cell viability through its mitochondrial reduction to formazan [56]. The absorbance was measured at 540 nm by using a microplate reader. RAW 264.7 cell viability was calculated by comparison of the absorbance of the control group with treated groups.

3.12. Statistical Analysis

The data were presented as means $\pm$ SD ($n = 3$). Differences between the means of the individual groups were assessed by one-way ANOVA with Duncan's multiple range tests. Differences were considered significant at $p < 0.05$. The statistical software package, SPSS v.16 (SPSS Inc., Chicago, IL, USA), was used for the analysis.

4. Conclusions

Green seaweed hydrolysates, *C. racemosa* and *U. lactuca*, were prepared via HWE and SWE. Compared to HWE, the SWE process showed higher extraction yields, bioactive compounds and antioxidant activities of seaweed hydrolysates. In addition, six phenolic acids, including gallic acids, chlorogenic acid, gentisic acid, procatechuic acid, *p*-hydroxybenzoic acid and vanillic acid were identified in *U. lactuca* hydrolysates obtained by SWE at 230 °C.

The SWE-enabled recovery of bioactive compounds from *C. racemosa* and *U. lactuca* with hydrolysis temperature at 230 °C was found to be the most optimum conditions to obtain bioactive materials with good radical scavenging activities, making it a potential candidate for antioxidant compounds. Collectively, this study provides the foundations for exploring under-exploited tropical green seaweeds and filling the gaps for future research in the development of nutraceuticals and cosmeceuticals from sea grape and sea lettuces.

Author Contributions: Conceptualization, R.P.; methodology, R.P., M.H.; analysis, R.P., M.H.; resources, P.R.; writing—original draft preparation, R.P.; writing—review and editing, R.P., P.R., M.H., B.-S.C.; supervision, B.-S.C.; project administration, B.-S.C., P.R.; funding acquisition, B.-S.C., P.R. All authors have read and agreed to the published version of the manuscript.

Funding: This research was supported by the National Research Foundation (Rep. of Korea) and National Research Priority (PRN)-MALSAI from the Indonesian Institute of Sciences (LIPI), National Research and Innovation Agency (BRIN) and Indonesia Endowment Fund for Education (LPDP), Rep. of Indonesia.

Institutional Review Board Statement: Not applicable.

Informed Consent Statement: Not applicable.

Acknowledgments: The authors would like to thank the National Research Foundation (South Korea) for the Postdoctoral fellowship awards and Pukyong National University for the research supports. The authors also acknowledge Deputy for Earth Science LIPI (2015-2019) Zainal Arifin, and Chairman of Research Organizations for Earth Sciences BRIN Ocky K. Radjasa for all the support.

Conflicts of Interest: The authors declare no conflict of interest.

References

1. Shannon, E.; Abu-Ghannam, N. Seaweeds as nutraceuticals for health and nutrition. *Phycologia* **2019**, *58*, 563–577. [CrossRef]
2. Mouritsen, O.G.; Rhatigan, P.; Cornish, M.L.; Critchley, A.T.; Pérez-Lloréns, J.L. Saved by seaweeds: Phyconomic contributions in times of crises. *J. Appl. Phycol.* **2021**, *33*, 443–458. [CrossRef]
3. Pangestuti, R.; Kim, S.-K. Biological activities and health benefit effects of natural pigments derived from marine algae. *J. Func. Foods* **2011**, *3*, 255–266. [CrossRef]
4. Pangestuti, R.; Siahaan, E.; Kim, S.-K. Photoprotective Substances Derived from Marine Algae. *Mar. Drugs* **2018**, *16*, 399. [CrossRef]
5. Pangestuti, R.; Getachew, A.T.; Siahaan, E.A.; Chun, B.-S. Characterization of functional materials derived from tropical red seaweed *Hypnea musciformis* produced by subcritical water extraction systems. *J. Appl. Phycol.* **2019**, *31*, 2517–2528. [CrossRef]
6. Hutomo, M.; Moosa, M.K. Indonesian marine and coastal biodiversity: Present status. *Indian. J. Mar. Sci.* **2005** *34*, 88–97.
7. Hung, Y.-H.R.; Chen, G.-W.; Pan, C.-L.; Lin, H.-T.V. Production of Ulvan Oligosaccharides with Antioxidant and Angiotensin-Converting Enzyme-Inhibitory Activities by Microbial Enzymatic Hydrolysis. *Fermentation* **2021**, *7*, 160. [CrossRef]
8. Harikrishnan, R.; Devi, G.; Van Doan, H.; Balasundaram, C.; Arockiaraj, J.; Jagruthi, C. Efficacy of ulvan on immune response and immuno-antioxidant gene modulation in Labeo rohita against columnaris disease. *Fish Shellfish Immunol.* **2021**, *117*, 262–273. [CrossRef] [PubMed]
9. Guidara, M.; Yaich, H.; Amor, I.B.; Fakhfakh, J.; Gargouri, J.; Lassoued, S.; Blecker, C.; Richel, A.; Attia, H.; Garna, H. Effect of extraction procedures on the chemical structure, antitumor and anticoagulant properties of ulvan from *Ulva lactuca* of Tunisia coast. *Carbohydr. Polym.* **2021**, *253*, 117283. [CrossRef]
10. Pangestuti, R.; Shin, K.-H.; Kim, S.-K. Anti-Photoaging and Potential Skin Health Benefits of Seaweeds. *Mar Drugs* **2021**, *19*, 172. [CrossRef] [PubMed]
11. Taher, M.; Ruslan, F.S.; Susanti, D.; Noor, N.M.; Aminudin, N.I. Bioactive Compounds, Cosmeceutical And Nutraceutical Applications of Green Seaweed Species (Chlorophyta). *Squalen Bull. Mar. Fish. Postharvest Biotechnol.* **2021**, *16*, 41–55. [CrossRef]
12. Saravana, P.S.; Cho, Y.-N.; Woo, H.-C.; Chun, B.-S. Green and efficient extraction of polysaccharides from brown seaweed by adding deep eutectic solvent in subcritical water hydrolysis. *J. Clean. Prod.* **2018**, *198*, 1474–1484. [CrossRef]
13. Saravana, P.S.; Getachew, A.T.; Cho, Y.-J.; Choi, J.H.; Park, Y.B.; Woo, H.C.; Chun, B.S. Influence of co-solvents on fucoxanthin and phlorotannin recovery from brown seaweed using supercritical CO_2. *J. Supercrit. Fluids* **2017**, *120*, 295–303. [CrossRef]
14. Alboofetileh, M.; Rezaei, M.; Tabarsa, M.; Rittà, M.; Donalisio, M.; Mariatti, F.; You, S.; Lembo, D.; Cravotto, G. Effect of different non-conventional extraction methods on the antibacterial and antiviral activity of fucoidans extracted from *Nizamuddinia zanardinii*. *Int. J. Biol. Macromol.* **2019**, *124*, 131–137. [CrossRef]
15. Rasyid, A. Evaluation of nutritional composition of the dried seaweed *Ulva lactuca* from Pameungpeuk waters, Indonesia. *Trop. Life Sci. Res.* **2017**, *28*, 119. [CrossRef] [PubMed]

16. Abdel-Khaliq, A.; Hassan, H.; Rateb, M.E.; Hammouda, O. Antimicrobial activity of three Ulva species collected from some Egyptian Mediterranean seashores. *Int. J. Eng. Res. Gen. Sci.* **2014**, *2*, 648–669.
17. Ortiz, J.; Romero, N.; Robert, P.; Araya, J.; Lopez-Hernández, J.; Bozzo, C.; Navarrete, E.; Osorio, A.; Rios, A. Dietary fiber, amino acid, fatty acid and tocopherol contents of the edible seaweeds *Ulva lactuca* and *Durvillaea antarctica*. *Food Chem.* **2006**, *99*, 98–104. [CrossRef]
18. Mak, W.; Hamid, N.; Liu, T.; Lu, J.; White, W. Fucoidan from New Zealand *Undaria pinnatifida*: Monthly variations and determination of antioxidant activities. *Carbohydr. Polym.* **2013**, *95*, 606–614. [CrossRef]
19. Pangestuti, R.; Kurnianto, D. Green Seaweeds-Derived Polysaccharides Ulvan: Occurrence, Medicinal Value and Potential Applications. In *Seaweed Polysaccharides*; Elsevier: Amsterdam, The Netherland, 2017; pp. 205–221.
20. Wijesekara, I.; Pangestuti, R.; Kim, S.K. Biological activities and potential health benefits of sulfated polysaccharides derived from marine algae. *Carbohydr. Polym.* **2010**, *84*, 14–21. [CrossRef]
21. Kidgell, J.T.; Magnusson, M.; de Nys, R.; Glasson, C.R. Ulvan: A systematic review of extraction, composition and function. *Algal. Res.* **2019**, *39*, 101422. [CrossRef]
22. Cindana Mo'o, F.R.; Wilar, G.; Devkota, H.P.; Wathoni, N. Ulvan, a polysaccharide from macroalga *Ulva* sp.: A review of chemistry, biological activities and potential for food and biomedical applications. *Appl. Sci.* **2020**, *10*, 5488. [CrossRef]
23. D'Armas, H.; Jaramillo, C.; D'Armas, M.; Echavarría, A.; Valverde, P. Proximate composition of several macroalgae from the coast of Salinas Bay, Ecuador. *Rev. Biol. Trop.* **2019**, *67*, 61–68.
24. Paul, N.A.; Neveux, N.; Magnusson, M.; De Nys, R. Comparative production and nutritional value of "sea grapes"—the tropical green seaweeds *Caulerpa lentillifera* and *C. racemosa*. *J. Appl. Phycol.* **2014**, *26*, 1833–1844. [CrossRef]
25. Simopoulos, A.P. An increase in the omega-6/omega-3 fatty acid ratio increases the risk for obesity. *Nutrients* **2016**, *8*, 128. [CrossRef] [PubMed]
26. Kim, S.K.; Pangestuti, R.; Rahmadi, P. Sea Lettuces: Culinary Uses and Nutritional Value. *Adv. Food Nutr. Res.* **2011**, *64*, 57–70. [PubMed]
27. Saravana, P.S.; Choi, J.H.; Park, Y.B.; Woo, H.C.; Chun, B.S. Evaluation of the chemical composition of brown seaweed (*Saccharina japonica*) hydrolysate by pressurized hot water extraction. *Algal. Res.* **2016**, *13*, 246–254. [CrossRef]
28. Park, J.-S.; Jeong, Y.-R.; Chun, B.-S. Physiological activities and bioactive compound from laver (*Pyropia yezoensis*) hydrolysates by using subcritical water hydrolysis. *J. Supercrit. Fluids* **2019**, *148*, 130–136. [CrossRef]
29. Hao, G.; Hu, Y.; Shi, L.; Chen, J.; Cui, A.; Weng, W.; Osako, K. Physicochemical characteristics of chitosan from swimming crab (*Portunus trituberculatus*) shells prepared by subcritical water pretreatment. *Sci. Rep.* **2021**, *11*, 1–9. [CrossRef]
30. Goss, R.; Jakob, T. Regulation and function of xanthophyll cycle-dependent photoprotection in algae. *Photosyn. Res.* **2010**, *106*, 103–122. [CrossRef]
31. Wiraguna, A.A.G.P.; Pangkahila, W.; Astawa, I.N.M. Antioxidant properties of topical *Caulerpa* sp. extract on UVB-induced photoaging in mice. *Derm. Rep.* **2018**, *10*, 7597. [CrossRef]
32. Liew, S.Q.; Teoh, W.H.; Tan, C.K.; Yusoff, R.; Ngoh, G.C. Subcritical water extraction of low methoxyl pectin from pomelo (*Citrus grandis* (L.) Osbeck) peels. *Int. J. Biologic. Macromol.* **2018**, *116*, 128–135. [CrossRef]
33. Pourali, O.; Asghari, F.S.; Yoshida, H. Production of phenolic compounds from rice bran biomass under subcritical water conditions. *Chem. Eng. J.* **2010**, *160*, 259–266. [CrossRef]
34. Essien, S.; Young, B.; Baroutian, S. Subcritical water extraction for selective recovery of phenolic bioactives from kānuka leaves. *J. Supercrit. Fluids* **2020**, *158*, 104721. [CrossRef]
35. Jeong, Y.-R.; Park, J.-S.; Nkurunziza, D.; Cho, Y.-J.; Chun, B.-S. Valorization of blue mussel for the recovery of free amino acids rich products by subcritical water hydrolysis. *J. Supercrit. Fluids* **2021**, *169*, 105135. [CrossRef]
36. Kramer, R.M.; Shende, V.R.; Motl, N.; Pace, C.N.; Scholtz, J.M. Toward a Molecular Understanding of Protein Solubility: Increased Negative Surface Charge Correlates with Increased Solubility. *Biophys. J.* **2012**, *102*, 1907–1915. [CrossRef] [PubMed]
37. Watchararuji, K.; Goto, M.; Sasaki, M.; Shotipruk, A. Value-added subcritical water hydrolysate from rice bran and soybean meal. *Bioresour. Technol.* **2008**, 6207–6213. [CrossRef] [PubMed]
38. Robin, A.; Chavel, P.; Chemodanov, A.; Israel, A.; Golberg, A. Diversity of monosaccharides in marine macroalgae from the Eastern Mediterranean Sea. *Algal Res.* **2017**, *28*, 118–127. [CrossRef]
39. Yaich, H.; Garna, H.; Besbes, S.; Paquot, M.; Blecker, C.; Attia, H. Chemical composition and functional properties of *Ulva lactuca* seaweed collected in Tunisia. *Food Chem.* **2011**, *128*, 895–901. [CrossRef]
40. Roleda, M.Y.; Lage, S.; Aluwini, D.F.; Rebours, C.; Brurberg, M.B.; Nitschke, U.; Gentili, F.G. Chemical profiling of the Arctic sea lettuce *Ulva lactuca* (Chlorophyta) mass-cultivated on land under controlled conditions for food applications. *Food Chem.* **2021**, *341*, 127999. [CrossRef] [PubMed]
41. Narita, Y.; Inouye, K. High antioxidant activity of coffee silverskin extracts obtained by the treatment of coffee silverskin with subcritical water. *Food Chem.* **2012**, *135*, 943–949. [CrossRef]
42. Meillisa, A.; Woo, H.-C.; Chun, B.-S. Production of monosaccharides and bio-active compounds derived from marine polysaccharides using subcritical water hydrolysis. *Food Chem.* **2015**, *171*, 70–77. [CrossRef]
43. Ko, M.-J.; Nam, H.-H.; Chung, M.-S. Subcritical water extraction of bioactive compounds from *Orostachys japonicus* A. Berger (Crassulaceae). *Sci. Rep.* **2020**, *10*, 1–10. [CrossRef]

44. Fabian, C.; Tran-Thi, N.Y.; Kasim, N.S.; Ju, Y.H. Release of phenolic acids from defatted rice bran by subcritical water treatment. *J. Sci. Food Agric.* **2010**, *90*, 2576–2581. [CrossRef]
45. Khuwijitjaru, P.; Plerrjit, J.; Suaylam, B.; Samuhaseneetoo, S.; Pongsawatmanit, R.; Adachi, S. Degradation kinetics of some phenolic compounds in subcritical water and radical scavenging activity of their degradation products. *Can. J. Chem. Eng.* **2014**, *92*, 810–815. [CrossRef]
46. Premarathna, A.D.; Wijesekera, S.K.; Jayasooriya, A.P.; Waduge, R.N.; Wijesundara, R.R.M.K.K.; Tuvikene, R.; Harishchandra, D.L.; Ranahewa, T.H.; Perera, N.A.N.D.; Wijewardana, V.; et al. In vitro and in vivo evaluation of the wound healing properties and safety assessment of two seaweeds (*Sargassum ilicifolium* and *Ulva lactuca*). *Biochem. Biophys. Rep.* **2021**, *26*, 100986.
47. Uddin, S.A.; Akter, S.; Hossen, S.; Rahman, M. Antioxidant, antibacterial and cytotoxic activity of *Caulerpa racemosa* (Forsskål) J. Agardh and *Ulva (Enteromorpha) intestinalis* L. *Bangladesh J. Sci. Ind. Res.* **2020**, *55*, 237–244. [CrossRef]
48. Benítez García, I.; Dueñas Ledezma, A.K.; Martínez Montaño, E.; Salazar Leyva, J.A.; Carrera, E.; Osuna Ruiz, I. Identification and quantification of plant growth regulators and antioxidant compounds in aqueous extracts of *Padina durvillaei* and *Ulva lactuca*. *Agronomy* **2020**, *10*, 866. [CrossRef]
49. Airanthi, M.W.A.; Hosokawa, M.; Miyashita, K. Comparative antioxidant activity of edible Japanese brown seaweeds. *J. Food Sci.* **2011**, *76*, C104–C111. [CrossRef]
50. Siahaan, E.A.; Pangestuti, R.; Pratama, I.S.; Putra, Y.; Kim, S.-K. Chapter 27—Beneficial Effects of Astaxanthin in Cosmeceuticals with Focus on Emerging Market Trends. In *Global Perspectives on Astaxanthin*; Ravishankar, G.A., Ranga Rao, A., Eds.; Academic Press: Cambridge, MA, USA, 2021; pp. 557–568.
51. AOAC. *Official Methods of Analysis*; Association of Official Analytical Chemists: Arlington, VA, USA, 1990.
52. Ajandouz, E.; Tchiakpe, L.; Ore, F.D.; Benajiba, A.; Puigserver, A. Effects of pH on caramelization and Maillard reaction kinetics in fructose-lysine model systems. *J. Food Sci.* **2001**, *66*, 926–931. [CrossRef]
53. Ozsoy, N.; Can, A.; Yanardag, R.; Akev, N. Antioxidant activity of Smilax excelsa L. leaf extracts. *Food Chem.* **2008**, *110*, 571–583. [CrossRef]
54. Matanjun, P.; Mohamed, S.; Mustapha, N.M.; Muhammad, K.; Ming, C.H. Antioxidant activities and phenolics content of eight species of seaweeds from north Borneo. *J. Appl. Phycol.* **2008**, *20*, 367. [CrossRef]
55. Hansen, M.; Nielsen, S.; Berg, K. Re-examination and further development of a precise and rapid dye method for measuring cell growth/cell kill. *J. Immunol. Methods* **1989**, *119*, 203–210. [CrossRef]
56. Kamiloglu, S.; Sari, G.; Ozdal, T.; Capanoglu, E. Guidelines for cell viability assays. *Food Front.* **2020**, *1*, 332–349. [CrossRef]

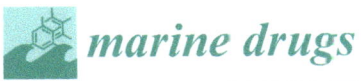

Article

Marine Ingredients for Sensitive Skin: Market Overview

Marta Salvador Ferreira [1,2,†], Diana I. S. P. Resende [3,4,†], José M. Sousa Lobo [1,2], Emília Sousa [3,4] and Isabel F. Almeida [1,2,*]

1. Associate Laboratory i4HB-Institute for Health and Bioeconomy, Faculty of Pharmacy, University of Porto, 4050-313 Porto, Portugal; msbferreira@ff.up.pt (M.S.F.); slobo@ff.up.pt (J.M.S.L.)
2. UCIBIO–Applied Molecular Biosciences Unit, MedTech, Laboratory of Pharmaceutical Technology, Department of Drug Sciences, Faculty of Pharmacy, University of Porto, 4050-313 Porto, Portugal
3. CIIMAR–Centro Interdisciplinar de Investigação Marinha e Ambiental, Avenida General Norton de Matos, S/N, 4450-208 Matosinhos, Portugal; cresende@ff.up.pt (D.I.S.P.R.); esousa@ff.up.pt (E.S.)
4. Laboratório de Química Orgânica e Farmacêutica, Departamento de Ciências Químicas, Faculdade de Farmácia, Universidade do Porto, 4050-313 Porto, Portugal
* Correspondence: ifalmeida@ff.up.pt; Tel.: +351-220-428
† These authors contributed equally to this work.

Abstract: Marine ingredients are a source of new chemical entities with biological action, which is the reason why they have gained relevance in the cosmetic industry. The facial care category is the most relevant in this industry, and within it, the sensitive skin segment occupies a prominent position. This work analyzed the use of marine ingredients in 88 facial cosmetics for sensitive skin from multinational brands, as well as their composition and the scientific evidence that supports their efficacy. Marine ingredients were used in 27% of the cosmetic products for sensitive skin and included the species *Laminaria ochroleuca*, *Ascophyllum nodosum* (brown macroalgae), *Asparagopsis armata* (red macroalgae), and *Chlorella vulgaris* (microalgae). Carotenoids, polysaccharides, and lipids are the chemical classes highlighted in these preparations. Two ingredients, namely the *Ascophyllum nodosum* extract and *Asparagopsis armata* extracts, present clinical evidence supporting their use for sensitive skin. Overall, marine ingredients used in cosmetics for sensitive skin are proposed to reduce skin inflammation and improve the barrier function. Marine-derived preparations constitute promising active ingredients for sensitive skin cosmetic products. Their in-depth study, focusing on the extracted metabolites, randomized placebo-controlled studies including volunteers with sensitive skin, and the use of extraction methods that are more profitable may provide a great opportunity for the cosmetic industry.

Keywords: marine ingredients; algae; sensitive skin; cosmetics

1. Introduction

The largely unexplored marine environment harbors unique biodiversity and represents the vastest resource for the discovery of novel chemical entities with novel modes of action that cover a biologically relevant chemical space. These new scaffolds derived from various marine organisms offer valuable bioactive properties with great relevance in medical, pharmaceutical, and cosmetic fields [1–6]. Although synthetic strategies towards natural products have evolved tremendously over the last years, natural marine products are still preferred against their synthetic counterparts since they have better physicochemical, biochemical, and rheological characteristics, maintaining their stability at different pH and temperature ranges [7]. Among marine organisms, algae are recognized as one of the richest sources of new bioactive compounds [7]. The unique diversity of bioactive compounds contained in algae, such as vitamins, minerals, amino acids, sugars, lipids, and other biologically active compounds, is translated into numerous attractive properties for various industries [8], including the food, pharmaceutical, and cosmetic industries, as evidenced by the appearance in the market of various cosmetic products derived from these

Citation: Ferreira, M.S.; Resende, D.I.S.P.; Lobo, J.M.S.; Sousa, E.; Almeida, I.F. Marine Ingredients for Sensitive Skin: Market Overview. *Mar. Drugs* 2021, 19, 464. https://doi.org/10.3390/md19080464

Academic Editors: María Lourdes Mourelle, Herminia Domínguez and Jose Luis Legido

Received: 2 August 2021
Accepted: 14 August 2021
Published: 17 August 2021

Publisher's Note: MDPI stays neutral with regard to jurisdictional claims in published maps and institutional affiliations.

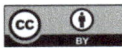

Copyright: © 2021 by the authors. Licensee MDPI, Basel, Switzerland. This article is an open access article distributed under the terms and conditions of the Creative Commons Attribution (CC BY) license (https://creativecommons.org/licenses/by/4.0/).

compounds [9]. Cosmetic products are stable substances or substance mixtures intended to clean, protect, perfume, and/or change the appearance of the external parts of the human body, teeth, and mucous membranes of the oral cavity, keeping them in good condition or correcting body odors [10]. They result from a formulation of raw materials which are categorized as active ingredients, excipients, and additives [11]. Cosmetic products may be categorized as body care, hair care, sun care, decorative cosmetics, oral care, and skin care, which is the largest cosmetic product category worldwide [12,13]. Skin care comprises a wide variety of products that should meet expectations of consumers with different skin types and organoleptic preferences. Sensitive skin is a condition characterized by multiple symptoms such as tightness, stinging, burning, or pruritus, which affects about 71% of the general adult population, being more frequent in the facial area [14–16]. Erythema, dryness, and desquamation are typically absent, but they may also occur [17]. Therefore, the sensitive skin segment allows meeting the needs of consumers who suffer from this condition [18]. Sensitive skin manifests in the presence of stimuli such as cold, heat, sun, pollution, cosmetics, or moisture which are not expected to produce unpleasant sensations, and the pathophysiological mechanisms involved in sensitive skin remain unknown [18]. Genetics, poor mental health, and microbiome imbalances have been proposed as contributing factors for this condition [19–21]. There are three hypotheses appointed in scientific literature for explaining the pathophysiology of this condition, namely the hyperactivity of the somatosensory and vascular systems, increased stratum corneum permeability, and an exacerbated immune response [22]. The hypothesis of an abnormal response from the somatosensory system is gaining increasing relevance. The skin contains sensory nerve fibers which are activated upon contact with physical and chemical stimuli such as heat, low pH solutions, or known irritants such as capsaicin, resulting in the release of neuropeptides, namely substance P or calcitonin gene-related peptide (CGRP). These neuropeptides cause a burning pain sensation through the activation of keratinocytes, mast cells, antigen-presenting cells, and T cells [23]. Neurosensory defects may lead to abnormalities in the communication with the central nervous system, resulting in a lower sensitivity threshold [15,16]. For example, an overexpression of transient receptor potential vanilloid type 1 (TRPV1), which is activated by heat and capsaicin, is thought to be involved in the pathophysiology of sensitive skin by increasing neuronal excitability [24,25]. Moreover, vascular hyperreactivity has been proposed in the pathophysiology of sensitive skin despite the absence of skin erythema [26]. The immune system is also associated with sensitive skin due to its interaction with nerve fibers, producing neurogenic inflammation. Neuropeptides activate keratinocytes, mast cells, antigen-presenting cells, and T cells, resulting in an inflammatory response [25]. Conversely, defects in the skin barrier function may be due to a derangement of intercellular lipids, due to a decrease in the ceramide content, a thinner stratum corneum with smaller corneocytes, as well as lower levels of pyrrolidone carboxylic acid (PCA) from the natural moisturizing factor (NMF), bleomycin hydrolase (BH), which is responsible for profilaggrin conversion, and transglutaminase (TG), which is essential for catalyzing the cross-linking between proteins and lipids during the corneocyte maturation process [22,27,28]. This may result in an increased permeability of the stratum corneum, which allows for the penetration of environmental aggressors [20]. More recently, this hypothesis has been questioned due to a study which failed to find significant differences in stratum corneum thickness, fatty acids, and the ceramide content, transepidermal water loss, or natural moisturizing factors between individuals with or without sensitive skin [29].

Recently, we have characterized the trends in the use of peptides in the sensitive skin care segment, reviewing their synthetic pathways and the scientific evidence that supports their efficacy [30]. We were able to conclude that three out of seven peptides have a neurotransmitter-inhibiting mechanism of action, while another three are signal peptides. As an example, palmitoyl tripeptide-8 may be a prime candidate for the development of pharmaceuticals aimed at alleviating the signs and symptoms of rosacea [30].

Given the variety of molecular targets involved in the sensitive skin pathophysiology, the chemical diversity of the marine ecosystem is a promising source for cosmetic ingredients for managing its symptoms. Our group has previously analyzed the market impact of marine ingredients in anti-aging cosmetics from multinational brands [31]. However, the use of these active ingredients in cosmetic products for sensitive skin remains unexplored. This study aims to unveil the state-of-the-art of marine ingredients in this segment by documenting their prevalence, as well as the most relevant species, their composition, and the scientific evidence that supports their efficacy for sensitive skin care.

2. Trends in the Use of Marine Ingredients in Cosmetic Formulations for Sensitive Skin

The analysis of the presence of marine ingredients in all of the studied 88 cosmetic formulations for sensitive skin (19 multinational brands) indicated that 27% of them contain marine-derived ingredients. Interestingly, a more detailed analysis regarding the origin of these ingredients (Table 1) revealed that they all derive from algae, mainly macroalgae. Although over the last decades mariculture and aquaculture techniques have been developed towards the sustainable supply of other marine organisms, such as fish, sponges, corals, mollusks, echinoderms, *Artemia*, plankton, and microorganisms [5,11,32–38], their potential is not translated in the number of cosmetic formulations for sensitive skin that have been commercialized in the Portuguese market and contained the referred ingredients. The constraints related to reduced biomass availability of these marine organisms and difficulties regarding their production/cultivation at larger scales still represent a major bottleneck in the sustainable supply of the desired natural ingredients for the cosmetic industry [32].

Table 1. Analysis of the prevalence and categorization of marine ingredients from the analyzed cosmetic products for sensitive skin (2019).

INCI [1]	Category	n	%
Laminaria ochroleuca extract	Brown algae	11	12.5
Ascophyllum nodosum extract	Brown algae	4	4.5
Asparagopsis armata extract	Red algae	4	4.5
Chlorella vulgaris extract	Green microalgae	3	3.4
Algae extract	Undefined	2	2.3

[1] INCI—International Nomenclature of Cosmetic Ingredients.

On the other hand, algae are emerging as one of the most promising long-term, sustainable sources of bioactive ingredients to be used in the formulation of cosmetic and skin care products, with a large number and wide variety of benefits associated with their secondary metabolites [2]. Their biodiversity, easy cultivation, and growth modulation are the main reasons for their increased use in a variety of industries [2]. Depending on their size, they can be divided into macroalgae, which are seaweeds and other benthic marine algae that are generally visible to the naked eye, and microalgae, which require a microscope to be observed [39]. Additionally, macroalgae can be divided into three groups based on their dominant pigments: Rhodophyceae (red algae), Phaeophyceae (brown algae), and Chlorophyceae (green algae) [40]. Bioactive substances derived from these algae have diverse functional roles as a secondary metabolite and these properties can be applied to the development of novel cosmetic products. Brown algae account for approximately 59% of the total macroalgae cultivated in the world, followed by red algae at 40% and green algae at less than 1% [40]. Hence, it is interesting to notice that the wider availability of brown and red algae is clearly translated to their use as ingredients amongst the 88 studied cosmetic formulations for sensitive skin (Figure 1). Additionally, red algae are represented in 17% of the cosmetic formulations, and none of them contained green algae, probably due to their limited availability and, therefore, associated cost to the cosmetic industry. Microalgae are also well-represented, with 13% of the studied formulations containing these marine ingredients (Figure 1).

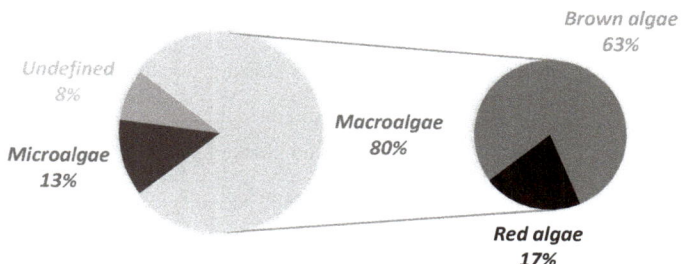

Figure 1. Categorization of the marine ingredients present in cosmetic formulations for sensitive skin commercialized in the Portuguese market (2019).

For several years, the use of the designation "algae extract" as a marine ingredient present in several cosmetic formulations with no specification of the species was permitted and included in the European Commission database for information on cosmetic ingredients contained in cosmetics (CosIng) [41]. Nowadays, the Commission requires that the new name assignment should be based on the current genus and species name of the specific alga. However, for an interim period of time, trade name assignments formerly published with the INCI name "algae extract" were retained. In this study, 2.3% of the 88 studied cosmetic formulations contained algae extract as a marine ingredient (Table 1, marked in Figure 1 as "undefined"); since the type of algae was not specified, a further detailed analysis could not be performed.

3. Efficacy of Algae-Containing Formulations on Sensitive Skin

The search results are summarized below (Figure 2):

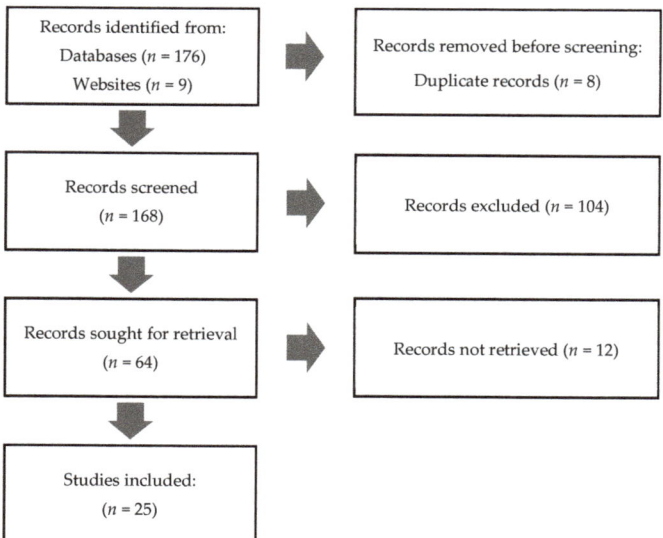

Figure 2. Flowchart of the selected articles according to four different parts of the search process: identification, screening, eligibility, and inclusion.

3.1. Brown Macroalgae

Brown seaweeds belonging to two different taxonomic orders, Fucales (*Ascophyllum Nodosum*) and Laminariales (*Laminaria ochroleuca*), were used as ingredients in 17% of the studied cosmetic formulations. The brown color presented by these species results from the dominance of the pigment fucoxanthin (Figure 3), which masks the other pigments (chlorophyll *a* and *c*, β-carotene, and other carotenoids) and, as reserve substances, oils and polysaccharides [31]. The main polysaccharide found in the brown seaweeds is alginic acid, while laminarins (up to 32–35% dry weight) and fucoidans appear as sulfated polysaccharides (Figure 3).

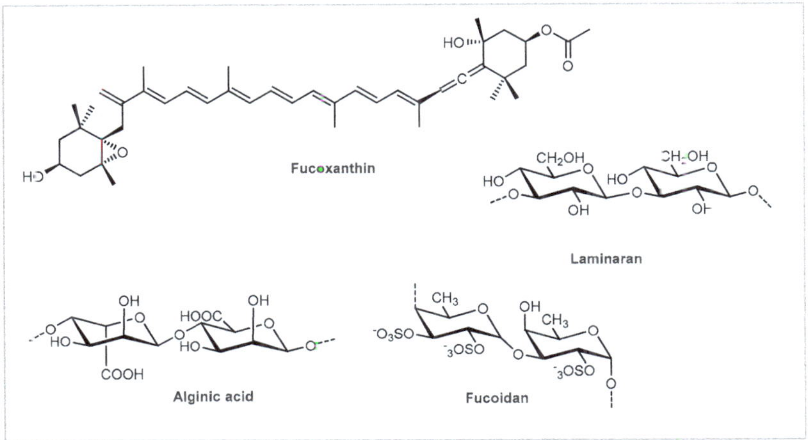

Figure 3. Bioactive constituents of brown seaweeds.

Although these main constituents are common to both taxonomic orders Fucales and Laminariales, studies focused on the discovery of other secondary metabolites of *Ascophyllum nodosum* and *Laminaria ochroleuca* complemented with studies on the biological activity of these metabolites have also been developed and are analyzed below. The scientific and marketing evidence of the application of active ingredients from *Ascophyllum nodosum* and *Laminaria ochroleuca* in cosmetic formulations for sensitive skin was also compiled and analyzed.

Laminaria ochroleuca is a yellow brown digitate kelp presently distributed from Morocco to southwest England in the United Kingdom [42]. This species is highly sensitive to temperature, which models their growth and performance, and the recent ocean warming has led to a proliferation of *Laminaria ochroleuca* by extension of their geographical ranges to new habitats [43]. Due to these temperature and geographical changes, along with other variables such as habitat, season of harvesting, and environmental conditions (light, temperature, and salinity), this species experiences major shifts in their composition. An interesting study on the effect of different harvesting times, depths, and growth conditions of *Laminaria ochroleuca* revealed considerable differences in both qualitative and quantitative pigment profiles [44]. Significant seasonal variations in the photosynthetic pigment composition of *Laminaria ochroleuca* were observed which point to the occurrence of a photoprotective mechanism in the algae that deflects energetic resources to pigment biosynthesis. The samples collected in months with higher sun exposure (June–October) exhibited higher amounts of zeaxanthin, β-carotene, and chlorophyll *c* (Figure 4), with some species presenting nearly twice the levels of pigments, amongst which carotenoids were the most prevalent (56.1% of the total quantified) [44]. Another study dealing with the determination of phenolic compounds in *Laminaria ochroleuca* for human consumption revealed epigallocatechin (Figure 4) as the main polyphenol (760.2 ± 52 µg/g dry weight), followed by epicatechin (28.7 ± 2.0 µg/g dry weight), catechin gallate (21.4 ± 5.7 µg/g dry weight), epicatechin gallate (11.2 ± 1.6 µg/g dry weight), and epigallocatechin gallate (9.7 ± 1.3 µg/g dry weight) [45]. These polyphenols have been shown to provide an antioxidant, anti-inflammatory, and UVB protective action [46,47]. Other phenolic derivatives include linear phlorethols, containing either ortho, meta-, or para-oriented (or even a combination) C–O–C oxidative phenolic couplings (Figure 4) as exemplified in tetraphlorethols A and B [48].

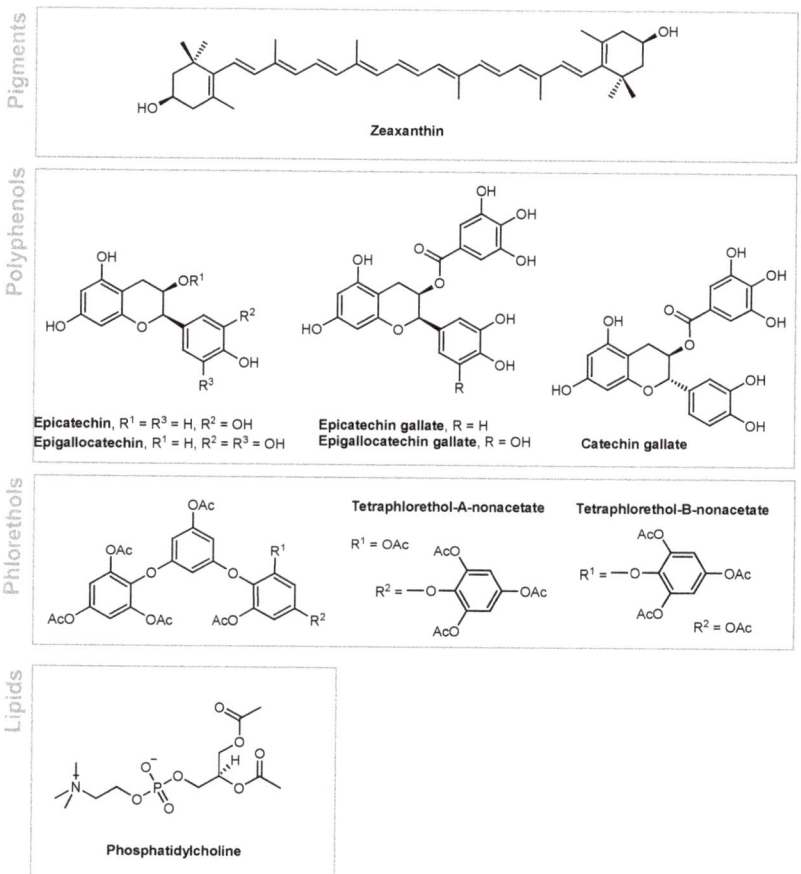

Figure 4. Bioactive metabolites of *Laminaria ochroleuca*.

A similar study was performed regarding fatty acid patterns of *Laminaria ochroleuca* [49]. This species exhibits a complex fatty acid profile, characterized mainly by the presence of medium and long fatty acyl chains (14–22 carbon atoms), with different degrees of unsaturation. The specimens from winter exhibited the lowest fatty acid concentrations (1255–1477 mg/kg of dry algae) whereas those harvested in warmer months presented higher fatty acid levels (1760 mg/kg of dry algae) [49].

Extracts of *Laminaria ochroleuca* have been incorporated in makeup, cleansers, moisturizers, and self-tanners, among other cosmetic products [50]. This extract is considered a natural skin soothing ingredient on several levels since it acts as an anti-inflammatory agent for skin irritations by boosting the skin's immune response and protects the DNA from UV damage [51].

One raw materials supplier performed a transcriptomic analysis by mRNA extraction and evaluation of expression makers by RT-qPCR on reconstituted human epidermis (RHE model, 11 days old), after a single application of a lipidic *Laminaria ochroleuca* extract (3 mg/cm^2) for 24 h [52]. An increase in the expression of proteins from the innate immune system was found, namely for toll-like receptor 4 (TLR 4), psoriasin (S 100 A7), RNAse 7, as well as upregulation of the enzymes linked to cellular homeostasis and oxidative stress, metallothioneins 1 (MT-1) and extracellular superoxide dismutase (SOD). Moreover, there was downregulation in the expression of proinflammatory cytokines IL-1α and IL-6, metalloproteinases 1, 3, and 9 (MMPs), as well as in plasminogen activator urokinase (PLAU), which are involved in the dermis' extracellular matrix degradation.

The same supplier also performed a clinical study including 10 volunteers, who were exposed to a fixed irradiation dose of the minimal erythema dose (minimum dosage of radiation that produces skin erythema) × 1.5. Then, a gel formulation containing 2% Laminaria ochroleuca extract was applied to the test area, and another irradiated area was left untreated. The test area and the amount of product which was applied are not disclosed. Skin erythema was measured after product application and in the next 30, 60 and 120 min. The gel reduced skin erythema by 6.07% after 30 min, presenting the greatest difference in comparison to the control, and it kept reducing skin erythema over time. Statistical significance was not assessed.

Another lipidic Laminaria ochroleuca extract was evaluated by a distinct raw materials supplier regarding its biological activity in in vitro studies using reconstituted skin which was subject to epidermal trauma. After the extract application, an anti-inflammatory effect was observed through the inhibition of IL-1α and IL-6, as previously stated [52], but also through PGE_2 release by epidermal cells and corneocyte degradation reduction, improving epidermal quality. Moreover, there was an increase in epidermal lipid content through phosphatidylcholine deposition, which contributes to reinforcing the epidermal barrier, thus reducing the penetration of environmental aggressors [53].

The anti-inflammatory activity of a lipidic Laminaria ochroleuca extract (Antileukine 6), which is mainly composed of phosphatidylcholine (Figure 4) derivatives, was evaluated in a murine model (C57BL/6 mice) [53,54]. Both ears were pretreated for 3 days twice a day with a Laminaria ochroleuca extract (2% in acetone/olive oil (4:1)) or the vehicle alone. Then, skin inflammation was induced by the application of 0.3% 2,4-dinitro-fluorobenzene (DNFB, hapten) in mouse ears, and the inflammatory response in terms of ear swelling (in μm) was scored at 0, 3, 6, 9, and 24 h in comparison with the vehicle applied at the other ear. The Laminaria ochroleuca extract reduced the inflammatory response as early as after 3 h, reaching the maximum effect at 6 h, with statistical significance, and showing a lasting effect up to 24 h. This anti-inflammatory effect may be due to the reduced DNFB penetration and/or a decrease in epidermal cytokines synthesis [54]. Having these results in mind, a Laminaria ochroleuca extract may be useful for reducing the symptoms associated with sensitive skin by improving the skin barrier function while modulating the neurogenic inflammation cascade by reducing the release of proinflammatory cytokines by mast cells, namely of IL-1 and prostaglandin E_2 (PGE_2). The metabolites which are responsible for these biological actions remain undisclosed.

Ascophyllum nodosum is an intertidal species characterized by its olive-brown fronds commonly detected around the periphery of the North Atlantic Ocean [55]. This intertidal fucoid has been extensively analyzed and studied for its chemical composition [55]. The most important constituents are the polysaccharides alginic acid, laminarins, and fucoidans (Figure 3), while other significant constituents like lipids, mannitol, ascophyllan, proteins, fibers, pigments, and phenols (Figure 5) [56–58], as well as vitamins, hormones, and enzymes are also present [55]. Ascophyllum nodosum has been used in bath oils, tablets, salts, as well as in skin cleansing and moisturizing cosmetics [50]. It has been shown to provide an antioxidant and photoprotective activity while inhibiting elastase and lipase [59–62]. While alginic acid or alginates have several applications in cosmetic formulations thanks to their thickening, gelling, emulsifying, and stabilizing abilities, fucoidans have been shown to reduce the intensity of the inflammatory response and promote a more rapid tissue healing, especially after wound or surgical trauma [55]. Fucoidans are fucans, sulfated polysaccharides with a fucose backbone, originating from seaweeds [29]. They have been shown to reduce the production of IgE by B cells which have been stimulated by allergens, thus blocking signals mediated by NFκB-p52. Furthermore, they have a free radical scavenging capacity, which may contribute to ameliorating skin inflammation [63,64]. Together, these properties make fucoidans a promising active ingredient for cosmetics intended to aid in the management of itching, stinging, and rashes [63]. One study evaluated the ability of this compound to reduce the inflammatory response using BALB/c mice as the murine model for atopic dermatitis and a DNFB solution (acetone/olive oil, 4:1) as the hapten [65]. Atopic dermatitis was induced in BALB/c mice by sensitization of the pre-shaved abdomen, with further challenge on the abdomen and ears after four, five, and nine days. Then, the treatment group received 50 µL of 0.2% fucoidan (from *Fucus vesiculosus*), while the negative control group received an acetone/olive oil vehicle, and the positive control group was given 0.1% dexamethasone. Fucoidan has been shown to ameliorate atopic dermatitis by decreasing inflammatory cell infiltration, splenocytes proliferation, and the CD4+ T cell response. However, fucoidans from *Ascophyllum nodosum* are distinct from those from *Fucus vesiculosus*, and their mechanisms of action are not expected to be effective on sensitive skin, based on what is known regarding the pathophysiology of this condition.

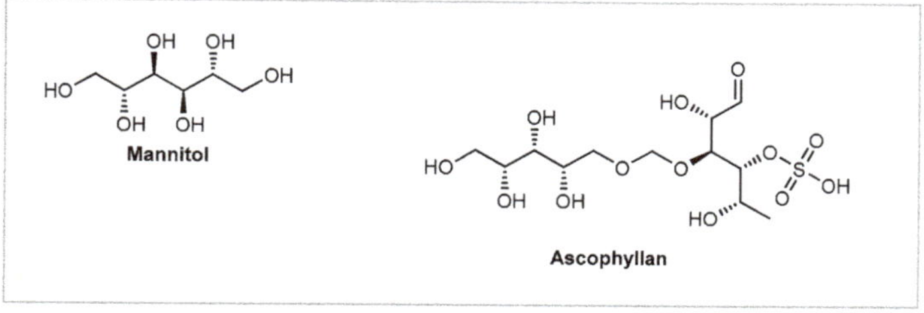

Figure 5. Bioactive metabolites of *Ascophyllum nodosum*.

Ascophyllan has been shown to inhibit MMP expression, reduce the production of NO, tumor necrosis factor-α (TNF-α), and granulocyte colony-stimulating factor (G-CSF) more markedly than fucoidan and provide an antioxidant action [66,67]. No studies were found regarding its benefits for sensitive skin or inflammatory conditions.

One raw materials supplier evaluated the efficacy of a cosmetic formulation containing *Ascophyllum nodosum* and *Asparagopsis armata* (red algae) extracts [68]. Keratinocytes were exposed to phorbol myristate acetate (PMA), a tumor promoter and proinflammatory substance, and incubated with 0.2% of the active ingredient (methods are not further described) [69]. The incubated keratinocytes have shown a very significant reduction both in the vascular endothelial growth factor (VEGF) and PGE_2 levels. VEGF stimulates the growth and dilation of capillaries, which may result in increased skin redness [17]. This combination also inhibited MMP-2 activity in a dose-dependent manner, reaching 37% inhibition at the concentration of 0.5%. Additionally, a clinical study was performed by the same supplier. Fifty-six volunteers presenting wrinkles and dry sensitive skin applied a formulation with 0.4% of this ingredient twice a day for 28 days. Then, their perception of the products was registered. Reduced tingling sensations, improved resiliency, immediate relief, and skin comfort were reported by 58%, 59%, 70%, and 71% of the volunteers, respectively. Although these results reveal a potential application of this ingredient for sensitive skin, it is not possible to conclude that *Ascophyllum nodosum* can be useful for this purpose as the tested ingredient also contains the algae *Asparagopsis armata*.

3.2. Red Macroalgae

Asparagopsis armata is a red seaweed which can be found in European coasts and in the Northeast Atlantic [70]. The main photosynthetic pigments of red algae are chlorophyll *a*, carotenoids (lutein, zeaxanthin, β-carotene) and phycobilins (phycocyanin and phycoerythrin), water-soluble pigments localized in the phycobilisomes, which give red algae their distinctive color [71]. Phycocyanin has been shown to provide anti-inflammatory, antioxidant, and wound-healing properties [72]. Besides photosynthetic pigments, red algae are also constituted of other interesting bioactive compounds (Figure 6), including agar [39], sulfated polysaccharides (carrageenans and porphyrans) [73,74], and mycosporine-like amino acids (MAA) [75–78].

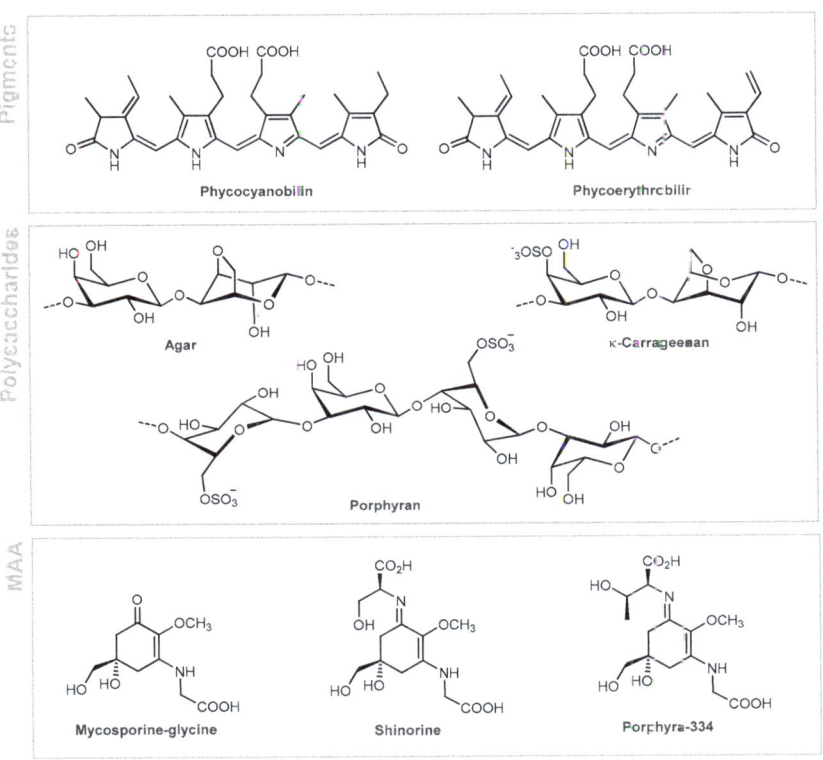

Figure 6. Bioactive constituents of red algae.

The wide practical uses of these polysaccharides are based on their ability to form gels in aqueous solutions and act as a stabilizer, being generally used in creams, sticks, soaps, shampoos, lotions, foams, and gels [79]. On the other hand, MAAs are used in cosmetic formulations due to their photoprotective potential, antioxidant and skin protective properties [9,80,81]. They constitute a group of low-molecular-weight water-soluble molecules that can absorb UV radiation and disperse the absorbed energy as heat without generating reactive oxygen species (ROS), being a natural promising UV-absorbing alternative [82]. Examples of the most abundant MAAs in red macroalgae are mycosporine-glycine, shinorine, and porphyra-334 (Figure 6) [83]. The anti-inflammatory effects of these MAAs on the expression of genes associated with inflammation in response to UV irradiation was investigated using the human fibroblast cell line, HaCaT [82]. Mycosporine-glycine was able to suppress the expression of an inflammation marker gene, COX-2, in a concentration-dependent manner [82,83].

One raw materials supplier reported the cytostimulatory action of an *Asparagopsis armata* extract on human fibroblasts (WI 38), reaching the maximum level at 0.1%. No further details are provided [84].

Other studies including the use of an *Asparagopsis armata* extract in cosmetic formulations for sensitive skin were already disclosed [68,69]. However, these formulations contain not only *Asparagopsis armata*, but also *Ascophyllum nodosum*, and were previously described in Section 3.1.

3.3. Microalgae

Marine microalgae also constitute an innovative source of bioactive compounds such as polyunsaturated fatty acids, tocopherols and sterols, vitamins and minerals, antioxidants, and pigments (e.g., chlorophyll and carotenoids), with great relevance in medical, pharmaceutical, and cosmetic fields [85]. Due to their unicellular or simple multicellular structure, they can grow rapidly and live under harsh conditions and environmental stressors such as heat, cold, anaerobiosis, salinity, photooxidation, osmotic pressure, and exposure to ultraviolet radiation [85]. The microalgae usually commercialized and used in biotechnology belong to the green algae, Chlorophyceae (such as *Chlorella vulgaris*, *Haematococcus pluvialis*, *Dunaliella salina*, and cyanobacteria) [85]. Their composition varies according to species and culture environments such as light intensity, temperature, pH, salinity, and medium [86]. *Chlorella vulgaris* is mainly constituted by proteins (43–58%), lipids (5–58%), carbohydrates (12–55%), pigments (chlorophyll (1–2%) and carotenoids (0.4%, astaxanthin, lutein, β-carotene, lycopene, canthaxanthin, see Figure 7 for examples)), vitamins (vitamins A, B, C, and E), and minerals (calcium, potassium, magnesium, and zinc) [86].

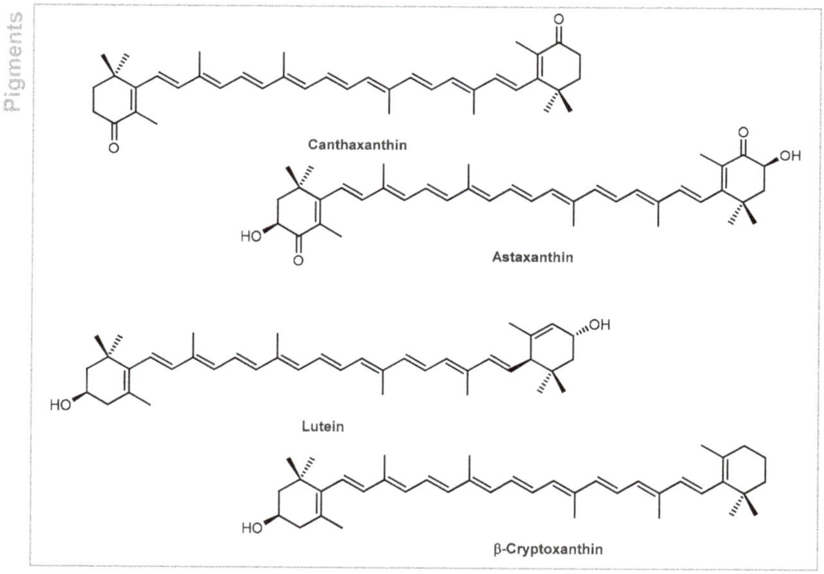

Figure 7. Pigments of *Chlorella vulgaris*.

Sulfated polysaccharides from *Chlorella vulgaris* exhibited a capacity to prevent the accumulation and activity of free radicals and reactive chemical species, acting as protecting systems against these oxidative and radical stress agents [87]; in addition, peptides have been shown to reduce the matrix metalloproteinase-1 (MMP-1) expression in human skin cell fibroblasts, responsible for the breakdown of collagen [88]. The fact that a *Chlorella vulgaris* extract is able to stimulate collagen synthesis in the skin makes it suitable to be used in anti-aging cosmetics, as well as in wound-healing products [89,90].

Several studies report beneficial effects of extracts of *Chlorella vulgaris* for skin health. One study found that a *Chlorella vulgaris* extract was able to attenuate *Dermatophagoides farinae* (DFE)-induced atopic dermatitis (AD) in NC/Nga mice by oral administration [91], reducing 12-dimethylbenz[a]anthracene (DMBA)-induced tumor size and number by upregulating the sulfhydryl (-SH) and glutathione S-transferase (GST) levels in skin tissues [92]. These findings indicate *Chlorella vulgaris* could be useful as a preventive and therapeutic agent for various inflammatory skin diseases.

The evidence of the use of extracts of this microalga in cosmetic formulations for sensitive skin is limited. One cosmetic product was tested for its angiogenic inhibiting ability against positive and negative controls (suramide and VEGF, respectively) by using the in vitro model AngioKit™ (TCS Cellworks), which allows following the development of the angiogenic process [93]. The formulation contained rhamnose, shea butter, argan oil, polyphenols, dextran sulfate, *Laminaria digitata*, caprapenols, *Chlorella vulgaris*, glycosaminoglycans, and UV filters (SPF 20). The formulation presented an antiangiogenic effect comparing to the positive control in the concentration range of 0.7–0.8 mg/mL, thus being useful for patients presenting rosacea. In spite of these results and *Chlorella vulgaris*' potential to modulate the inflammatory response involved in sensitive skin, the composition of this formulation does not allow drawing conclusions regarding *Chlorella vulgaris*' efficacy for treating this condition.

4. Materials and Methods

4.1. Data Collection

The composition of a pool of skin care facial cosmetic products from multinational manufacturers marketed in Portuguese parapharmacies and pharmacies was collected in 2019 in order to access the most used active ingredients in formulations for sensitive skin. Skin care products were included in the study if they exhibited in the label one of the following expressions: "sensitive skin" or "reactive skin" or "intolerant skin". All the information available in the product labels was collected, along with the information available on the manufacturers' websites.

4.2. Data Analysis

The marine ingredients contained in cosmetic products for sensitive skin were listed according to the International Nomenclature of Cosmetic Ingredients (INCI). Afterwards, the data were analyzed with respect to the following parameters:

4.2.1. Marine Ingredients Use

The relative amount of cosmetic products for sensitive skin containing marine ingredients was evaluated and expressed in percentage.

4.2.2. Top Marine Ingredients for Sensitive Skin

Marine ingredients were identified from INCI lists and ranked in the descending order of occurrence to disclose the top. Their categorization was also performed based on their marine organism species.

4.2.3. Scientific Evidence Supporting the Efficacy of Marine Ingredients in Sensitive Skin Care

The efficacy data for each marine ingredient were searched in the online databases PubMed, Scopus, KOSMET, and SciFinder. Due to the lack of studies regarding the applicability of active ingredients in cosmetics for sensitive skin, a broader search was performed, using the keywords ("INCI name" OR "synonyms" when applicable) AND ("skin" OR "topical).

5. Conclusions

Sensitive skin affects a significant proportion of the population worldwide, making it an appealing segment for the cosmetics industry. Marine organisms possess unique chemical pathways that are able to produce unprecedented scaffolds.

Marine ingredients were present in 27% of the analyzed cosmetic products for sensitive skin. Noteworthy, macroalgae are the prime marine ingredient used probably due to the easiness of cultivation allied with the development of a cutting-edge technology. These are easily cultivated either in a pond or a photobioreactor, in nonarable lands with minimal use of freshwater, or even in seawater or wastewater. It is also worth highlighting that among macroalgae, brown algae represent the main type of algae used in the analyzed cosmetic formulations.

Two preparations from brown algae (a *Laminaria ochroleuca* extract and an *Ascophyllum nodosum* extract), one—from red algae (an *Asparagopsis armata* extract), and one—from green microalgae (an *Chlorella vulgaris* extract) were found. The scientific evidence regarding the efficacy of these ingredients on sensitive skin is limited, especially due to the lack of clinical studies including volunteers with this condition. Noteworthily, there is one study that meets these requirements referring to a combination of an *Ascophyllum nodosum* extract and an *Asparagopsis armata* extract, which was found to reduce a tingling sensation, resiliency, and skin comfort in volunteers with sensitive skin. On the other hand, an *Laminaria ochroleuca* extract has a potential for improving the skin barrier function due to its lipid content and for reducing neurogenic inflammation by decreasing the release of pro-inflammatory cytokines by mast cells while increasing the production of antioxidant enzymes such as MT-1 and SOD. As for a *Chlorella vulgaris* extract, the in vivo evidence supporting its use in inflammatory conditions is still preliminary.

It is interesting to notice that efforts amongst the scientific community towards the identification of the active ingredient responsible for a certain property in the analyzed cosmetic formulation are still scarce. Usually, the entire extract is applied without further understanding of which chemical entity is associated with the bioactivity. Hence, research and development strategies should be employed both to identify the specific compounds responsible for the observed activities and determine their mechanisms of action. Among the chemical substances that can be found in these ingredients, carotenoids, sulfated polysaccharides, amino acids, and lipids are the most abundant. Of those, certain compounds usually isolated from marine organisms could be of interest for managing the symptoms of sensitive skin. Fucoidans from brown algae present evidence for managing inflammatory conditions, and they have been proposed to reduce itching and stinging symptoms. Additionally, mycosporine-like amino acids provide an antioxidant and anti-inflammatory activity by modulating the expression of the fibroblasts' genes associated with inflammation. New strategies to increase the profitability of the extraction process are also needed in order to increase the cosmetic industry interest. Biotechnology may present advantages in this regard by reducing the environmental impact from the exploitation of these resources. The preliminary studies described herein are a major step towards the design of more innovative target-oriented ingredients by the cosmetic industry, providing efficacious products for sensitive skin. Overall, marine ingredients are already used in the sensitive skin segment, and they have a great potential to keep growing. Their in-depth study and the further investigation of other organisms, such as fish, sponges, corals, mollusks, echinoderms, *Artemia*, plankton, and microorganisms, constitute a great opportunity for formulators, cosmetic companies with R&D departments, and raw materials suppliers from the cosmetic industry.

Author Contributions: Conceptualization: I.F.A.; Data collection and analysis: M.S.F.; Writing—original draft preparation and final manuscript: M.S.F. and D.I.S.P.R.; Supervision: J.M.S.L.; Writing—review and editing: I.F.A. and E.S. All authors have read and agreed to the published version of the manuscript.

Funding: This work is financed by national funds from FCT—Fundação para a Ciência e a Tecnologia, I.P., in the scope of the project UIDP/04378/2020 and UIDB/04378/2020 of the Research Unit on Applied Molecular Biosciences—UCIBIO and the project LA/P/0140/2020 of the Associate Laboratory Institute for Health and Bioeconomy—i4HB." This research was also supported by national funds through FCT (Foundation for Science and Technology) within the scope of UIDB/04423/2020, UIDP/04423/2020 (Group of Natural Products and Medicinal Chemistry—CIIMAR), and under the project PTDC/SAU-PUB/28736/2017 (reference POCI-01-0145-FEDER-028736), co-financed by COMPETE 2020, Portugal 2020 and the European Union through the ERDF and by FCT through national funds, as well as structured program of R&D&I ATLANTIDA (NORTE-01-0145-FEDER-000040), supported by NORTE2020, through ERDF, and CHIRALBIO ACTIVE-PI-3RL-IINFACTS-2019.

Institutional Review Board Statement: Not applicable.

Informed Consent Statement: Not applicable.

Data Availability Statement: Data sharing not applicable.

Acknowledgments: Not applicable.

Conflicts of Interest: The authors declare no conflict of interest. The funders had no role in the design of the study; in the collection, analyses, or interpretation of data; in the writing of the manuscript, or in the decision to publish the results.

Limitations: This study was performed for the Portuguese cosmetic market, which is dominated by multinational cosmetic brands. Therefore, this may result in discrepancies when comparing the data with other markets. Many ingredients found in cosmetic products from the market lack scientific literature regarding their efficacy. Therefore, some of the information used in this study was collected in technical documents and patents from suppliers.

References

1. Kim, J.H.; Lee, J.-E.; Kim, K.H.; Kang, N.J. Beneficial effects of marine algae-derived carbohydrates for skin health. *Mar. Drugs* **2018**, *16*, 459. [CrossRef] [PubMed]
2. Kim, S.-K.; Pangestuti, R. Biological properties of cosmeceuticals derived from marine algae. In *Marine Cosmeceuticals: Trends and Prospects*; Kim, S.-K., Ed.; CRC Press: Boca Raton, FL, USA, 2012; p. 191.
3. Lochhead, R.Y. Chapter 13-The use of polymers in cosmetic products. In *Cosmetic Science and Technology*; Sakamoto, K., Lochhead, R.Y., Maibach, H.I., Yamashita, Y., Eds.; Elsevier: Amsterdam, The Netherlands, 2017; pp. 171–221.
4. Sathasivam, R.; Radhakrishnan, R.; Hashem, A.; Abd_Allah, E.F. Microalgae metabolites: A rich source for food and medicine. *Saudi J. Biol. Sci.* **2019**, *26*, 709–722. [CrossRef] [PubMed]
5. Brunt, E.G.; Burgess, J.G. The promise of marine molecules as cosmetic active ingredients. *Int. J. Cosmet. Sci* **2018**, *40*, 1–15. [CrossRef] [PubMed]
6. Kim, S.K.; Ravichandran, Y.D.; Khan, S.B.; Kim, Y.T. Prospective of the cosmeceuticals derived from marine organisms. *Biotechnol. Bioprocess Eng.* **2008**, *13*, 511–523. [CrossRef]
7. Bayona, K.C.D.; Navarro, S.M.; Lara, A.D.; Colorado, J.; Atehortua, L.; Martínez, A. Activity of sulfated polysaccharides from microalgae Porphyridium cruentum over degenerative mechanisms of the skin. *Int. J. Adv. Sci. Technol.* **2012**, *2*, 85–92.
8. Leandro, A.; Pereira, L.; Gonçalves, A.M.M. Diverse applications of marine macroalgae. *Mar. Drugs* **2020**, *18*, 17. [CrossRef]
9. Drouart, C.; SEPPIC. Ingredients and Formulas. Available online: https://www.seppic.com/ (accessed on 3 May 2021).
10. The European Parliament and The Council of the European Union. Regulation (EC) No 1223/2009 of the European Parliament and of the Council of 30 November 2009 on cosmetic products. *Off. J. Eur. Union L* **2009**, *342*, 59.
11. Guillerme, J.-B.; Couteau, C.; Coiffard, L. Applications for marine resources in cosmetics. *Cosmetics* **2017**, *4*, 35. [CrossRef]
12. Cosmetic Products. Available online: https://cosmeticseurope.eu/cosmetic-products/ (accessed on 1 June 2021).
13. 2020 Annual Report-Cosmetics Market. Available online: https://www.loreal-finance.com/en/annual-report-2020/cosmetics-market-2-1-0/ (accessed on 1 June 2021).
14. Chen, W.; Dai, R.; Li, L. The prevalence of self-declared sensitive skin: A systematic review and meta-analysis. *J. Eur. Acad. Dermatol. Venereol.* **2020**, *34*, 1779–1788. [CrossRef]
15. Farage, M.A. The prevalence of sensitive skin. *Front. Med.* **2019**, *6*, 98. [CrossRef]
16. Misery, L. Neuropsychiatric factors in sensitive skin. *Clin. Dermatol.* **2017**, *35*, 281–284. [CrossRef]
17. Berardesca, E.; Farage, M.; Maibach, H. Sensitive skin: An overview. *Int. J. Cosmet. Sci.* **2013**, *35*, 2–8. [CrossRef]
18. Misery, L. Sensitive skin, reactive skin. *Ann. Dermatol. Venereol.* **2019**, *146*, 585–591. [CrossRef]
19. Farage, M.A.; Jiang, Y.; Tiesman, J.P.; Fontanillas, P.; Osborne, R. Genome-wide association study identifies loci associated with sensitive skin. *Cosmetics* **2020**, *7*, 49. [CrossRef]
20. Verhoeven, E.W.; de Klerk, S.; Kraaimaat, F.W.; van de Kerkhof, P.C.; de Jong, E.M.; Evers, A.W. Biopsychosocial mechanisms of chronic itch in patients with skin diseases: A review. *Acta Derm. Venereol.* **2008**, *88*, 211–218. [CrossRef] [PubMed]
21. Zheng, Y.; Liang, H.; Li, Z.; Tang, M.; Song, L. Skin microbiome in sensitive skin: The decrease of Staphylococcus epidermidis seems to be related to female lactic acid sting test sensitive skin. *J. Dermatol. Sci.* **2020**, *97*, 225–228. [CrossRef] [PubMed]
22. Misery, L.; Weisshaar, E.; Brenaut, E.; Evers, A.W.M.; Huet, F.; Stander, S.; Reich, A.; Berardesca, E.; Serra-Baldrich, E.; Wallengren, J.; et al. Pathophysiology and management of sensitive skin: Position paper from the special interest group on sensitive skin of the International Forum for the Study of Itch (IFSI). *J. Eur. Acad. Dermatol. Venereol.* **2020**, *34*, 222–229. [CrossRef] [PubMed]
23. Misery, L.; Loser, K.; Stander, S. Sensitive skin. *J. Eur. Acad. Dermatol. Venereol.* **2016**, *30* (Suppl. 1), 2–8. [CrossRef]
24. Richters, R.; Falcone, D.; Uzunbajakava, N.; Verkruysse, W.; van Erp, P.; van de Kerkhof, P. What is sensitive skin? A systematic literature review of objective measurements. *Skin Pharmacol. Physiol.* **2015**, *28*, 75–83. [CrossRef] [PubMed]

25. Ferrer-Montiel, A.; Camprubí-Robles, M.; García-Sanz, N.; Sempere, A.; Valente, P.; Nest, W.V.D.; Carreño, C. The contribution of neurogenic inflammation to sensitive skin: Concepts, mechanisms and cosmeceutical intervention. *Int. J. Cosmet. Sci.* **2009**, *11*, 311–315. [CrossRef]
26. Roussaki-Schulze, A.V.; Zafiriou, E.; Nikoulis, D.; Klimi, E.; Rallis, E.; Zintzaras, E. Objective biophysical findings in patients with sensitive skin. *Drugs Exp. Clin. Res.* **2005**, *31*, 17–24. [PubMed]
27. Raj, N.; Voegeli, R.; Rawlings, A.V.; Doppler, S.; Imfeld, D.; Munday, M.R.; Lane, M.E. A fundamental investigation into aspects of the physiology and biochemistry of the stratum corneum in subjects with sensitive skin. *Int. J. Cosmet. Sci.* **2017**, *39*, 2–10. [CrossRef] [PubMed]
28. Cho, H.J.; Chung, B.Y.; Lee, H.B.; Kim, H.O.; Park, C.W.; Lee, C.H. Quantitative study of stratum corneum ceramides contents in patients with sensitive skin. *J. Dermatol.* **2012**, *39*, 295–300. [CrossRef]
29. Richters, R.J.; Falcone, D.; Uzunbajakava, N.E.; Varghese, B.; Caspers, P.J.; Puppels, G.J.; van Erp, P.E.; van de Kerkhof, P.C. Sensitive Skin: Assessment of the skin barrier using confocal raman microspectroscopy. *Skin Pharmacol. Physiol.* **2017**, *30*, 1–12. [CrossRef] [PubMed]
30. Resende, D.I.S.P.; Ferreira, M.S.; Sousa-Lobo, J.M.; Sousa, E.; Almeida, I.F. Usage of Synthetic Peptides in Cosmetics for Sensitive Skin. *Pharmaceuticals* **2021**, *14*, 702. [CrossRef]
31. Resende, D.I.S.P.; Ferreira, M.; Magalhães, C.; Sousa Lobo, J.M.; Sousa, E.; Almeida, I.F. Trends in the use of marine ingredients in anti-aging cosmetics. *Algal Res.* **2021**, *55*, 102273. [CrossRef]
32. Martins, A.; Vieira, H.; Gaspar, H.; Santos, S. Marketed marine natural products in the pharmaceutical and cosmeceutical industries: Tips for success. *Mar. Drugs* **2014**, *12*, 1066–1101. [CrossRef]
33. Siahaan, E.A.; Pangestuti, R.; Munandar, H.; Kim, S.-K. Cosmeceuticals properties of sea cucumbers: Prospects and trends. *Cosmetics* **2017**, *4*, 26. [CrossRef]
34. Domloge, N.; Bauza, E.; Cucumel, K.; Peyronel, D.; Dal Farra, C. Artemia extract toward more extensive sun protection. *Cosmet. Toilet.* **2002**, *2002*, 67–78.
35. Cho, M.G.; Han, G.T.; Han, S.I.; Kang, J.G.; Lee, G.H.; Lee, Y.S.; Oh, J.Y.; Park, M.S. Wrinkle Resisting Cosmetic Composition Containing Plankton Artemia Salina (Brine Shrimp) Extract, and Its Preparation Method. KR Patent KR 2002073725-A, September 2002.
36. Vaseli-Hagh, N.; Deezagi, A.; Shahraki, M.K. Anti-aging effects of the proteins fromartemia extract on human fibroblasts cell proliferation and collagen expression in induced aging conditions. *Ann. Biotechnol.* **2018**, *3*, 1015.
37. Kim, S.-K.; Wijesekara, I. Cosmeceuticals from marine resources: Prospects and commercial trends. In *Marine Cosmeceuticals: Trends and Prospects*; Kim, S.-K., Ed.; CRC Press: Boca Raton, FL, USA, 2012; pp. 1–10.
38. Alves, A.L.; Marques, A.L.P.; Martins, E.; Silva, T.H.; Reis, R.L. Cosmetic potential of marine fish skin collagen. *Cosmetics* **2017**, *4*, 39. [CrossRef]
39. Pereira, L. Seaweeds as source of bioactive substances and skin care therapy—cosmeceuticals, algotheraphy, and thalassotherapy. *Cosmetics* **2018**, *5*, 68. [CrossRef]
40. Wang, H.-M.D.; Chen, C.-C.; Huynh, P.; Chang, J.-S. Exploring the potential of using algae in cosmetics. *Bioresour. Technol.* **2015**, *184*, 355–362. [CrossRef]
41. CosIng. Available online: https://ec.europa.eu/growth/tools-databases/cosing/ (accessed on 17 June 2021).
42. Smale, D.A.; Wernberg, T.; Yunnie, A.L.E.; Vance, T. The rise of *Laminaria ochroleuca* in the Western English Channel (UK) and comparisons with its competitor and assemblage dominant Laminaria hyperborea. *Mar. Ecol.* **2015**, *36*, 1033–1044. [CrossRef]
43. Pessarrodona, A.; Foggo, A.; Smale, D.A. Can ecosystem functioning be maintained despite climate-driven shifts in species composition? Insights from novel marine forests. *J. Ecol.* **2019**, *107*, 91–104. [CrossRef]
44. Fernandes, F.; Barbosa, M.; Oliveira, A.P.; Azevedo, I.C.; Sousa-Pinto, I.; Valentão, P.; Andrade, P.B. The pigments of kelps (Ochrophyta) as part of the flexible response to highly variable marine environments. *J. App. Phycol.* **2016**, *28*, 3689–3696. [CrossRef]
45. Rodríguez-Bernaldo de Quirós, A.; Lage-Yusty, M.A.; López-Hernández, J. Determination of phenolic compounds in macroalgae for human consumption. *Food Chem.* **2010**, *121*, 634–638. [CrossRef]
46. Katiyar, S.K.; Ahmad, N.; Mukhtar, H. Green tea and skin. *Arch. Dermatol.* **2000**, *136*, 989–994. [CrossRef] [PubMed]
47. Katiyar, S.K.; Elmets, C.A.; Agarwal, R.; Mukhtar, H. Protection against ultraviolet-B radiation-induced local and systemic suppression of contact hypersensitivity and edema responses in C3H/HeN mice by green tea polyphenols. *Photochem. Photobiol.* **1995**, *62*, 855–861. [CrossRef]
48. Koch, M.; Glombitza, K.-W.; Eckhard, G. Phlorotannins of phaeophycea *Laminaria ochroleuca*. *Phytochemistry* **1980**, *19*, 1821–1823. [CrossRef]
49. Barbosa, M.; Fernandes, F.; Pereira, D.M.; Azevedo, I.C.; Sousa-Pinto, I.; Andrade, P.B.; Valentão, P. Fatty acid patterns of the kelps Saccharina latissima, Saccorhiza polyschides and *Laminaria ochroleuca*: Influence of changing environmental conditions. *Arab. J. Chem.* **2020**, *13*, 45–58. [CrossRef]
50. Safety Assessment of Brown Algae-Derived Ingredients as Used in Cosmetics. Available online: https://www.cir-safety.org/sites/default/files/Brown%20Algae_1.pdf (accessed on 1 June 2021).
51. Algotherm. *Laminaria ochroleuca*. Available online: https://algotherm.ua/en/algae/laminaria-ochroleuca/ (accessed on 5 May 2021).
52. OCEA DEFENCE® Marine Skin Immunity Booster. Available online: http://www.biosiltech.com/pdf/gelyma/OCEA%20DEFENCE%20-%20LEAFLET.pdf (accessed on 3 June 2021).

53. ANTILEUKINE 6—Global Defense Active Ingredient. Available online: https://www.seppic.com/en/antileukine-6 (accessed on 1 June 2001).
54. Bonneville, M.; Saint-Mezard, P.; Benetiere, J.; Hennino, A.; Pernet, I.; Denis, A.; Nicolas, J. *Laminaria ochroleuca* extract reduces skin inflammation. *J. Eur. Acad. Dermatol. Venereol.* 2007, 21, 1124–1125. [CrossRef]
55. Pereira, L.; Morrison, L.; Shukla, P.S.; Critchley, A.T. A concise review of the brown macroalga *Ascophyllum nodosum* (Linnaeus) Le Jolis. *J. Appl. Phycol.* 2020, 32, 3561–3584. [CrossRef]
56. Audibert, L.; Fauchon, M.; Blanc, N.; Hauchard, D.; Ar Gall, E. Phenolic compounds in the brown seaweed *Ascophyllum nodosum*: Distribution and radical-scavenging activities. *Phytochem. Anal.* 2010, 21, 399–405. [CrossRef]
57. Holdt, S.L.; Kraan, S. Bioactive compounds in seaweed: Functional food applications and legislation. *J. Appl. Phycol.* 2011, 23, 543–597. [CrossRef]
58. Bahar, B.; O'Doherty, J.V.; Smyth, T.J.; Sweeney, T. A comparison of the effects of an *Ascophyllum nodosum* ethanol extract and its molecular weight fractions on the inflammatory immune gene expression in-vitro and ex-vivo. *Innov. Food Sci. Emerg. Technol.* 2016, 37, 276–285. [CrossRef]
59. Senni, K.; Gueniche, F.; Foucault-Bertaud, A.; Igondjo-Tchen, S.; Fioretti, F.; Colliec-Jouault, S.; Durand, P.; Guezennec, J.; Godeau, G.; Letourneur, D. Fucoidan a sulfated polysaccharide from brown algae is a potent modulator of connective tissue proteolysis. *Arch. Biochem. Biophys.* 2006, 445, 56–64. [CrossRef]
60. Quéguineur, B.; Goya, L.; Ramos, S.; Martín, M.A.; Mateos, R.; Guiry, M.D.; Bravo, L. Effect of phlorotannin-rich extracts of *Ascophyllum nodosum* and Himanthalia elongata (Phaeophyceae) on cellular oxidative markers in human HepG2 cells. *J. App. Phycol.* 2013, 25, 1–11. [CrossRef]
61. Guinea, M.; Franco, V.; Araujo-Bazán, L.; Rodríguez-Martín, I.; González, S. In vivo UVB-photoprotective activity of extracts from commercial marine macroalgae. *Food Chem. Toxicol.* 2012, 50, 1109–1117. [CrossRef]
62. Chater, P.I.; Wilcox, M.; Cherry, P.; Herford, A.; Mustar, S.; Wheater, H.; Brownlee, I.; Seal, C.; Pearson, J. Inhibitory activity of extracts of Hebridean brown seaweeds on lipase activity. *J. App. Phycol.* 2016, 28, 1303–1313. [CrossRef]
63. SHIK, B.J.; SIK, J.; SOOK, K.Y.; PIL, P.K. A discoloration method of fucoidan containing solution, discolorized fucoidan containing solution and cosmetic compositions for sensitive skins containing the same. KR101025903B1, 2009.
64. Oomizu, S.; Yanase, Y.; Suzuki, H.; Kameyoshi, Y.; Hide, M. Fucoidan prevents Cε germline transcription and NFκB p52 translocation for IgE production in B cells. *Biochem. Biophys. Res. Commun.* 2006, 350, 501–507. [CrossRef] [PubMed]
65. Tian, T.; Chang, H.; He, Y.; Ni, Y.; Li, C.; Hou, M.; Chen, L.; Xu, Z.; Chen, B.; Ji, M. Fucoidan from seaweed Fucus vesiculosus inhibits 2,4-dinitrochlorobenzene-induced atopic dermatitis. *Int. Immunopharmacol.* 2019, 75, 105823. [CrossRef]
66. Abu, R.; Jiang, Z.; Ueno, M.; Isaka, S.; Nakazono, S.; Okimura, T.; Cho, K.; Yamaguchi, K.; Kim, D.; Oda, T. Anti-metastatic effects of the sulfated polysaccharide ascophyllan isolated from *Ascophyllum nodosum* on B16 melanoma. *Biochem. Biophys. Res. Commun.* 2015, 458, 727–732. [CrossRef] [PubMed]
67. Jiang, Z.; Okimura, T.; Yamaguchi, K.; Oda, T. The potent activity of sulfated polysaccharide, ascophyllan, isolated from *Ascophyllum nodosum* to induce nitric oxide and cytokine production from mouse macrophage RAW264.7 cells: Comparison between ascophyllan and fucoidan. *Nitric Oxide* 2011, 25, 407–415. [CrossRef] [PubMed]
68. Aldavine™ 5X Algae Polysaccharides Complex. Available online: http://ulprospector.com/documents/1428707.pdf?bs=4499&b=124731&st=20&r=eu&ind=personalcare (accessed on 4 June 2021).
69. Chang, S.N.; Dey, D.K.; Oh, S.T.; Kong, W.H.; Cho, K.H.; Al-Olayar, E.M.; Hwang, B.S.; Kang, S.C.; Park, J.G. Phorbol 12-Myristate 13-acetate induced toxicity study and the role of tangeretin in abrogating HIF-1α-NF-κB crosstalk In vitro and in vivo. *Int. J. Mol. Sci.* 2020, 21, 9261. [CrossRef] [PubMed]
70. Pinteus, S.; Lemos, M.F.L.; Alves, C.; Neugebauer, A.; Silva, J.; Thomas, O.P.; Botana, L.M.; Gaspar, H.; Pedrosa, R. Marine invasive macroalgae: Turning a real threat into a major opportunity-the biotechnological potential of *Sargassum muticum* and *Asparagopsis armata Algal Res.* 2018, 34, 217–234. [CrossRef]
71. Gantt, E.; Grabowski, B.; Cunningham, F.X. Antenna systems of red algae: Phycobilisomes with photosystem II and chlorophyll complexes with photosystem I. In *Light-Harvesting Antennas in Photosynthesis*; Green, B.R., Parson, W.W., Eds.; Springer: Dordrecht, The Netherlands, 2003; pp. 307–322.
72. Ragusa, I.; Nardone, G.N.; Zanatta, S.; Bertin, W.; Amadio, E. Spirulina for skin care: A bright blue future. *Cosmetics* 2021, 8, 7. [CrossRef]
73. Pimentel, F.B.; Alves, R.C.; Rodrigues, F.; P. P. Oliveira, M.B. Macroalgae-derived ingredients for cosmetic industry—An update. *Cosmetics* 2018, 5, 2 [CrossRef]
74. Carvalhal, F.; Cristelo, R.R.; Resende, D.I.S.P.; Pinto, M.M.M.; Sousa, E.; Correia-da-Silva, M. Antithrombotics from the sea: Polysaccharides and beyond. *Mar. Drugs* 2019, 17, 170. [CrossRef]
75. Shick, J.M.; Dunlap, W.C. Mycosporine-like amino acids and related gadusols: Biosynthesis, accumulation, and UV-protective functions in aquatic organisms. *Annu. Rev. Physiol.* 2002, 64, 223–262. [CrossRef]
76. Reef, R.; Kaniewska, P.; Hoegh-Guldberg, O. Coral skeletons defend against ultraviolet radiation. *PLoS ONE* 2009, 4, e7995. [CrossRef]
77. Bedoux, G.; Hardouin, K.; Burlot, A.S.; Bourgougnon, N. Chapter Twelve-Bioactive components from seaweeds: Cosmetic applications and future development. In *Advances in Botanical Research*; Bourgougnon, N., Ed.; Academic Press: Cambridge, MA, USA, 2014; Volume 71, pp. 345–378.

78. Pereira, L. Seaweed flora of the european north atlantic and mediterranean. In *Springer Handbook of Marine Biotechnology*; Kim, S.-K., Ed.; Springer: Berlin/Heidelberg, Germany, 2015; pp. 65–178.
79. Pangestuti, R.; Kim, S.-K. Chapter Seven-Biological activities of carrageenan. In *Advances in Food and Nutrition Research*; Kim, S.-K., Ed.; Academic Press: Cambridge, MA, USA, 2014; Volume 72, pp. 113–124.
80. Hartmann, A.; Gostner, J.; Fuchs, J.E.; Chaita, E.; Aligiannis, N.; Skaltsounis, L.; Ganzera, M. Inhibition of collagenase by mycosporine-like amino acids from marine sources. *Planta Med.* **2015**, *81*, 813–820. [CrossRef]
81. Chrapusta, E.; Kaminski, A.; Duchnik, K.; Bober, B.; Adamski, M.; Bialczyk, J. Mycosporine-like amino acids: Potential health and beauty ingredients. *Mar. Drugs* **2017**, *15*, 326. [CrossRef]
82. Kageyama, H.; Waditee-Sirisattha, R. Antioxidative, anti-inflammatory, and anti-aging properties of mycosporine-like amino acids: Molecular and cellular mechanisms in the protection of skin-aging. *Mar. Drugs* **2019**, *17*, 222. [CrossRef] [PubMed]
83. Suh, S.-S.; Hwang, J.; Park, M.; Seo, H.H.; Kim, H.-S.; Lee, J.H.; Moh, S.H.; Lee, T.-K. Anti-inflammation activities of mycosporine-like amino acids (MAAs) in response to UV radiation suggest potential anti-skin aging activity. *Mar. Drugs* **2014**, *12*, 5174–5187. [CrossRef]
84. Phykosil 2000. Available online: https://www.ulprospector.com/documents/1055240.pdf?bs=4655&b=132140&st=20&r=na&ind=personalcare (accessed on 15 June 2021).
85. Christaki, E.; Eleftherios, B.; Ilias, G.; Panagiota, F.P. Functional properties of carotenoids originating from algae. *J. Sci. Food Agric.* **2013**, *93*, 5–11. [CrossRef] [PubMed]
86. Ru, I.T.K.; Sung, Y.Y.; Jusoh, M.; Wahid, M.E.A.; Nagappan, T. *Chlorella vulgaris*: A perspective on its potential for combining high biomass with high value bioproducts. *App. Phycol.* **2020**, *1*, 2–11. [CrossRef]
87. Raposo, M.F.d.J.; De Morais, R.M.S.C.; Bernardo de Morais, A.M.M. Bioactivity and applications of sulphated polysaccharides from marine microalgae. *Mar. Drugs* **2013**, *11*, 233–252. [CrossRef] [PubMed]
88. Chen, C.-L.; Liou, S.-F.; Chen, S.-J.; Shih, M.-F. Protective effects of Chlorella-derived peptide on UVB-induced production of MMP-1 and degradation of procollagen genes in human skin fibroblasts. *Regul. Toxicol. Pharmacol.* **2011**, *60*, 112–119. [CrossRef]
89. de Melo, R.G.; de Andrade, A.F.; Bezerra, R.P.; Viana Marques, D.d.A.; da Silva, J.V.A.; Paz, S.T.; de Lima Filho, J.L.; Porto, A.L.F. Hydrogel-based *Chlorella vulgaris* extracts: A new topical formulation for wound healing treatment. *J. Appl. Phycol.* **2019**, *31*, 3653–3663. [CrossRef]
90. Machmud, E.; Ruslin, M.; Waris, R.; Asse, R.A.; Qadafi, A.M.; Achmad, H. Effect of the Application of *Chlorella vulgaris* Ointment to the Number of Fibroblast Cells as an Indicator of Wound Healing in the Soft Tissue of Pig Ears. *Pesqui. Bras. Odontopediatria Clin. Integr.* **2020**, *20*, 5012. [CrossRef]
91. Kang, H.; Lee, C.H.; Kim, J.R.; Kwon, J.Y.; Seo, S.G.; Han, J.G.; Kim, B.G.; Kim, J.-E.; Lee, K.W. *Chlorella vulgaris* attenuates dermatophagoides farinae-induced atopic dermatitis-like symptoms in NC/Nga mice. *Int. J. Mol. Sci.* **2015**, *16*, 21021–21034. [CrossRef] [PubMed]
92. Singh, A.; Singh, S.P.; Bamezai, R. Inhibitory potential of *Chlorella vulgaris* (E-25) on mouse skin papillomagenesis and xenobiotic detoxication system. *Anticancer Res.* **1999**, *19*, 1887–1891. [PubMed]
93. Cornejo Navarro, P. Inhibición de la angiogénesis por un producto destinado a la prevención y cuidado del enrojecimiento facial y sus aplicaciones cosméticas. *Piel* **2016**, *31*, 321–324. [CrossRef]

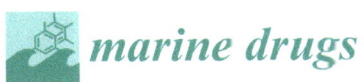

Article

Characterization of Neoagarooligosaccharide Hydrolase BpGH117 from a Human Gut Bacterium *Bacteroides plebeius*

Yerin Jin †, Sora Yu †, Dong Hyun Kim, Eun Ju Yun and Kyoung Heon Kim *

Department of Biotechnology, Graduate School, Korea University, Seoul 02841, Korea; dpfls96@korea.ac.kr (Y.J.); sora30715@korea.ac.kr (S.Y.); goodsoul4u@korea.ac.kr (D.H.K.); jdjddcld@korea.ac.kr (E.J.Y.)
* Correspondence: khekim@korea.ac.kr
† These authors contributed equally to this work.

Abstract: α-Neoagarobiose (NAB)/neoagarooligosaccharide (NAO) hydrolase plays an important role as an exo-acting 3,6-anhydro-α-(1,3)-L-galactosidase in agarose utilization. Agarose is an abundant polysaccharide found in red seaweeds, comprising 3,6-anhydro-L-galactose (AHG) and D-galactose residues. Unlike agarose degradation, which has been reported in marine microbes, recent metagenomic analysis of *Bacteroides plebeius*, a human gut bacterium, revealed the presence of genes encoding enzymes involved in agarose degradation, including α-NAB/NAO hydrolase. Among the agarolytic enzymes, BpGH117 has been partially characterized. Here, we characterized the exo-acting α-NAB/NAO hydrolase BpGH117, originating from *B. plebeius*. The optimal temperature and pH for His-tagged BpGH117 activity were 35 °C and 9.0, respectively, indicative of its unique origin. His-tagged BpGH117 was thermostable up to 35 °C, and the enzyme activity was maintained at 80% of the initial activity at a pre-incubation temperature of 40 °C for 120 min. K_m and V_{max} values for NAB were 30.22 mM and 54.84 U/mg, respectively, and k_{cat}/K_m was 2.65 s^{-1} mM^{-1}. These results suggest that His-tagged BpGH117 can be used for producing bioactive products such as AHG and agarotriose from agarose efficiently.

Keywords: α-neoagarooligosaccharide hydrolase; exo-acting 3,6-anhydro-α-(1,3)-L-galactosidase; BpGH117; 3,6-anhydro-L-galactose; human gut bacterium; *Bacteroides plebeius*; agarose

Citation: Jin, Y.; Yu, S.; Kim, D.H.; Yun, E.J.; Kim, K.H. Characterization of Neoagarooligosaccharide Hydrolase BpGH117 from a Human Gut Bacterium *Bacteroides plebeius*. *Mar. Drugs* **2021**, *19*, 271. https://doi.org/10.3390/md19050271

Academic Editors: Herminia Domínguez, María Lourdes Mourelle and Jose Luis Legido

Received: 1 March 2021
Accepted: 10 May 2021
Published: 13 May 2021

Publisher's Note: MDPI stays neutral with regard to jurisdictional claims in published maps and institutional affiliations.

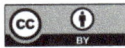

Copyright: © 2021 by the authors. Licensee MDPI, Basel, Switzerland. This article is an open access article distributed under the terms and conditions of the Creative Commons Attribution (CC BY) license (https://creativecommons.org/licenses/by/4.0/).

1. Introduction

Diet plays an important role in gut microbiome formation, and dietary changes show transient but significant microbial population changes in the gut [1]. Among various dietary components, non-digestible carbohydrates such as resistant starch and fiber cannot be decomposed in the small intestine. Instead, when non-digestible carbohydrates reach the large intestine, they are utilized by resident microorganisms. Therefore, diet can change intestinal microflora and consequently affect overall host health [2–4].

Marine red macroalgae, one of the representative non-digestible diets, especially in East Asia, has received much attention as an important food resource [5,6]. Most enzymes required to degrade red macroalgae are known to originate from marine microorganisms [7–9]. However, recent studies have revealed that human gut microbes also carry genes encoding Carbohydrate-Active enZymes (CAZymes), which can hydrolyze marine polysaccharides, including agarose [10–12]. Additionally, it was suggested that the genes encoding CAZymes involved in agarose degradation have been transferred from the marine bacterium *Zobellia galactanivorans* to the human gut bacterium *Bacteroides plebeius*, which was isolated from the microbiota of Japanese individuals [10,13]. This implies that human gut microbes may help humans utilize red seaweeds that cannot be degraded by the innate enzymes found in humans.

Agar, a major polysaccharide in the cell wall of marine red macroalgae, comprises agarose and porphyran [13,14]. Agarose, which occupies 70–80% of agar, is a neutral and linear polysaccharide composed of alternating 3,6-anhydro-L-galactose (AHG) and

D-galactose by α-1,3- and β-1,4-glycosidic linkages [15]. Agarases have been extensively studied for the cleavage of the β-1,4 bonds in agarose [16,17]. However, little is known about the biochemical characteristics of 3,6-anhydro-α-(1,3)-L-galactosidases, including α-neoagarobiose hydrolase (α-NABH) and α-neoagarooligosaccharide hydrolase (α-NAOH) belonging to the glycoside hydrolase 117 family (GH117), compared to agarases [18]. Since all agarolytic bacteria contain at least one conserved GH117 enzyme, GH117 appears to be the major evolutionary solution for cleaving α-1,3 glycosidic bonds in agarose [19]. This suggests that GH117 enzymes are important for polysaccharide utilization in agarolytic bacteria.

B. plebeius was shown to have an exo-acting 3,6-anhydro-α-(1,3)-L-galactosidase, *Bp*GH117, which belongs to GH117 and removes AHG from the non-reducing end of neoagarooligosaccharide (NAO) of agarose [19]. *Bp*GH117 decomposes neoagarotetraose (NeoDP4) into AHG and agarotriose (AgaDP3), and also neoagarobiose (NeoDP2) into AHG and galactose [19]. Lately, AgaDP3 has been found to have various health-benefiting effects. AgaDP3 is suggested to be a prebiotic since it is utilized by probiotic strains *Bifidobacterium infantis* and *Bifidobacterium adolescentis* [11]. Additionally, in vitro anti-colon cancer activity of AgaDP3 has been revealed recently [20]. In addition, AHG has been shown to have skin whitening, anticariogenic, and anti-inflammatory effects [21,22]. Although *Bp*GH117 has the potential to be used to produce high value-added products from agarose, it has only been partially characterized. Enzymatic properties such as optimal pH and temperature, and kinetic parameters of His-tagged *Bp*GH117, remain unknown.

In this study, we characterized His-tagged *Bp*GH117 originating from a human gut bacterium, *B. plebeius*. The characteristics of His-tagged *Bp*GH117 were comparatively studied with those of previously characterized 3,6-anhydro-α-(1,3)-L-galactosidases, and His-tagged *Bp*GH117 was investigated to determine whether this enzyme is optimal for the human gut environment. The results of this study can be used to utilize His-tagged *Bp*GH117 for industrial use.

2. Results

2.1. Analysis of the Enzymatic Reaction Products by Thin-Layer Chromatography (TLC) and High-Performance Liquid Chromatography (HPLC)

To reveal the mode of enzymatic action of *Bp*GH117, the purified His-tagged *Bp*GH117 was prepared to react with NeoDP2 and NeoDP4. The His-tagged *Bp*GH117 overexpressed without a signal sequence was identified by sodium dodecyl sulfate–polyacrylamide gel electrophoresis (SDS-PAGE) using a theoretical molar mass of 44.5 kDa (Figure 1). The reaction products formed after the treatment of NeoDP2 or NeoDP4 with His-tagged *Bp*GH117 were analyzed by TLC and HPLC (Figure 2). First, the products formed after the treatment of NAOs, NeoDP2 and NeoDP4, with His-tagged *Bp*GH117, were visualized by TLC. According to the TLC analysis results, NeoDP2 was hydrolyzed into AHG and galactose, and NeoDP4 was hydrolyzed into AgaDP3 and AHG by enzymatic reactions with His-tagged *Bp*GH117, respectively, while NeoDP2 and NeoDP4 remained due to the negative control reaction (Figure 2A,B).

In addition, the enzymatic reaction mixtures of His-tagged *Bp*GH117 were analyzed using HPLC. When NeoDP2 was used as the substrate, a peak corresponding to NeoDP2 disappeared, while a peak corresponding to galactose and AHG appeared after 2 h reaction with His-tagged *Bp*GH117 (Figure 2C). Similarly, when using NeoDP4 as the substrate, a peak corresponding to NeoDP4 disappeared, and peaks corresponding to AgaDP3 and AHG appeared after the His-tagged *Bp*GH117 enzymatic reaction (Figure 2D). These results confirmed that *Bp*GH117 is an α-NAOH that can cleave α-1,3-glycosidic bonds in both NeoDP2 and NeoDP4.

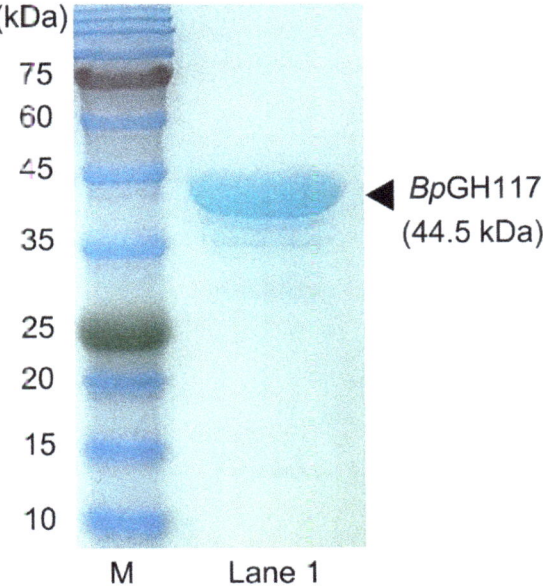

Figure 1. Sodium dodecyl sulfate-polyacrylamide gel electrophoresis (SDS-PAGE) analysis of purified His-tagged BpGH117. Lanes: M, protein marker; Lane 1, purified His-tagged BpGH117.

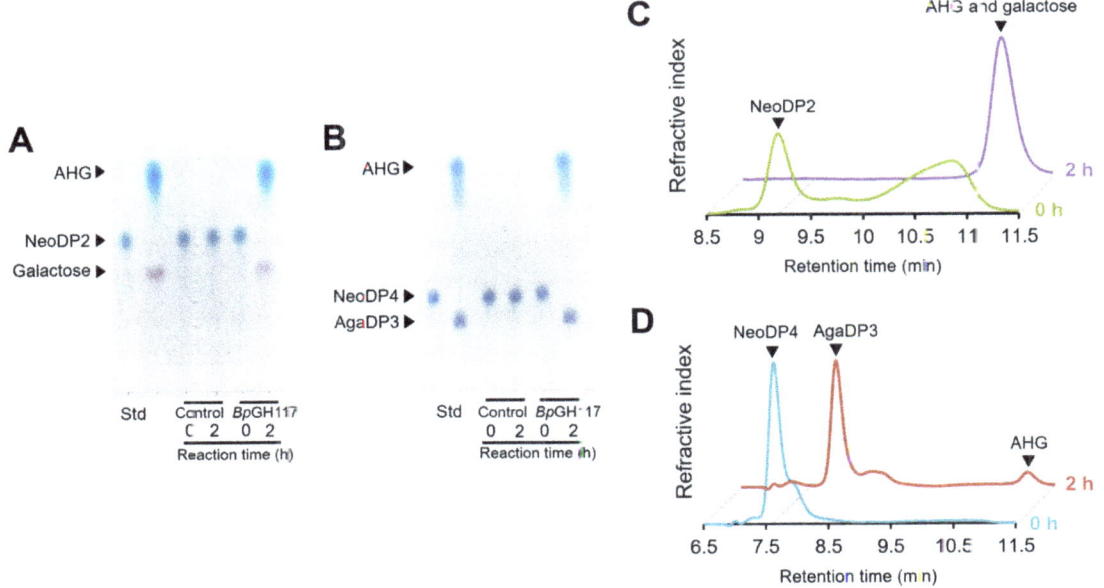

Figure 2. Product analyses of His-tagged BpGH117 with neoagarobiose (NeoDP2) and neoagarotetraose (NeoDP4) by (**A**,**B**) thin-layer chromatography and (**C**,**D**) overlaid high-performance liquid chromatography. All reactions were carried out with 2 mg/mL NeoDP2 or NeoDP4 in 50 mM Tris-HCl (pH 9.0) buffer at 35 °C. Control: negative control containing the same volume of 50 mM Tris-HCl buffer (pH 9.0) instead of BpGH117. AgaDP3, agarotriose; AHG, 3,6-anhydro-L-galactose; Std, standard.

2.2. Optimal pH and Temperature of BpGH117

To determine the optimal pH and temperature for the enzymatic reaction of His-tagged BpGH117, the enzymatic reactions were performed at various pH values and temperatures. First, the effect of pH on His-tagged BpGH117 activity was evaluated by performing enzymatic reactions at pH 4.0–10.0 (Figure 3). His-tagged BpGH117 showed the highest enzymatic activity at pH 9.0. Additionally, 50% of the maximum activity was maintained at pH 8.0, and 44, 41, and 36% of the maximum activity was maintained at pH 6.5, 7.5, and 10.0, respectively.

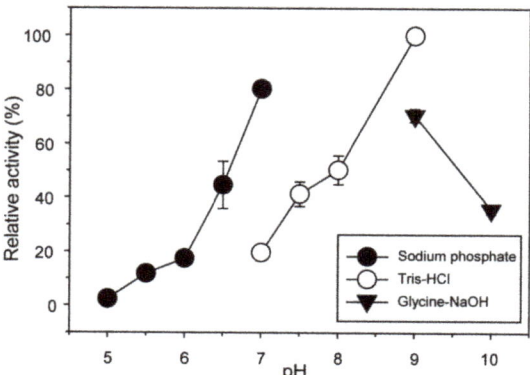

Figure 3. Effect of pH on His-tagged BpGH117 activity. To assess the effect of pH, the reactions were performed at 35 °C for 10 min in different buffers: 50 mM sodium citrate buffer (pH 4.0), 50 mM sodium phosphate buffer (pH 5.0–7.0), 50 mM Tris-HCl buffer (pH 7.0–9.0), and 50 mM glycine-NaOH buffer (pH 9.0–10.0).

Similarly, the effect of temperature on His-tagged BpGH117 activity was determined by measuring the enzyme activities at 10–70 °C (Figure 4). The highest activity of His-tagged BpGH117 was observed at 35 °C. In addition, 97, 70, and 48% of the maximal activity were maintained at 30, 40, and 45 °C, respectively. However, the relative activity of His-tagged BpGH117 decreased below 33% at $\leq$25 °C, and also decreased below 20% at $\geq$50 °C.

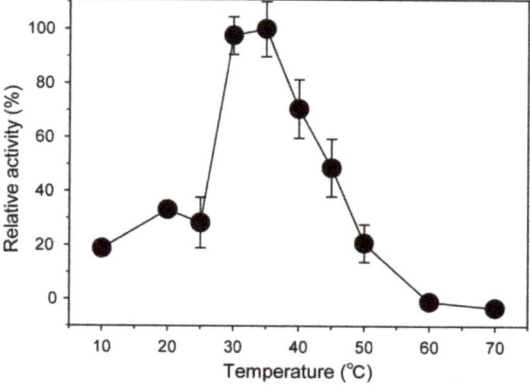

Figure 4. Effect of temperature on His-tagged BpGH117 activity. To determine the optimal temperature of His-tagged BpGH117, the reactions were performed at 10–70 °C in 50 mM Tris-HCl buffer at pH 9.0 for 10 min.

2.3. Thermostability of BpGH117

To determine the thermostability of His-tagged BpGH117, the enzyme was pre-incubated at 35–60 °C for 0–120 min (Figure 5) before reacting with 2 mg/mL NeoDP4 in 50 mM Tris-HCl buffer (pH 9.0) at 35 °C for 10 min. His-tagged BpGH117 maintained 100% of its initial activity for up to 120 min at 35 °C. Even though the residual relative activity of His-tagged BpGH117 slightly decreased, more than 80% of its initial activity was maintained after pre-incubating for 120 min at 40 °C. However, the enzymatic activity after pre-incubating for 120 min at 45 °C or higher was only about 25% of the initial activity.

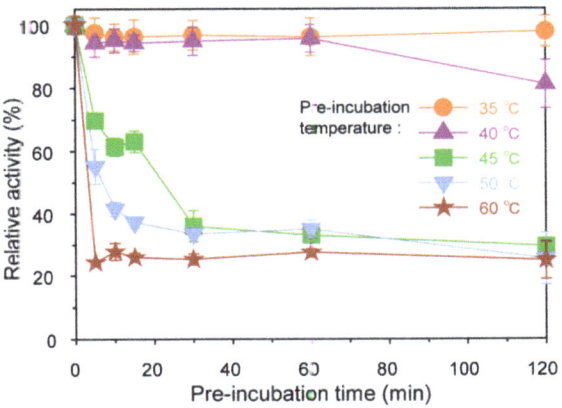

Figure 5. Thermostability of His-tagged BpGH117. To determine the thermostability of His-tagged BpGH117, His-tagged BpGH117 was pre-incubated at 35–60 °C for 0–120 min before the enzymatic reaction at 35 °C for 10 min.

2.4. Effect of Metal Ions and EDTA on the Activity of BpGH117

The effect of various metal ions and a chelating agent, EDTA, on the enzymatic activity of His-tagged BpGH117, was tested by measuring the enzyme activity in reaction mixtures containing 1 mM of the metal ions in the form of chloride salts or EDTA. The results revealed that His-tagged BpGH117 activity was not affected by any metal ions tested in this study or EDTA (Table 1).

Table 1. Effect of metal ions and EDTA on His-tagged BpGH117 activity. The enzyme activity was determined with various metal ions in the form of chloride salts or EDTA at the final concentration of 1 mM. The enzyme activity without metal ions or EDTA was considered as 100%.

	Relative Activity (%)
Control	100.0 ± 4.3
Metal ion in the form of chloride salt	
KCl	92.6 ± 11.6
NaCl	102.7 ± 8.7
NH_4Cl	98.8 ± 5.6
LiCl	95.5 ± 12.7
$CaCl_2$	80.0 ± 4.2
$MgCl_2$	100.3 ± 7.4
$RbCl_2$	100.9 ± 7.9
$MnCl_2$	98.6 ± 7.9
Chelating agent	
EDTA	98.1 ± 0.7

2.5. Kinetic Parameters of BpGH117

The kinetic parameters of His-tagged BpGH117 toward NeoDP2 and NeoDP4 were determined from the Lineweaver–Burk plot. The K_m, V_{max}, and k_{cat} values of His-tagged BpGH117 toward NeoDP2 were 30.22 mM, 54.84 U/mg, and 80.1 s^{-1}, respectively, while those toward NeoDP4 were 14.16 mM, 26.98 U/mg, and 40 s^{-1}, respectively. Therefore, His-tagged BpGH117 showed a lower K_m value toward NeoDP4 than NeoDP2, which implies that His-tagged BpGH117 may exhibit a higher substrate affinity toward NeoDP4 than toward NeoDP2.

The kinetic parameters, K_m and V_{max} values of His-tagged BpGH117, were also compared with those of previously characterized α-NABH and α-NAOH toward NeoDP2 (Table 2). His-tagged BpGH117 had the highest K_m value among the characterized α-NABH and α-NAOH enzymes. In addition, His-tagged BpGH117 had the fourth highest V_{max} value among the 14 enzymes listed in Table 2.

2.6. Amino Acid Sequence Analysis of BpGH117

The BACPLE_01671 gene has 1206 base pairs and is translated into a 402-amino acid protein, BpGH117. A BLAST search for available sequence databases suggested that the amino acid sequence of BpGH117 was quite similar to that of several GH117 enzymes known to exhibit α-NABH or α-NAOH activity [25]. Protein sequence alignment of BpGH117 showed several domains that were highly conserved with other known GH117 enzymes (Figure 6). BpGH117 carries the SxAxxR motif, the signature motif of the GH117 family, which represents the basal requirement for the multimerization of GH117 enzymes and is known to be present in several GH117 enzymes [25,29,30]. The acidic amino acids Asp-90, Asp-245, and Glu-303 are probably involved in the coordination with an NAO substrate [19]. The conserved residues Trp-128, Thr-165, Gln-180, His-244, and His-302 are assumed to act as the catalytic sites of GH117 enzymes [29,30].

Table 2. Comparison of characterized α-neoagarobiose/neoagarooligosaccharide hydrolases. K_m and V_{max} values are toward neoagarobiose (NeoDP2). n.a., not available, Identity (%), a number that describes how similar the query sequence is to the target sequence (how many characters in each sequence are identical).

Strain (Enzyme)	Molar Mass of Subunit (kDa)	Monomer/ Multimer	Location of Protein	Effect of Metal Ion Activation	Effect of Metal Ion Inhibition	Optimum Temp. (°C)	Optimum pH	K_m (mM)	V_{max} (U/mg)	Substrate	Identity (%)	Reference
Bacteroides plebeius (BpGH117)	45.6	Dimer	Extracellular	n.a.	n.a.	35	9.0	30.22	54.84	NeoDP2/4/6		This study, [19]
Streptomyces coelicolor A3(2) (ScJC117)	41	n.a.	Extracellular	Mg^{2+}	Ba^{2+}, Ca^{2+}, Co^{2+}, Fe^{3+}, Zn^{2+}, Ni^{2+}	30	6.0	11.57	n.a.	NeoDP2/4/6	51.8	[23]
Gayadomonas joobiniege GJ (Ahg558)	40.8	Dimer	n.a.	Mn^{2+}	Cu^{2+}, Mg^{2+}	30	9.0	0.01	133.33	NeoDP2/4/6	59.9	[24]
Gayadomonas joobiniege (Ahg786)	45.18	Dimer	Extracellular	Mn^{2+}	Cu^{2+}, Mg^{2+}, Zn^{2+}, Ni^{2+}	15	7.0	4.5	1.33	NeoDP2/4/6	56.9	[18]
Cellulophaga sp. W5C (AhgI)	45	Octamer	Extracellular	Ca^{2+}	n.a.	20–30	7.0	1.03	10.22	NeoDP2/4/6	68.1	[25]
Celltrbrio sp. WU-0601	42	Dimer	Cytosolic	Mn^{2+}, Mg^{2+}	Ag^+, Hg^{2+}, Cu^{2+}, Ni^{2+}	25	6.0	5.8	60	NeoDP2/4/6	58.5	[26]
Agarivorans gilvus WH0801 (AgaWH117)	41	n.a.	Cytosolic	n.a.	n.a.	30	6.0	6.45	6.98	NeoDP2/4	59.0	[27]
Celltrbrio sp. OA-2007	40	Dimer	Cytosolic	n.a.	n.a.	32	7.0–7.2	6	19	NeoDP2/4/6	57.0	[28]
Saccharophagus degradans 2-40T (SdNABH)	41.6	Dimer	Cytosolic	n.a.	Zn^{2+}, Ni^{2+}, Cu^{2+}, Co^{2+}	42	6.5	3.5	n.a.	NeoDP2/4/6	60.3	[29]
Zobellia galactanivorans (AhgA)	41	Dimer	Extracellular	n.a.	n.a.	n.a.	n.a.	n.a.	n.a.	NeoDP4/6	69.1	[30]
Bacillus sp. MK03	42	Octamer	Extracellular	Mg^{2+}	Ag^+, Ni^{2+}, Cu^{2+}, Hg^{2+}	30	6.1	n.a.	22.2	NeoDP2/4/6	n.a.	[31]
Vibrio sp. JT0107	42	Dimer	Cytosolic	n.a.	n.a.	30	7.7	5.37	92	NeoDP2/4/6	n.a.	[32]
Cytophaga flevensis	n.a.	n.a.	Cytosolic	n.a.	Ag^+, Hg^{2+}, Zn^{2+}, Pb^{2+}	25	6.75	n.a.	n.a.	NeoDP2	n.a.	[33]
Pseudomonas atlantica	10	n.a.	Periplasmic	Na^+	n.a.	n.a.	7.3–8.0	n.a.	n.a.	NeoDP2	n.a.	[34]

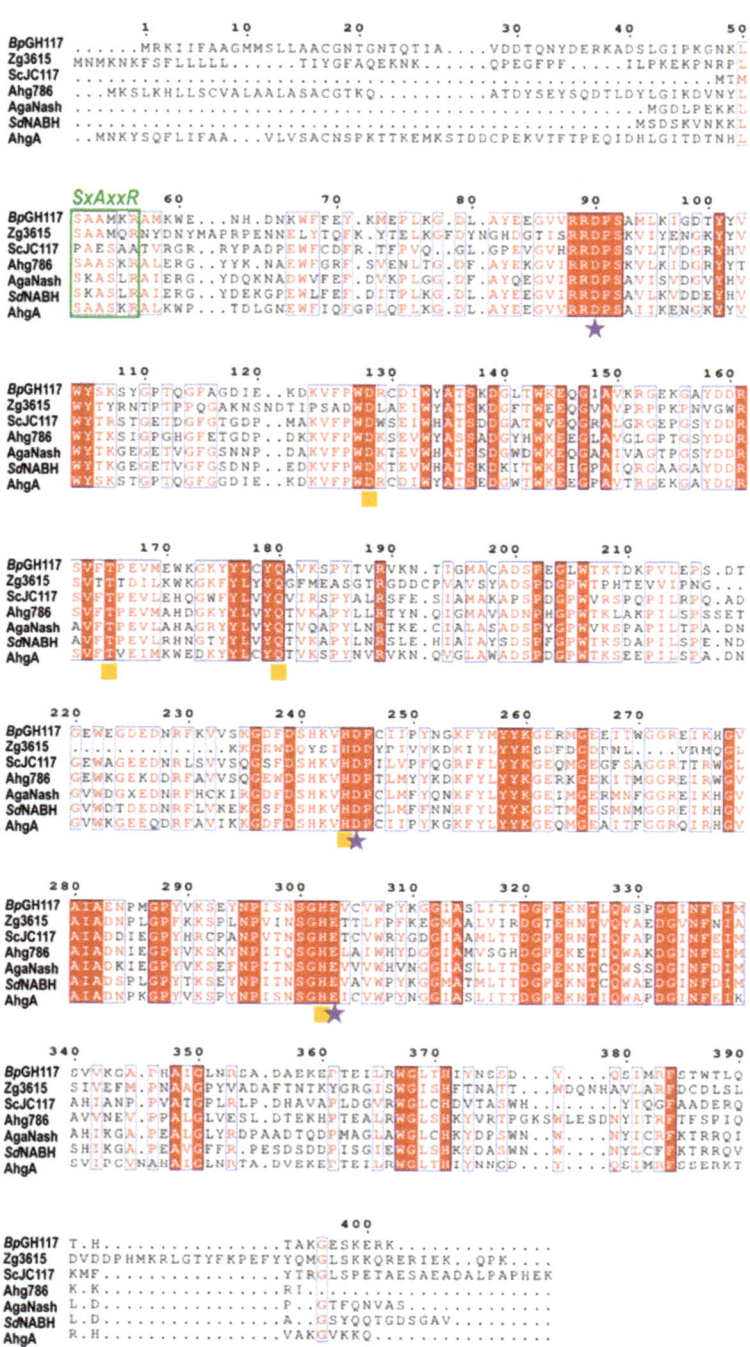

Figure 6. Amino acid alignment of *Bp*GH117 with other GH117 family members. Stars (★) denote catalytic residues and squares (■) indicate residues involved in substrate binding.

3. Discussion

α-NAOH has been suggested to play an important role in breaking down agar, a non-digestible carbohydrate [19]. Most agarolytic microorganisms are known to be marine microorganisms [7–9]. However, a human gut bacterium, B. plebeius, was recently found to have enzymes that can hydrolyze agar [10–12]. Agarooligosaccharides have been shown to promote the growth of beneficial strains in the intestine, suggesting their possibility as prebiotics [11]. Thus, by studying enzymes derived from the human gut bacterium, it becomes possible to further understand the processes or enzymes which decompose agarose in the intestine, and how prebiotics would be produced from agarose. Additionally, through this information, the GH117 enzyme BpGH117, could be applied to a wider variety of fields, such as producing prebiotics derived from marine macroalgae. Therefore, it is important to study B. plebeius-derived enzymes to understand how agarose, which is usually not degraded by innate enzymes in humans, is metabolized in the intestine. However, only crystallographic studies have been performed on the BpGH117 enzyme and its biochemical characteristics have been partially studied to date [19]. Thus, we characterized the enzymatic properties of His-tagged BpGH117, an α-NAOH isolated from B. plebeius.

In this study, His-tagged BpGH117 was found to be alkaline α-NAOH and α-NABH, which showed the highest activity at pH 9.0 (Figure 3). It is noteworthy that His-tagged BpGH117 has optimal activity in an alkaline environment, unlike most 3,6-anhydro-α-(1,3)-L-galactosidases which showed optimal activity in a neutral environment (pH 6.0–8.0) (Table 2). The highest activity of His-tagged BpGH117 was observed at 35 °C, which is similar to human body temperature, while most GH117 enzymes except SdNABH exhibited the maximum activity below 30 °C (Figure 4 and Table 2). These results are attributed to the origin of His-tagged BpGH117, which is B. plebeius isolated from the human gut.

Regarding cofactors, α-NAOH and α-NABH enzymes do not have a common metal ion requirement (Table 2). For example, ScJC117, Ahg786, SdNABH, and neoagarobiose hydrolase from *Cytophaga flevensis* were inhibited by Zn^{2+} [18,23,29,33]. Ahg558, Ahg786, α-NAOH from *Cellvibrio* sp. WU-0601, SdNABH, and α-NAOH from *Bacillus* sp. MK03 were inhibited by Cu^{2+} [18,24,26,29,31]. Crystallographic data for BpGH117 showed that the protein binds to Mg^{2+} ions [19]. However, it was revealed that metal ions do not affect His-tagged BpGH117 activity in vitro.

To date, the k_{cat}/K_m values of α-NABH and α-NAOH toward NeoDP2 have been reported for only four enzymes, most of them, except Ahg558, being less than $1\ s^{-1}\ mM^{-1}$, whereas k_{cat}/K_m of His-tagged BpGH117 was $2.65\ s^{-1}$/mM [23,24,26,27]. The high k_{cat}/K_m value of BpGH117 suggests that the enzyme has high catalytic efficiency. This implies that His-tagged BpGH117 may hydrolyze NAOs, including NeoDP4 and NeoDP2, more efficiently than most other GH117 enzymes.

In this study, His-tagged BpGH117 was found to cleave the α-1,3-glycosidic linkage from the non-reducing ends of NAOs, including NeoDP2 and NeoDP4. More specifically, when His-tagged BpGH117 hydrolyzes NeoDP4, AgaDP3 and AHG are produced. Odd-numbered agarooligosaccharides have been reported to have prebiotic effects by showing that probiotic strains, B. infantis and B. adolescentis, decompose AgaDP3 and grow with AgaDP3 as the sole carbon source [11]. In addition, AHG has been known to have various physiological activities such as anti-inflammatory, skin whitening, and anticariogenic activities [21,22]. Therefore, His-tagged BpGH117 enzyme would be advantageous in producing high value-added products such as AHG and AgaDP3 from agarose, owing to its higher k_{cat}/K_m value than most other α-NABH and α-NAOH enzymes. In conclusion, BpGH117 originating from B. plebeius was characterized as a GH117 enzyme from human gut bacterium in this study. In particular, His-tagged BpGH117 derived from human gut bacterium has unique optimal conditions for enzymatic activity at 35 °C and pH 9.0. Furthermore, His-tagged BpGH117 showed the second highest k_{cat}/K_m value toward NeoDP2 among the characterized GH117 enzymes. Notably, His-tagged BpGH117 can produce value-added products including AgaDP3 and AHG when NAOs such as NeoDP2 and NeoDP4 are given as a substrate. Therefore, *Bp*GH117 can be used to produce bioactive agar-derived products, and information about its optimal enzymatic reaction conditions revealed in this study can also be utilized for its industrial processes.

4. Materials and Methods

4.1. Overexpression and Purification of Recombinant BpGH117

The gene BACPLE_01671 encoding *Bp*GH117 without a signal sequence (1–54 bp) was cloned into the pET-21α(+) vector (Novagen, Madison, WI, USA), and the recombinant plasmid was transformed into *Escherichia coli* BL21(DE3) (Novagen). To produce recombinant His-tagged *Bp*GH117, recombinant *E. coli* BL21(DE3) harboring the *Bp*GH117 gene was incubated in Luria–Bertani (LB; BD; San Jose, CA, USA) broth medium containing 100 µg/mL of ampicillin (Sigma-Aldrich, St. Louis, MO, USA) at 37 °C until the culture reached the mid-exponential phase of growth.

When the optical density at 600 nm (OD_{600}) reached 0.5, 0.5 mM isopropyl-β-D-1-thiogalactopyranoside (IPTG; Sigma-Aldrich, St. Louis, MO, USA) was added to the culture medium to induce recombinant His-tagged *Bp*GH117. After incubation for 16 h at 16 °C, the cells were harvested by centrifugation at 10,000 × *g* for 30 min at 4 °C. The cell pellet was resuspended in ice-cold lysis buffer (20 mM Tris-HCl, pH 7.4) and the cell suspension was disrupted using a sonicator (Branson, Gunpo, Korea). The supernatant containing the soluble protein was collected by centrifugation at 15,000 × *g* for 40 min at 4 °C. The recombinant His-tagged *Bp*GH117 was purified by affinity chromatography using a His-Trap column (GE Healthcare, Piscataway, NJ, USA) and the eluent buffer containing 0.5 M NaCl and 0.1 M imidazole in 20 mM sodium phosphate buffer (pH 7.4). The purified His-tagged *Bp*GH117 was concentrated using an Amicon ultrafiltration membrane (MW cutoff 30 kDa; Millipore, Billerica, MA, USA). The protein concentration was determined using a bicinchoninic acid (BCA) protein assay kit (Thermo Fisher Scientific, Waltham, MA, USA).

4.2. Enzyme Activity Measurement Using 3,5-Dinitrosalicylic Acid (DNS) Assay

The enzyme activity of His-tagged *Bp*GH117 was determined by measuring the amount of released reducing sugar in the reaction mixture using the DNS method with D-galactose as a monomeric sugar standard [35]. To prepare NeoDP2 and NeoDP4 as the substrates for reactions by His-tagged *Bp*GH117, we carried out the enzymatic degradation of agarose, followed by purification. For the degradation of agarose, two in-house recombinant enzymes were used: an endo-type β-agarase, *Bp*GH16A, which produces NeoDP4 as the major product from agarose [36], and an exo-type β-agarase, Aga50D, which produces NeoDP2 from agarose. NeoDP2 and NeoDP4 were purified from each reaction product by gel filtration chromatography using Bio-Gel P-2 Gel polyacrylamide (Bio-Rad, Hercules, CA, USA) and distilled water as an eluent. The enzymatic reaction mixture containing 0.05 mg/mL recombinant His-tagged *Bp*GH117 and 2 mg/mL NeoDP2 or NeoDP4 in 50 mM Tris-HCl buffer (pH 9.0) was incubated at 35 °C for 10 min. As a negative control, the same volume of 50 mM Tris-HCl buffer (pH 9.0) was incubated instead of the enzyme. The reaction mixture was incubated in boiling water for 5 min to terminate the enzymatic reaction. To determine the amount of total reducing sugar produced, 60 µL of the DNS solution was added to 60 µL of the enzymatic reaction mixture. The mixture was incubated at 95 °C for 5 min and cooled at 4 °C for 5 min. The absorbance at 540 nm was recorded using a microplate spectrophotometer (xMark; Bio-Rad, Hercules, CA, USA) to measure the concentration of reducing sugars. One unit (U) of *Bp*GH117 activity was defined as the amount of enzyme required to release 1 µmol of reducing sugar per minute under the above reaction conditions.

4.3. TLC and HPLC Analyses of Enzymatic Reaction Products

For analyzing the products generated after the substrate was completely reacted, the enzymatic reaction was performed for 2 h under the same conditions as when the

DNS analysis was performed. First, the products formed by treating NeoDP2 or NeoDP4 with His-tagged BpGH117 were analyzed by TLC. An aliquot of 1 µL from each reaction sample was spotted on silica gel 60 TLC plates (Merck, Darmstadt, Germany), which were developed with water: ethanol: n-butanol (1:1: 3, v/v). The plates loaded with samples were visualized by spraying 10% (v/v) H_2SO_4 in ethanol and 0.2% (w/v) naphthoresorcinol in ethanol [21]. The reaction products were also analyzed by HPLC (Agilent Technologies, Santa Clara, CA, USA) system with an Aminex HPX-87H column (Bio-Rad) and a refractive index detector (Agilent Technologies). HPLC analysis was performed at 65 °C using 0.005 N H_2SO_4 as the mobile phase at a flow rate of 0.5 mL/min.

4.4. Biochemical Characterization of BpGH117

The optimal pH of His-tagged BpGH117 activity was determined by incubating 0.05 mg/mL His-tagged BpGH117 with 2 mg/mL NeoDP4 at 35 °C for 10 min at pH 4.0–10.0 using different buffers, depending on the pH: 50 mM sodium citrate buffer for pH 4.0, 50 mM sodium phosphate buffer for pH 5.0–7.0, 50 mM Tris-HCl buffer for pH 7.0–9.0, and 50 mM glycine-NaOH buffer for pH 9.0–10.0. To determine the optimal temperature of His-tagged BpGH117 activity, 0.05 mg/mL His-tagged BpGH117 was incubated with 2 mg/mL NeoDP4 in 50 mM Tris-HCl buffer (pH 9.0) for 10 min at 10–70 °C.

To measure the thermostability of His-tagged BpGH117, prior to the enzymatic reaction, 0.05 mg/mL His-tagged BpGH117 in 50 mM Tris-HCl buffer (pH 9.0) was pre-incubated at 30–70 °C for 0–120 min. After pre-incubation, the enzymatic reaction was performed by adding 2 mg/mL NeoDP4 to the pre-incubated mixture and incubating at 35 °C for 10 min. After pre-incubation, residual enzyme activity was determined, and His-tagged BpGH117 activity without pre-incubation was considered as 100%.

To study the effect of metal ions and a chelating agent, EDTA, on His-tagged BpGH117 activity, various metal ions in the form of chloride salts, Na^+, K^+, NH_4^+, Li^+, Ca^{2+}, Mg^{2+}, Mn^{2+}, and Rb^{2+}, and EDTA were used. The enzymatic reaction was performed by incubating 0.05 mg/mL His-tagged BpGH117 with 2 mg/mL NeoDP4 in 50 mM Tris-HCl buffer (pH 9.0) containing 1 mM of each ion or EDTA at 35 °C for 10 min. BpGH117 activity measured in the absence of metal ions or EDTA was considered to be 100%.

4.5. Determination of the Kinetic Parameters of BpGH117

The kinetic parameters of His-tagged BpGH117 were determined by the enzymatic reactions of 0.05 mg/mL His-tagged BpGH117 with 0.5–4 mg/mL NeoDP2 or NeoDP4 at 35 °C in 50 mM Tris-HCl buffer (pH 9.0) for 10 min. The V_{max}, K_m, and k_{cat} values were calculated from the Lineweaver–Burk plot based on the Michaelis–Menten kinetics (Figure S1 in the Supplementary Materials) [37].

4.6. Amino Acid Sequence Analysis of BpGH117 for Comparison with other GH117 Enzymes

The amino acid sequence of BpGH117 was compared using the BLAST program of the National Center for Biotechnology Information (NCBI; https://blast.ncbi.nlm.nih.gov/Blast.cgi, accessed on 12 June 2020) and UniProt (http://www.uniprot.org/blast/, accessed on: 12 June 2020). Espript and Clustal omega were used for multiple sequence alignment of the BpGH117 amino acid sequence [38,39].

Supplementary Materials: The following are available online at https://www.mdpi.com/article/10.3390/md19050271/s1, Figure S1: Lineweaver-Burk plot of BpGH117.

Author Contributions: Y.J. designed and performed the experiments, analyzed the data, and wrote the manuscript. S.Y. designed the project and experiments, analyzed the data, and wrote the manuscript. E.J.Y. and D.H.K. analyzed the data and wrote the manuscript. K.H.K. conceived the project, designed the experiments, analyzed the data, and wrote the manuscript. All authors have read and agreed to the published version of the manuscript.

Funding: This work was supported by the Mid-career Researcher Program (2020R1A2B5B02002631) through the National Research Foundation of Korea (NRF), the Ministry of Oceans and Fisheries of

Korea (20200367), and by the Korea Institute of Planning and Evaluation for Technology in Food, Agriculture, Forestry, and Fisheries, funded by the Ministry of Agriculture, Food, and Rural Affairs (321036051SB010). D.H.K. acknowledges the grant support from the NRF (2020R1C1C1008196). This work was performed at the Institute of Biomedical and Food Safety at the CJ Food Safety Hall, Korea University.

Institutional Review Board Statement: Not applicable.

Informed Consent Statement: Not applicable.

Data Availability Statement: The datasets used and/or analyzed during the current study are available from the corresponding author upon reasonable request.

Conflicts of Interest: The authors declare no conflict of interest.

References

1. David, L.A.; Maurice, C.F.; Carmody, R.N.; Gootenberg, D.B.; Button, J.E.; Wolfe, B.E.; Ling, A.V.; Devlin, A.S.; Varma, Y.; Fischbach, M.A. Diet rapidly and reproducibly alters the human gut microbiome. *Nature* **2014**, *505*, 559–563. [CrossRef]
2. Lozupone, C.; Faust, K.; Raes, J.; Faith, J.J.; Frank, D.N.; Zaneveld, J.; Gordon, J.I.; Knight, R. Identifying genomic and metabolic features that can underlie early successional and opportunistic lifestyles of human gut symbionts. *Genome Res.* **2012**, *22*, 1974–1984. [CrossRef] [PubMed]
3. Pistollato, F.; Sumalla Cano, S.; Elio, I.; Masias Vergara, M.; Giampieri, F.; Battino, M. Role of gut microbiota and nutrients in amyloid formation and pathogenesis of Alzheimer disease. *Nutr. Rev.* **2016**, *74*, 624–634. [CrossRef]
4. Sonnenburg, E.D.; Sonnenburg, J.L. Starving our microbial self: The deleterious consequences of a diet deficient in microbiota-accessible carbohydrates. *Cell Metab.* **2014**, *20*, 779–786. [CrossRef] [PubMed]
5. Hehemann, J.-H.; Correc, G.; Thomas, F.; Bernard, T.; Barbeyron, T.; Jam, M.; Helbert, W.; Michel, G.; Czjzek, M. Biochemical and structural characterization of the complex agarolytic enzyme system from the marine bacterium *Zobellia galactanivorans*. *J. Biol. Chem.* **2012**, *287*, 30571–30584. [CrossRef]
6. Kolb, N.; Vallorani, L.; Milanović, N.; Stocchi, V. Evaluation of marine algae wakame (*Undaria pinnatifida*) and kombu (*Laminaria digitata japonica*) as food supplements. *Food Technol. Biotechnol.* **2004**, *42*, 57–61.
7. Hu, Z.; Lin, B.K.; Xu, Y.; Zhong, M.; Liu, G.M. Production and purification of agarase from a marine agarolytic bacterium *Agarivorans* sp. HZ105. *J. Appl. Microbiol.* **2009**, *106*, 181–190. [CrossRef]
8. Shan, D.; Ying, J.; Li, X.; Gao, Z.; Wei, G.; Shao, Z. Draft genome sequence of the carrageenan-degrading bacterium *Cellulophaga* sp. strain KL-A, isolated from decaying marine algae. *Genome. Announc.* **2014**, *2*, e00145-14. [CrossRef] [PubMed]
9. Yagi, H.; Fujise, A.; Itabashi, N.; Ohshiro, T. Purification and characterization of a novel alginate lyase from the marine bacterium *Cobetia* sp. NAP1 isolated from brown algae. *Biosci. Biotechnol. Biochem.* **2016**, *80*, 2338–2346. [CrossRef]
10. Hehemann, J.-H.; Kelly, A.G.; Pudlo, N.A.; Martens, E.C.; Boraston, A.B. Bacteria of the human gut microbiome catabolize red seaweed glycans with carbohydrate-active enzyme updates from extrinsic microbes. *Proc. Natl. Acad. Sci. USA* **2012**, *109*, 19786–19791. [CrossRef]
11. Li, M.; Li, G.; Zhu, L.; Yin, Y.; Zhao, X.; Xiang, C.; Yu, G.; Wang, X. Isolation and characterization of an agaro-oligosaccharide (AO)-hydrolyzing bacterium from the gut microflora of Chinese individuals. *PLoS ONE* **2014**, *9*, e91106. [CrossRef] [PubMed]
12. Li, M.; Shang, Q.; Li, G.; Wang, X.; Yu, G. Degradation of marine algae-derived carbohydrates by Bacteroidetes isolated from human gut microbiota. *Mar. Drugs* **2017**, *15*, 92. [CrossRef] [PubMed]
13. Hehemann, J.-H.; Correc, G.; Barbeyron, T.; Helbert, W.; Czjzek, M.; Michel, G. Transfer of carbohydrate-active enzymes from marine bacteria to Japanese gut microbiota. *Nature* **2010**, *464*, 908–912. [CrossRef] [PubMed]
14. Correc, G.; Hehemann, J.-H.; Czjzek, M.; Helbert, W. Structural analysis of the degradation products of porphyran digested by *Zobellia galactanivorans* β-porphyranase A. *Carbohydr. Polym.* **2011**, *83*, 277–283. [CrossRef]
15. Araki, C. Structure of the agarose constituent of agar-agar. *Bull. Chem. Soc. Jpn.* **1956**, *29*, 543–544. [CrossRef]
16. Kloareg, B.; Quatrano, R. Structure of the cell walls of marine algae and ecophysiological functions of the matrix polysaccharides. *Oceanogr. Mar. Biol. Annu. Rev.* **1988**, *26*, 259–315.
17. Martens, E.C.; Koropatkin, N.M.; Smith, T.J.; Gordon, J.I. Complex glycan catabolism by the human gut microbiota: The Bacteroidetes Sus-like paradigm. *J. Biol. Chem.* **2009**, *284*, 24673–24677. [CrossRef]
18. Asghar, S.; Lee, C.-R.; Park, J.-S.; Chi, W.-J.; Kang, D.-K.; Hong, S.-K. Identification and biochemical characterization of a novel cold-adapted 1, 3-α-3, 6-anhydro-L-galactosidase, Ahg786, from *Gayadomonas joobiniege* G7. *Appl. Microbiol. Biotechnol.* **2018**, *102*, 8855–8866. [CrossRef]
19. Hehemann, J.-H.; Smyth, L.; Yadav, A.; Vocadlo, D.J.; Boraston, A.B. Analysis of keystone enzyme in agar hydrolysis provides insight into the degradation (of a polysaccharide from) red seaweeds. *J. Biol. Chem.* **2012**, *287*, 13985–13995. [CrossRef]
20. Yun, E.J.; Yu, S.; Kim, Y.-A.; Liu, J.-J.; Kang, N.J.; Jin, Y.-S.; Kim, K.H. In vitro prebiotic and anti-colon cancer activities of agar-derived sugars from red seaweeds. *Mar. Drugs* **2021**, *19*, 213. [CrossRef]

21. Yun, E.J.; Lee, S.; Kim, J.H.; Kim, B.B.; Kim, H.T.; Lee, S.H.; Pelton, J.G.; Kang, N.J.; Choi, I.-G.; Kim, K.H. Enzymatic production of 3,6-anhydro-L-galactose from agarose and its purification and in vitro skin whitening and anti-inflammatory activities. *Appl. Microbiol. Biotechnol.* **2013**, *97*, 2961–2970. [CrossRef]
22. Yun, E.J.; Lee, A.R.; Kim, J.H.; Cho, K.M.; Kim, K.H. 3,6-Anhydro-l-galactose, a rare sugar from agar, a new anticariogenic sugar to replace xylitol. *Food Chem.* **2017**, *221*, 976–983. [CrossRef] [PubMed]
23. Jiang, C.; Liu, Z.; Sun, J.; Mao, X. Characterization of a novel α-neoagarobiose hydrolase capable of preparation of medium- and long-chain agarooligosaccharides. *Front. Bioeng. Biotech.* **2020**, *7*, 470. [CrossRef] [PubMed]
24. Asghar, S.; Lee, C.-R.; Chi, W.-J.; Kang, D.-K.; Hong, S.-K. Molecular cloning and characterization of a novel cold-adapted alkaline 1,3-α-3,6-anhydro-l-galactosidase, Ahg558, from *Gayadomonas joobiniege* G7. *Appl. Biochem. Biotechnol.* **2019**, *188*, 1077–1095. [CrossRef]
25. Ramos, K.R.M.; Valdehuesa, K.N.G.; Maza, P.A.M.M.; Nisola, G.M.; Lee, W.-K.; Chung, W.-J. Overexpression and characterization of a novel α-neoagarobiose hydrolase and its application in the production of D-galactonate from *Gelidium amansii*. *Process Biochem.* **2017**, *63*, 105–112. [CrossRef]
26. Watanabe, T.; Kashimura, K.; Kirimura, K. Purification, characterization and gene identification of a α-neoagarooligosaccharide hydrolase from an alkaliphilic bacterium *Cellvibrio* sp. WU-0601. *J. Mol. Catal. B Enzym.* **2016**, *133*, S328–S336. [CrossRef]
27. Liu, N.; Yang, M.; Mao, X.; Mu, B; Wei, D. Molecular cloning and expression of a new α-neoagarobiose hydrolase from *Agarivorans gilvus* WH0801 and enzymatic production of 3,6-anhydro-l-galactose. *Biotechnol. Appl. Biochem.* **2016**, *63*, 230–237. [CrossRef]
28. Ariga, O.; Okamoto, N.; Harimoto, N.; Nakasaki, K. Purification and characterization of α-neoagarooligosaccharide hydrolase from *Cellvibrio* sp. OA-2007. *J. Microbiol. Biotechnol.* **2014**, *24*, 48–51. [CrossRef]
29. Ha, S.C.; Lee, S.; Lee, J.; Kim, H.T.; Ko, H.-J.; Kim, K.H.; Choi, I.-G. Crystal structure of a key enzyme in the agarolytic pathway, α-neoagarobiose hydrolase from *Saccharophagus degradans* 2–40. *Biochem. Biophys. Res. Commun.* **2011**, *412*, 238–244. [CrossRef]
30. Rebuffet, E.; Groisillier, A.; Thompson, A.; Jeudy, A.; Barbeyron, T.; Czjzek, M.; Michel, G. Discovery and structural characterization of a novel glycosidase family of marine origin. *Environ. Microbiol.* **2011**, *13*, 1253–1270. [CrossRef]
31. Suzuki, H.; Sawai, Y.; Suzuki, T.; Kawai, K. Purification and characterization of an extracellular α-neoagarooligosaccharide hydrolase from *Bacillus* sp. MK03. *J. Biosci. Bioeng.* **2002**, *93*, 456–463. [CrossRef]
32. Sugano, Y.; Kodama, H.; Terada, I.; Yamazaki, Y.; Noma, M. Purification and characterization of a novel enzyme, alpha-neoagarooligosaccharide hydrolase (alpha-NAOS hydrolase), from a marine bacterium, *Vibrio* sp. strain JT0107. *J. Bacteriol.* **1994**, *176*, 6812–6818. [CrossRef] [PubMed]
33. Van Der Meulen, H.; Harder, W. Characterization of the neoagarotetra-ase and neoagarobiase of *Cytophaga flevensis*. *Antonie Van Leeuwenhoek* **1976**, *42*, 81–94. [CrossRef]
34. Day, D.; Yaphe, W. Enzymatic hydrolysis of agar: Purification and characterization of neoagarobiose hydrolase and p-nitrophenyl α-galactoside hydrolases. *Can. J. Microbiol.* **1975**, *21*, 1512–1518. [CrossRef] [PubMed]
35. Miller, G.L. Use of dinitrosalicylic acid reagent for determination of reducing sugar. *Anal. Chem.* **1959**, *31*, 426–423. [CrossRef]
36. Park, N.J.; Yu, S.; Kim, D.H.; Yun, E.J.; Kim, K.H. Characterization of *Bp*GH16A of *Bacteroides plebeius*, a key enzyme initiating the depolymerization of agarose in the human gut. *Appl. Microbiol. Biotechnol.* **2021**, *105*, 617–625. [CrossRef] [PubMed]
37. Lineweaver, H.; Burk, D. The determination of enzyme dissociation constants. *J. Am. Chem. Soc.* **1934**, *56*, 658–666. [CrossRef]
38. Gouet, P.; Courcelle, E.; Stuart, D.I.; Metoz, F. ESPript: Analysis of multiple sequence alignments in PostScript. *Bioinformatics* **1999**, *15*, 305–308. [CrossRef]
39. Sievers, F.; Wilm, A.; Dineen, D.; Gibson, T.J.; Karplus, K.; Li, W.; Lopez, R.; McWilliam, H.; Remmert, M.; Söding, J. Fast, scalable generation of high-quality protein multiple sequence alignments using Clustal Omega. *Mol. Syst. Biol.* **2011**, *7*, 539. [CrossRef]

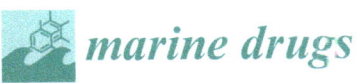

Article

In Vitro Prebiotic and Anti-Colon Cancer Activities of Agar-Derived Sugars from Red Seaweeds

Eun Ju Yun [1,2,†], Sora Yu [1,†], Young-Ah Kim [3], Jing-Jing Liu [2,4], Nam Joo Kang [3], Yong-Su Jin [2,4,*] and Kyoung Heon Kim [1,*]

1. Department of Biotechnology, Graduate School, Korea University, Seoul 02841, Korea; jdjddcld@korea.ac.kr (E.J.Y.); sora90715@korea.ac.kr (S.Y.)
2. Carl R. Woese Institute for Genomic Biology, University of Illinois at Urbana-Champaign, Urbana, IL 61801, USA; jingjing@sugarlogix.com
3. School of Food Science and Biotechnology, Kyungpook National University, Daegu 41566, Korea; yakim@o.cnu.ac.kr (Y.-A.K.); njkang@knu.ac.kr (N.J.K.)
4. Department of Food Science and Human Nutrition, University of Illinois at Urbana-Champaign, Urbana, IL 61801, USA
* Correspondence: ysjin@illinois.edu (Y.-S.J.); khekim@korea.ac.kr (K.H.K.)
† These authors contributed equally to this work.

Abstract: Numerous health benefits of diets containing red seaweeds or agar-derived sugar mixtures produced by enzymatic or acid hydrolysis of agar have been reported. However, among various agar-derived sugars, the key components that confer health-beneficial effects, such as prebiotic and anti-colon cancer activities, remain unclear. Here, we prepared various agar-derived sugars by multiple enzymatic reactions using an endo-type and an exo-type of β-agarase and a neoagarobiose hydrolase and tested their in vitro prebiotic and anti-colon cancer activities. Among various agar-derived sugars, agarotriose exhibited prebiotic activity that was verified based on the fermentability of agarotriose by probiotic bifidobacteria. Furthermore, we demonstrated the anti-colon cancer activity of 3,6-anhydro-L-galactose, which significantly inhibited the proliferation of human colon cancer cells and induced their apoptosis. Our results provide crucial information regarding the key compounds derived from red seaweeds that confer beneficial health effects, including prebiotic and anti-colon cancer activities, to the host.

Keywords: red seaweeds; agarose; agarotriose; 3,6-anhydro-L-galactose; prebiotics; anti-colon cancer activity

1. Introduction

Modern lifestyles have caused social and economic concerns regarding health disorders such as chronic diseases and metabolic dysfunction on a global level [1,2]. The human gut microbiome is known to play crucial roles in various human diseases, including chronic disorders and metabolic disease [3]. Additionally, diet, considered to be one of the major factors causing such diseases, has been hypothesized to modulate the functionality of the human microbiome [4]. Thus, there is increasing interest in dietary fiber as prebiotics that can selectively stimulate the growth of probiotics, conferring health benefits.

Marine macroalgae are considered to be good sources of prebiotics owing to their abundance in carbohydrates [1,5]. Red macroalgae are known to have higher carbohydrate content and lower amounts of recalcitrant substrates to saccharification, such as insoluble fiber, compared to other types of marine macroalgae [6]. Agarose—the major component of red macroalgae cell walls—consists of alternating units of D-galactose and 3,6-anhydro-L-galactose (AHG), which are linked alternately with α-1,3- and β-1,4-glycosidic linkages [7]. Agarose is distinct among red macroalgal polysaccharides since it can reach the large intestine, where it is degraded, fermented, and metabolized by gut microorganisms after consumption [8].

Citation: Yun, E.J.; Yu, S.; Kim, Y.-A.; Liu, J.-J.; Kang, N.J.; Jin, Y.-S.; Kim, K.H. In Vitro Prebiotic and Anti-Colon Cancer Activities of Agar-Derived Sugars from Red Seaweeds. *Mar. Drugs* **2021**, *19*, 213. https://doi.org/10.3390/md19040213

Academic Editors: María Lourdes Mourelle, Herminia Domínguez and Jose Luis Legido

Received: 4 March 2021
Accepted: 7 April 2021
Published: 12 April 2021

Publisher's Note: MDPI stays neutral with regard to jurisdictional claims in published maps and institutional affiliations.

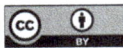

Copyright: © 2021 by the authors. Licensee MDPI, Basel, Switzerland. This article is an open access article distributed under the terms and conditions of the Creative Commons Attribution (CC BY) license (https://creativecommons.org/licenses/by/4.0/).

Agarose and oligosaccharides from agarose, including agarooligosaccharides (AOSs) and neoagarooligosaccharides (NAOSs), have been reported to have prebiotic effects that can promote the growth of beneficial gut bacteria and increase levels of short-chain fatty acids (SCFAs) [9,10]. However, most previous studies used agarose extracts containing heterogeneous components with various degrees of polymerization (DPs). Therefore, it is difficult to specify the exact source and cause of such prebiotic effects.

In addition to prebiotic effects, red macroalgae are known to possess various biological functions, including anti-inflammatory and antioxidant activities [11,12]. Additionally, clinical trials suggested that daily intake of seaweeds, including brown and red seaweeds, is associated with a lower risk of colon, colorectal, and breast cancers in Asian people who frequently consume red or brown seaweeds [13–15]. Fucoidan has been reported to be a key component for the anticancer activity of brown macroalgae and can induce apoptosis of cancer cells [16–18]. However, very little is known regarding which components are responsible for the anticancer effects of red macroalgae.

In this study, we produced agarose-derived sugars with various DPs by multiple enzymatic reactions and investigated the prebiotic effect of each agar-derived sugar. We also tested the in vitro anti-colon cancer activity of agar-derived sugars, which could be released from red seaweeds diets. This study can provide basic information about the health benefits, such as prebiotic and anti-colon cancer effects, that can be obtained from dietary red seaweed.

2. Results and Discussion
2.1. Enzymatic Production of Agar-Derived Sugars with Various DPs

Various agar-derived sugars were prepared by multiple enzymatic reactions using the purified recombinant enzymes Aga16B, Aga50D, and *Sd*NABH acting as an endo-type β-agarase, an exo-type β-agarase, and a neoagarobiose hydrolase, respectively (Figure 1A and Supplementary Materials Figure S1) [19–21]. Initially, the enzymatic liquefaction of agarose was performed using a thermostable endo-type β-agarase, Aga16B. Aga16B hydrolyzed agarose into NeoDP4 and NeoDP6 as the major reaction products, as described previously (Figure 1B) [21]. Then, the reaction products of Aga16B—which mainly comprised neoagarotetraose (NeoDP4) and neoagarohexaose (NeoDP6)—were hydrolyzed to AHG, agarotriose (AgaDP3), and agaropentaose (AgaDP5) by *Sd*NABH (Figure 1B) [19]. To produce neoagarobiose (NeoDP2), the reaction products of Aga16B—which mainly comprised NeoDP4 and NeoDP6—were further hydrolyzed to NeoDP2 by Aga50D (Figure 1B). After enzymatic production of agar-derived sugars from agarose, each sugar was purified by gel-permeation chromatography using a G-10 column (Figure 1C). Then, each purified sugar was used for testing in vitro prebiotic activity.

2.2. In Vitro Prebiotic Activity of Agar-Derived Sugars

A probiotic strain, *Bifidobacterium longum* ssp. *infantis* ATCC 15697, is known as a champion colonizer of the infant gut due to an extensive repertoire of bacterial genes that encode an array of glycosidases and oligosaccharide transporters not found in other gut bacteria [22]. The prebiotic effects of agar-derived sugars prepared in this study, AHG, NeoDP2, AgaDP3, NeoDP4, AgaDP5, and NeoDP6, were tested by examining their effects on the growth of *B. infantis* ATCC 15697 (Figure 2). Of the six agar-derived sugars tested in the present study, only AgaDP3 was utilized by *B. infantis* ATCC 15697 (Figure 2C). However, under AgaDP3, the cell growth of *B. infantis* ATCC 15697 was lower than that obtained under glucose, galactose, or 2'-fucosyllactose conditions (Figure 2G–I).

For the utilization of AgaDP3 by *B. infantis* ATCC 15697, it is presumed that *B. infantis* ATCC 15697 initially cleaves AgaDP3 into galactose and NeoDP2 by its β-galactosidase activity [23]. Galactose is utilized for the cell growth of *B. infantis* ATCC 15697. However, NeoDP2 is not utilized by *B. infantis* ATCC 15697 (Figure 2B). Therefore, incomplete utilization of AgaDP3 by *B. infantis* ATCC 15697 may cause the lower cell growth of

B. infantis ATCC 15697 under the AgaDP3 condition (Figure 2C) compared to glucose, galactose, or 2′-fucosyllactose conditions (Figure 2G–I).

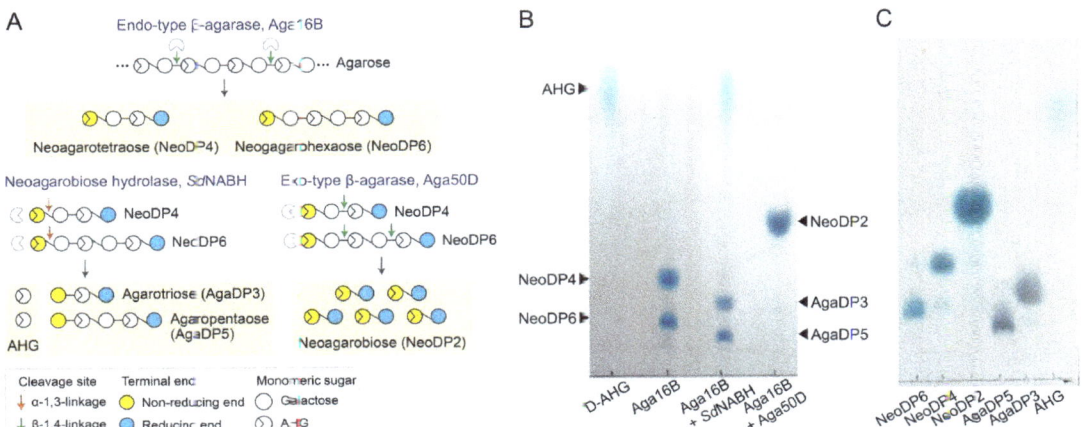

Figure 1. Enzymatic production of various agarose-derived sugars. (**A**) Schematic diagram illustrating the production of agar-derived sugars (i.e., AHG, NeoDP2, NeoDP4, NeoDP6, AgaDP3, and AgaDP5) by the enzymatic reactions of Aga16B, Aga50D, and *Sd*NABH. First, Aga16B produces NeoDP4 and NeoDP6 from agarose by the endolytic cleavage of agarose. *Sd*NABH subsequently produces AHG, AgaDP3, and AgaDP5 from the reaction products of Aga16B (mainly NeoDP4 and NeoDP6). Finally, Aga50D produces NeoDP2 from the reaction products of Aga16B. (**B**) Thin-layer chromatography analysis of the reaction products of Aga16B, Aga50D, and *Sd*NABH. (**C**) Purification of agar-derived sugars AHG, NeoDP2, NeoDP4, NeoDP6, AgaDP3, and AgaDP5 by gel-permeation chromatography of the reaction products of Aga16B, Aga50D, and *Sd*NABH.

Meanwhile, the cell growth of *B. infantis* ATCC 15697 was not observed under the AgaDP5 condition (Figure 2E); this may be because although *B. infantis* ATCC 15697 can cleave AgaDP5 into galactose and NeoDP4 by its β-galactosidase activity, NeoDP4 is not utilized by *B. infantis* ATCC 15697 (Figure 2D). Therefore, galactose released from AgaDP5 may not be enough to support the cell growth of *B. infantis* ATCC 15697 as much as AgaDP3.

2.3. Fermentation of AgaDP3 by Bifidobacteria

Interestingly, it was reported that *B. infantis* ATCC 15697 possesses β-galactosidases (i.e., Bga42A and Bga2A), which are active on various human milk oligosaccharides (HMOs) belonging to type-1 and -2 isomers of HMOs [23]. These two enzymes are expected to be associated with the degradation of AgaDP3 by *B. infantis* ATCC 15697. This implies that not only *B. infantis* ATCC 15697, but also other HMO-utilizing *Bifidobacterium* strains might utilize AgaDP3. To verify this, the fermentation profiles of other probiotic HMO-utilizing *Bifidobacterium* strains—*B. infantis* ATCC 17930 [24], *B. infantis* ATCC 15702 [24], *Bifidobacterium kashiwanohense* DSM 21854 [25], and *Bifidobacterium bifidum* DSM 20082 [24]—were evaluated under the AgaDP3 condition. We found that among the four different probiotic HMO-utilizing *Bifidobacterium* strains, *B. infantis* ATCC 17930, *B. infantis* ATCC 15702, and *B. kashiwanohense* DSM 21854 metabolized AgaDP3 as a carbon source (Figure 3A–H). These results indicated the possible high potential of AgaDP3 from red seaweeds as a prebiotic due to the utilization of AgaDP3, not only by *B. infantis* ATCC 15697, but also by other *Bifidobacterium* strains tested in this study.

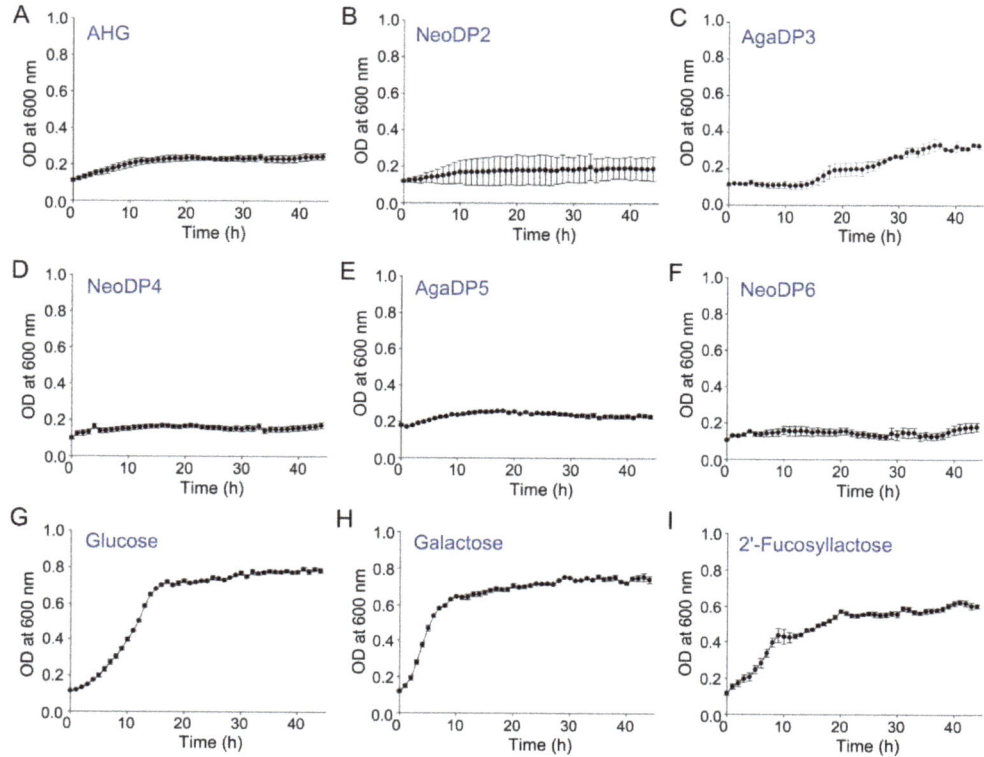

Figure 2. Screening of in vitro prebiotic effects of agar-derived sugars: (**A**) AHG, (**B**) NeoDP2, (**C**) AgaDP3, (**D**) NeoDP4, (**E**) AgaDP5, and (**F**) NeoDP6. *Bifidobacterium longum* ssp. *infantis* ATCC 15697 cells were cultured in synthetic de Man, Rogosa, and Sharpe broth supplemented with 5 g/L of each agar-derived sugar as a carbon source at 37 °C under anaerobic conditions. The positive control was 5 g/L (**G**) glucose, (**H**) galactose, or (**I**) 2′-fucosyllactose, which is a common prebiotic human milk oligosaccharide. During fermentation, the cell density was monitored by measuring optical absorbance at 600 nm using the Bioscreen C system.

The modes of action for the degradation of AgaDP3 exhibited by *B. infantis* ATCC 17930, *B. infantis* ATCC 15702, and *B. kashiwanohense* DSM 21854 can be explained as follows: AgaDP3 is initially transported into the cytosol of cells, and the intracellular β-galactosidases belonging to GH42 or GH2 cleave AgaDP3 into galactose and NeoDP2. Then, non-fermentable NeoDP2 is exported from the cells (Figure 3A–F).

In contrast, the degradation of AgaDP3 by *B. bifidum* DSM 20082 on AgaDP3 was different from that of the other strains (Figure 3G). *B. bifidum* DSM 20082 hydrolyzed AgaDP3 into galactose and NeoDP2 extracellularly, probably using secreted β-galactosidases [26]. However, *B. bifidum* DSM 20082 did not consume galactose (Figure 3G), which is fermentable by this strain [27]. Therefore, it was presumed that NeoDP2 accumulated in the culture medium might have inhibited the consumption of galactose (Figure 3G).

Next, the stability of AgaDP3 in simulated gastric fluid was tested because oral administration of AgaDP3 might lead to its decomposition in the stomach before reaching the intestine. As the incubation time increased, AgaDP3 was partially degraded to agarobiose and galactose due to the cleavage of the α1,3-glycosidic bond of AgaDP3 under low pH conditions (Supplementary Materials Figure S2) [28]. However, it was found that more than 80% of AgaDP3 was stably maintained in simulated gastric fluid at 37 °C for 3 h (Supplementary Materials Figure S2).

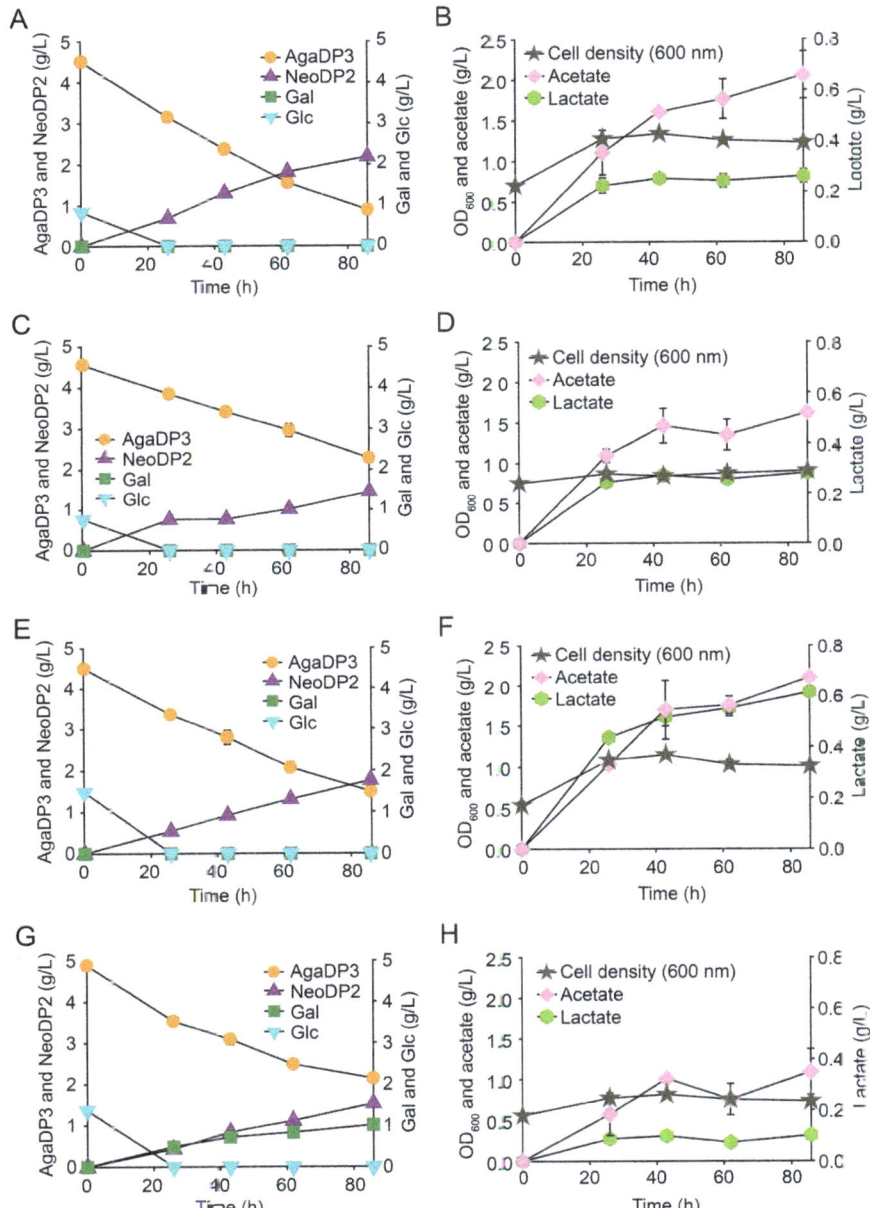

Figure 3. Fermentation of AgaDP3 by human milk oligosaccharide-utilizing *Bifidobacterium* strains. Fermentation profiles of AgaDP3 from various *Bifidobacterium* strains, namely, (**A**,**B**) *B. longum* ssp. *infantis* ATCC 17930, (**C**,**D**) *B. infantis* ATCC 15702, (**E**,**F**) *B. bifidum* DSM 20082, and (**G**,**H**) *B. kashiwanohense* DSM 21854. The *Bifidobacterium* strains were cultured in synthetic de Man, Rogosa and Sharpe broth supplemented with 5 g/L AgaDP3 as a carbon source at 37 °C under anaerobic conditions. During fermentation, cell density and the concentrations of AgaDP3, NeoDP2, galactose, glucose, acetate, and lactate were monitored.

2.4. In Vitro Anti-Colon Cancer Activity of AHG

We investigated the in vitro anti-colon cancer activity of monomeric and dimeric sugars, AHG, galactose, and NeoDP2, which can be released from agarose or AOSs by the actions of agarolytic marine or gut bacteria [29,30]. Our results showed that among the three different sugars, only AHG significantly inhibited the growth of HCT-116 human colon cancer cells (Figure 4A) and reduced their viability (Figure 4E). NeoDP2 and galactose neither inhibited cell growth (Figure 4A) nor reduced HCT-116 cell viability (Figure 4C,D). Intriguingly, AHG did not reduce the viability of CCD-18Co cells (human colon normal fibroblasts) (Figure 4B). Therefore, among the three different monomeric and dimeric sugars generated from agarose degradation (i.e., AHG, NeoDP2, and galactose), only AHG exhibited in vitro anti-colon cancer activity. Notably, AHG selectively inhibits the growth of HCT-116 human colon cancer cells but does not inhibit the growth of CCD-18Co cells, suggesting that AHG has a high potential for the development of anti-colon cancer agents.

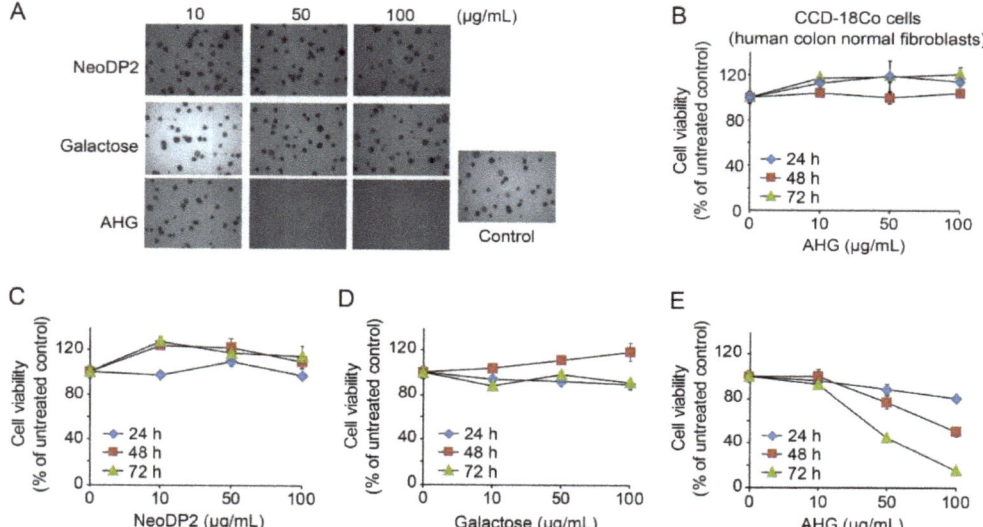

Figure 4. In vitro anti-colon cancer activity of AHG. (**A**) Inhibitory effects of NeoDP2, galactose, and AHG on the formation of HCT-116 human colon cancer cell colonies. (**B**) Effects of AHG on the viability of CCD-18Co cells, human colon normal fibroblasts. Error bars represent means ± SD. (**C–E**) Effects of NeoDP2 (**C**), galactose (**D**), and AHG (**E**) on the viability of HCT-116 cells. Error bars represent means ± SD.

DAPI staining results showed that upon HCT-116 cell treatment with AHG, apoptotic bodies typically observed in apoptosis were formed in the colon cancer cells (Figure 5A). Apoptosis is a form of programmed cell death (PCD) that is controlled by numerous apoptotic proteins [31]. Apoptosis is an energy-dependent process that requires the activation of a group of cysteine proteases (caspases). Initiator caspases-8, -9, or -10 activate executioner caspase-3. In AHG-treated HCT-116 cells, the expression levels of the active forms of caspase-3 and caspase-9 were both elevated (Figure 5B). Once caspases are activated, the execution phase of apoptosis is triggered. As expected, one of the execution pathway proteins, poly (ADP-ribose) polymerase (PARP), was cleaved and activated (Figure 5B). Apoptosis is a complex process that is controlled and regulated by B-cell lymphoma (Bcl)-2 family proteins. Accordingly, AHG reduced the expression levels of anti-apoptotic proteins Bcl-2 and Bcl-xL and enhanced the expression of the pro-apoptotic protein Bax in HCT-116 cells (Figure 5C,D). Interestingly, the tumor suppressor protein P53, which is involved in apoptosis, was also induced by AHG (Figure 5E).

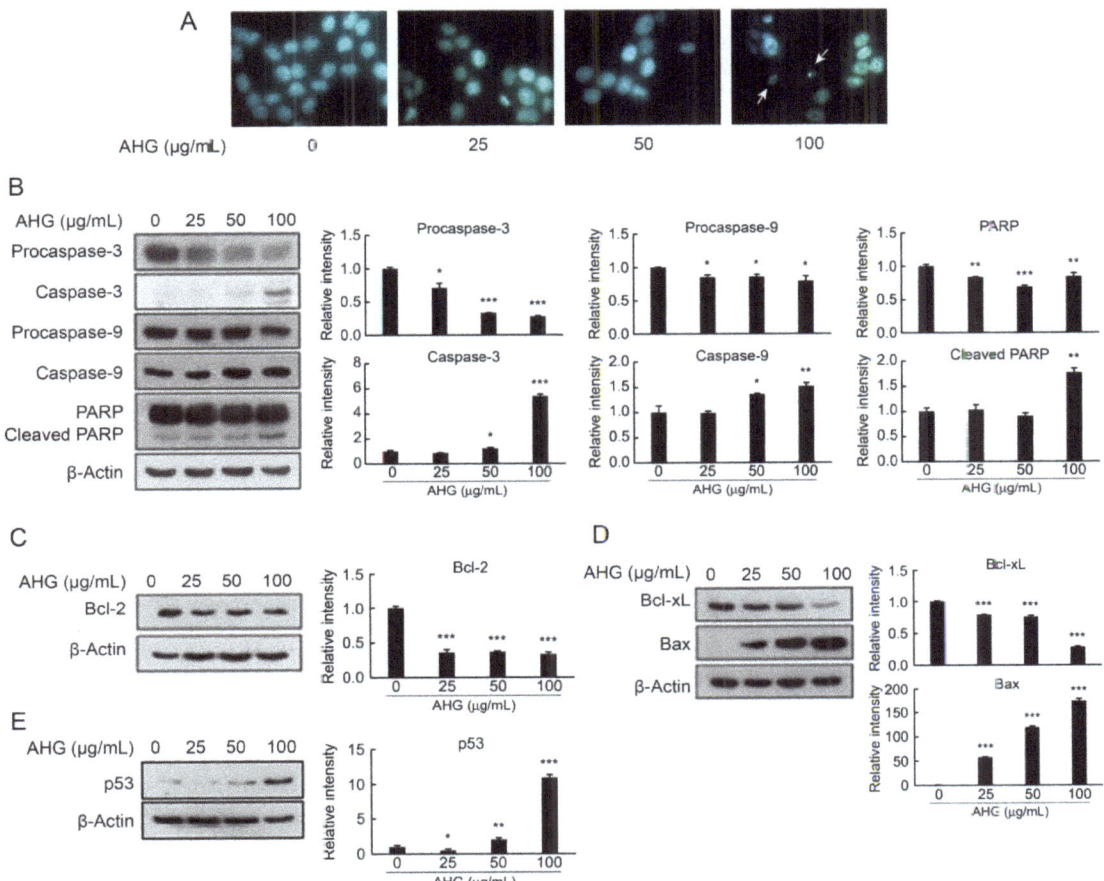

Figure 5. Induction of apoptosis in HCT-116 human colon cancer cells by AHG. (**A**) 4′,6-Diamidino-2-phenylindole (DAPI) staining of HCT-116 cells treated with AHG. (**B–E**) Western blot results showing the effects of AHG on expression of apoptosis-related proteins in cancer cells: procaspase-3 (**B**), caspase-3 (**B**), procaspase-9 (**B**), caspase-9 (**B**), poly(ADP-ribose) polymerase (PARP) (**B**), cleaved PARP (**B**), Bcl-2 (**C**), Bcl-xL (**D**), Bax (**D**), and p53 (**E**). β-actin was used as a control for all Western blot experiments. The relative intensities were quantified using an Image J program and normalized by the intensity of β-actin. Data are mean ± SD relative to the untreated group. *, $p < 0.05$; **, $p < 0.01$; ***, $p < 0.001$ vs. untreated control.

Taken together, we prepared agar-derived sugars with various DPs by multiple enzymatic reactions to investigate the physiological activities, especially prebiotic and anti-colon cancer activities, of each agar-derived sugar. We demonstrated in vitro prebiotic activity of AgaDP3 and in vitro anti-colon cancer activity of AHG. Our results suggest that marine macroalgae-derived oligosaccharides can be utilized as prebiotics. Moreover, the monosaccharides constituting marine macroalgae such as AHG can be utilized as potential anti-cancer agents.

3. Materials and Methods

3.1. Preparation of Agar-Derived Sugars by Enzymatic Hydrolysis of Agarose

Various agar-derived sugars were produced by multiple enzymatic reactions using Aga16B, Aga50D, and SdNABH. The recombinant purified enzymes were prepared following the previously described methods [19–21]. To produce NAOSs, including NeoDP4 and NeoDP6, 100 mL of a reaction mixture comprising 1 mg of a thermostable endo-type β-agarase, Aga16B [21], and 1% (*w/v*) agarose in 20 mM Tris-HCl (pH 7.0) was incubated at 50 °C and 200 rpm for 12 h. To produce AHG, AgaDP3, and AgaDP5, 2.5 mg of neoagarobiose hydrolase, *Sd*NABH [19], was added to 100 mL of the reaction products of Aga16B containing NeoDP4 and NeoDP6. The reaction mixture was then incubated at 30 °C and 200 rpm for 12 h. To produce NeoDP2, 10 mg of an exo-type β-agarase, Aga50D [20], was added to 100 mL of the reaction products of Aga16B, and the reaction mixture was incubated at 30 °C and 200 rpm for 12 h. All enzymatic reactions were terminated by heating the reaction samples in boiling water for 3 min. After terminating enzymatic reactions, the reaction products obtained from each sample were identified by thin-layer chromatography (TLC).

3.2. Purification of Agar-Derived Sugars by Size-Exclusion Chromatography

To purify the agar-derived sugars—that is, AHG, NeoDP2, NeoDP4, NeoDP6, AgaDP3, and AgaDP5—by gel-permeation chromatography, the reaction products obtained from the enzymatic reactions using Aga16B, Aga50D, and *Sd*NABH were loaded onto a Sephadex G-10 column (Sigma-Aldrich, St. Louis, MO, USA) equilibrated with water. Each 1.5 mL fraction was obtained by elution with water as the mobile phase, and only the fractions containing each sugar were collected; this was confirmed by TLC.

3.3. TLC Analysis

TLC analysis of the enzymatic reaction products was conducted on a silica gel 60 plate (Merck, Burlington, MA, USA), and the plate was developed with an *n*-butanol–ethanol–water mixture (3:1:1, *v/v/v*) for 1 h. The plate was then dried and visualized using a solution comprising 10% (*v/v*) sulfuric acid and 0.2% (*w/v*) 1,3-dihydroxynaphthalene (Sigma-Aldrich) in ethanol at 90 °C for 1 min.

3.4. Screening of In Vitro Prebiotic Effects of Agar-Derived Sugars

To screen for in vitro prebiotic effects of the agar-derived sugars—that is, AHG, NeoDP2, NeoDP4, NeoDP6, AgaDP3, and AgaDP5—we cultured one of the most common probiotic bacteria, *B. infantis* ATCC 15697 in 200 µL of synthetic de Man, Rogosa, and Sharpe (sMRS) broth supplemented with 5 g/L of each agar-derived sugar as a carbon source. The sMRS broth was composed of 10 g/L peptone, 5 g/L yeast extract, 2 g/L anhydrous dipotassium phosphate, 5 g/L anhydrous sodium acetate, 2 g/L tribasic ammonium citrate, 0.2 g/L magnesium sulfate heptahydrate, 0.05 g/L manganese (II) sulfate, 1 mL/L polysorbate 80, 0.5 g/L cysteine, and 5 g/L of a carbon source [32]. The positive control was 5 g/L glucose, galactose, or 2′-fucosyllactose, which is a common prebiotic human milk oligosaccharide. During fermentation, cell growth was monitored by measuring optical density at 600 nm (OD_{600}) using a Bioscreen C system (Labsystems, Helsinki, Finland).

3.5. Fermentation of AgaDP3 by Bifidobacteria

Five *Bifidobacterium* strains—namely, *B. infantis* ATCC 15697, *B. infantis* ATCC 17930, *B. infantis* ATCC 15702, *B. bifidum* DSM 20082, and *B. kashiwanohense* DSM 21854—were cultured in de Man, Rogosa and Sharpe (MRS; Sigma-Aldrich) or sMRS broth. The *Bifidobacterium* strains were cultured in a chamber with an anaerobic atmosphere comprising 90% N_2 and 10% CO_2, or 90% N_2, 5% H_2, and 5% CO_2 (Airgas, Radnor, PA, USA) at 37 °C. During fermentation, cell growth was monitored by measuring OD_{600}.

3.6. High-Performance Liquid Chromatography Analysis

A high-performance liquid chromatography (HPLC) system (1200 Series, Agilent Technologies, Santa Clara, CA, USA) equipped with an H^+ (8%) column (Rezex ROA-Organic Acid; Phenomenex, Torrance, CA, USA) and a refractive index (RI) detector were used for HPLC analysis. The flow rate of the 0.005 N H_2SO_4 mobile phase was set at 0.6 mL/min, and the column and RI detector temperatures were set at 50 °C.

For the quantitative analysis of AHG, NeoDP2, and AgaDP3, authentic standards of D-AHG, NeoDP2, and AgaDP3 were purchased from Carbosynth (Compton, Berkshire, UK) (Supplementary Materials Figure S3).

3.7. High-Performance Anion-Exchange Chromatography with Pulsed Amperometric Detection Analysis

A high-performance anion-exchange chromatography with pulsed amperometric detection (HPAEC-PAD) on a Dionex ICS-5000 system (Thermo Fisher Scientific, Waltham, MA, USA) equipped with a Dionex CarboPac PA100 column (250 mm × 2 mm; Thermo Fisher Scientific) was used for the quantitative analysis of NeoDP4, NeoDP6, and AgaDP5 [33]. At a flow rate of 0.25 mL/min, a gradient comprising the following mobile phases at 25 °C were used: (A) double-distilled water, (B) 0.1 M sodium hydroxide, (C) 0.1 M sodium hydroxide with 0.2 M sodium acetate, and (D) 0.25 M sodium hydroxide with 1 M sodium acetate. Before running samples, the column was washed with 100% D for 15 min, a linear gradient to 100% C for 10 min, and subsequently to 90% A and 10% B. Then, the column was equilibrated with 90% A and 10% B for 20 min. After sample injection, the following gradient was applied: 0 to 10 min, isocratic 90% A and 10% B; 10 to 20 min, linear to 100% B; 20 to 65 min, linear to 50% B and 50% C; 65 to 80 min, linear to 100% C; and 80 to 90 min, linear to 100% D. Cellotetraose (Sigma-Aldrich), cellopentaose (Sigma-Aldrich), and cellohexaose (Sigma-Aldrich) were used as standards for the quantitative analysis of NeoDP4, AgaDP5, and NeoDP6, respectively (Supplementary Materials Figure S3).

3.8. Stability Test of AgaDP3 on Simulated Gastric Fluid

To test the stability of AgaDP3 in gastric fluid, 1 g/L (w/v) AgaDP3 was incubated in a simulated gastric fluid comprising 0.2% (w/v) sodium chloride in 0.7% (v/v) hydrochloric acid (pH 1.11) at 37 °C for 4 h. Residual amounts of AgaDP3 were measured by HPLC every hour.

3.9. In Vitro Anti-Colon Cancer Activity Test of AHG Using Soft Agar Assay

To evaluate the inhibitory effects of NeoDP2, galactose, and AHG on colony formation by human colon cancer cells, HCT-116 cells (Korean Cell Line Bank, Seoul, Republic of Korea) were used. The HCT-116 cells were cultured on a 6-well soft agar plate for two weeks at 37 °C in the presence of various concentrations of NeoDP2, galactose, and AHG. Cell colonies were observed under a Nikon phase-contrast microscope (Nikon, Tokyo, Japan).

3.10. In Vitro Anti-Colon Cancer Activity Test of AHG by Using Cell Viability Assay

To estimate the effects of NeoDP2, galactose, and AHG on the viability of HCT-116 cells, cell proliferation was determined using a 3-(4,5-dimethylthiazol-2-yl)-2,5-diphenyltetrazolium bromide (MTT) assay [34]. One hundred microliters of Roswell Park Memorial Institute (RPMI) 1640 medium supplemented with 10% fetal bovine serum (FBS) was inoculated with 3×10^4 cells/mL of HCT-116 cells in each well of a 96-well plate. NeoDP2, galactose, and AHG were added to the culture medium at a final concentration of 10, 50, or 100 µg/mL. After culturing for 72 h, 20 µL of the MTT solution was added to each well. The cells were then incubated for 2 h at 37 °C in a 5% CO_2 incubator, and the optical absorbance of the cell culture was measured at 570 nm. CCD-18Co cells (American Type Culture Collection, Manassas, VA, USA) at 5×10^4 cell/mL in Eagle's Minimum Essential Medium (EMEM) with 10% FBS were cultured at 100 µL per well in a 96-well plate.

3.11. In Vitro Anti-Colon Cancer Activity Test of AHG by 4′,6-Diamidino-2-Phenylindole Staining

Apoptotic cell death was determined morphologically using the fluorescent nuclear dye 4′,6-diamidino-2-phenylindole (DAPI). HCT-116 cells (3×10^4/mL) were cultured in a 6 cm dish for 24 h, treated with AHG (0–100 µg/mL) for 72 h, and then fixed with 100% ethanol for 30 min. The fixed cells were washed with PBS and stained with the DNA-specific fluorochrome DAPI (1 mg/mL). After 10 min of incubation, the cells were washed with PBS, deposited onto microscope slides, and observed under a fluorescent microscope (Nikon) to detect apoptotic characteristics.

3.12. In Vitro Anti-Colon Cancer Activity Test of AHG by Western Blot

To investigate the possible mechanism by which AHG inhibits the growth of HCT-116 cells, Western blot analysis of changes in expression of genes involved in apoptosis was carried out.

To measure the expression levels of certain apoptosis-related proteins—that is, procaspase-3, caspase-3, procaspase-9, caspase-9, PARP, cleaved PARP, Bcl-2, p53, Bcl-xL, and Bax—HCT-116 cells were seeded in a 60 mm dish and incubated at 37 °C and 5% CO_2 for 24 h using RPMI 1640 medium supplemented with 10% FBS. After 24 h, the medium was replaced, but this time AHG at concentrations of 25, 50, and 100 µg/mL was included. The cells were then incubated under the same conditions described above, until at least approximately 80% of the bottom of each well was confluent with cells.

Western blot analysis was performed after incubation for 5 days. The cells were washed twice with phosphate-buffered saline, and the cells attached to the bottom of the well were collected using a lysis buffer comprising 20 mM Tris-HCl (pH 7.5), 150 mM NaCl, 1 mM ethylenediaminetetraacetic acid disodium salt (Na_2EDTA), 1 mM ethylene glycol-bis(β-aminoethyl ether)-N,N',N',N-tetraacetic acid (EGTA), 1% Triton X-100, 2.5 mM sodium pyrophosphate, 1 mM β-glycerophosphate, 1 mM Na_3VO_4, 1 µg/mL leupeptin, 1 mM phenylmethylsulfonyl fluoride (PMSF), and a protease inhibitor cocktail. The resuspended solution containing the cells was then centrifuged at $18,407 \times g$ for 10 min at 4 °C. After obtaining each supernatant, the protein concentration was quantified using a protein assay kit (Bio-Rad Laboratories, Hercules, CA, USA).

Each protein prepared (20–40 µg) was degenerated and separated by SDS-PAGE, then transferred to a polyvinylidene difluoride (PVDF) membrane presoaked in methanol at 100 V for 2 h. The PVDF membrane was then immersed for 2 h in TBST solution (a mixture of Tris-buffered saline (TBS) and polysorbate 20) containing 5% skim milk to block non-specific protein binding sites. Next, the following antibodies purchased from Cell Signaling Technology (Danvers, MA, USA) were used to determine expression levels of the indicated proteins: rabbit polyclonal anti-human caspase-3, rabbit polyclonal anti-human caspase-9, rabbit polyclonal anti-human PARP, rabbit polyclonal anti-human Bcl-2, rabbit polyclonal anti-human Bcl-xL, rabbit polyclonal anti-human Bax, rabbit monoclonal anti-human p53, and mouse monoclonal anti-β-actin. The antibodies described above were diluted in TBST containing 5% skim milk at a ratio of 1:1000, and the reaction was carried out at 4 °C overnight. Anti-rabbit IgG (Santa Cruz Biotechnology, Dallas, TX, USA) and anti-mouse IgG (Santa Cruz Biotechnology) were used as secondary antibodies at a dilution of 1:5000, and the reactions were performed at 25 °C for 2 h. The PVDF membranes were then washed 4 times with TBST and reacted for 1–3 min with an enhanced chemiluminescence (ECL) substrate (Amersham, Little Chalfont, BM, UK). The membranes were pre-sensitized to X-ray film in a dark room to determine expression levels of apoptosis-related proteins present in each sample. The band intensities were quantified using an Image J from NIH (Bethesda, MD, USA) and normalized by the intensity of the β-actin, a loading control. The protein expression levels were expressed as relative intensities (fold change) for the untreated group. Single statistical comparisons were performed using a Student's t-test. The data represented three independent experiments that gave similar results.

4. Conclusions

We prepared various agar-derived sugars through multiple enzymatic reactions and demonstrated the in vitro prebiotic and anti-colon cancer activities of agar-derived sugars. Specifically, AgaDP3 was consumed by HMO-utilizing probiotic bifidobacteria such as *B. infantis* and *B. kashiwanohense*. We also elucidated for the first time that AHG exhibits in vitro anti-colon cancer activity. Specifically, AHG significantly inhibited the proliferation of colon cancer cells, and induced apoptosis of such cells. Therefore, we conclude that

AgaDP3 and AHG are key compounds that confer various health benefits, especially prebiotic and anti-colon cancer effects, to the host. Our results provide crucial information regarding potential key compounds derived from red seaweeds that confer health-beneficial effects, such as prebiotic and anti-colon cancer activities in humans; it can be applied to discover new functional food ingredients derived from dietary fibers.

Supplementary Materials: The following are available online at https://www.mdpi.com/article/10.3390/md19040213/s1, Figure S1. Sodium dodecyl sulfate–polyacrylamide gel electrophoresis analysis of the purified recombinant proteins of Aga16B, Aga50D, and SdNABH. Lanes: M, protein markers; 1-3, (1) Aga16B, (2) Aga50D, and (3) SdNABH purified by His-tag affinity chromatography. Figure S2. Stability test of AgaDP3 in the presence of simulated gastric fluid. (A) AgaDP3 was incubated with simulated gastric fluid comprising 0.2% (w/v) sodium chloride in 0.7% (v/v) hydrochloric acid at 37 °C for 3 h. The concentration of AgaDP3 was monitored using HPLC. (B) Overlaid HPLC chromatograms profiling the partial degradation of AgaDP3 during incubation. Figure S3. Calibration curves of purified agar-derived sugars produced from agarose by the enzymatic reactions of Aga16B, Aga50D, and SdNABH. (A–C) Calibration curves of AHG, NeoDP2, and AgaDP3 for quantitative analyses by HPLC. (D–F) Calibration curves for cellotetraose, cellopentaose, and cellohexaose for quantitative analyses of NeoDP4, AgaDP5, and NeoDP6, respectively, by HPAEC-PAD.

Author Contributions: Conceptualization, E.J.Y., Y.-S.J. and K.H.K.; data curation, S.Y. and J.-J.L.; funding acquisition, K.H.K.; investigation, E.J.Y., S.Y., Y.-A.K. and N.J.K.; methodology, E.J.Y. and Y.-A.K.; supervision, N.J.K., Y.-S.J. and K.H.K.; visualization, E.J.Y. and Y.-A.K.; writing–original draft, E.J.Y., S.Y. and J.-J.L.; writing–review and editing, Y.-S.J. and K.H.K. All authors have read and agreed to the published version of the manuscript.

Funding: This work was supported by the Mid-career Researcher Program through the National Research Foundation (NRF) of Korea (2020R1A2B5B02002631); by the Ministry of Oceans and Fisheries, Korea (20200367); by the Korea Institute of Planning and Evaluation for Technology in Food, Agriculture, Forestry, and Fisheries (iPET), funded by the Ministry of Agriculture, Food, and Rural Affairs (321036051SB010); and by the Brain Pool Program through the Korean Federation of Science and Technology Societies funded by the Ministry of Science and ICT of Korea (2019H1D3A2A01100327). N.J.K. was supported by a grant from the NRF of Korea (2018R1A2B6005972).

Institutional Review Board Statement: Not applicable.

Informed Consent Statement: Not applicable.

Data Availability Statement: The datasets used and/or analyzed during the current study are available from the corresponding author upon reasonable request.

Acknowledgments: We also acknowledge the support of a KU-FRG grant by Korea University and the facility support of the Institute of Biomedical and Food Safety at CJ Food Safety Hall, Korea University.

Conflicts of Interest: The authors declare no conflict of interest.

References

1. de Borba Gurpilhares, D.; Cinelli, L.P.; Simas, N.K.; Pessoa, A., Jr.; Sette, L.D. Marine prebiotics: Polysaccharides and oligosaccharides obtained by using microbial enzymes. *Food Chem.* **2019**, *280*, 175–186. [CrossRef]
2. Maheshwari, G.; Sowrirajan, S.; Joseph, B. β-Glucan, a dietary fiber in effective prevention of lifestyle diseases–An insight. *Bioact. Carbohydr. Diet. Fibre* **2019**, *19*, 100187. [CrossRef]
3. Lozupone, C.; Faust, K.; Raes, J.; Faith, J.J.; Frank, D.N.; Zaneveld, J.; Gordon, J.I.; Knight, R. Identifying genomic and metabolic features that can underlie early successional and opportunistic lifestyles of human gut symbionts. *Genome Res.* **2012**, *22*, 1974–1984. [CrossRef] [PubMed]
4. Sonnenburg, J.L.; Bäckhed, F. Diet–microbiota interactions as moderators of human metabolism. *Nature* **2016**, *535*, 56–64. [CrossRef]
5. Wells, M.L.; Potin, P.; Craigie, J.S.; Raven, J.A.; Merchant, S.S.; Helliwell, K.E.; Smith, A.G.; Camire, M.E.; Brawley, S.H. Algae as nutritional and functional food sources: Revisiting our understanding. *J. Appl. Phycol.* **2017**, *29*, 949–982. [CrossRef] [PubMed]
6. Yun, E.J.; Kim, H.T.; Cho, K.M.; Yu, S.; Kim, S.; Choi, I.-G.; Kim, K.H. Pretreatment and saccharification of red macroalgae to produce fermentable sugars. *Bioresour. Technol.* **2016**, *199*, 311–318. [CrossRef]

7. Knutsen, S.; Myslabodski, D.; Larsen, B.; Usov, A. A modified system of nomenclature for red algal galactans. *Bot. Mar.* **1994**, *37*, 163–170. [CrossRef]
8. Shang, Q.; Jiang, H.; Cai, C.; Hao, J.; Li, G.; Yu, G. Gut microbiota fermentation of marine polysaccharides and its effects on intestinal ecology: An overview. *Carbohydr. Polym.* **2018**, *179*, 173–185. [CrossRef]
9. Ramnani, P.; Chitarrari, R.; Tuohy, K.; Grant, J.; Hotchkiss, S.; Philp, K.; Campbell, R.; Gill, C.; Rowland, I. In vitro fermentation and prebiotic potential of novel low molecular weight polysaccharides derived from agar and alginate seaweeds. *Anaerobe* **2012**, *18*, 1–6. [CrossRef]
10. Zhang, N.; Mao, X.; Li, R.; Hou, E.; Wang, Y.; Xue, C.; Tang, Q.-J. Neoagarotetraose protects mice against intense exercise induced fatigue damage by modulating gut microbial composition and function. *Mol. Nutr. Food Res.* **2017**, *61*, 1600585. [CrossRef]
11. Chen, H.; Yan, X.; Zhu, P.; Lin, J. Antioxidant activity and hepatoprotective potential of agaro-oligosaccharides in vitro and in vivo. *Nutr. J.* **2006**, *5*, 31. [CrossRef]
12. Enoki, T.; Okuda, S.; Kudo, Y.; Takashima, F.; Sagawa, H.; Kato, I. Oligosaccharides from agar inhibit pro-inflammatory mediator release by inducing heme oxygenase 1. *Biosci. Biotechnol. Biochem.* **2010**, *74*, 766–770. [CrossRef]
13. Kim, J.; Lee, J.; Oh, J.H.; Chang, H.J.; Sohn, D.K.; Shin, A.; Kim, J. Associations among dietary seaweed intake, c-MYC rs6983267 polymorphism, and risk of colorectal cancer in a Korean population: A case–control study. *Eur. J. Nutr.* **2020**, *59*, 1963–1974. [CrossRef] [PubMed]
14. Minami, Y.; Kanemura, S.; Oikawa, T.; Suzuki, S.; Hasegawa, Y.; Nishino, Y.; Fujiya, T.; Miura, K. Associations of Japanese food intake with survival of stomach and colorectal cancer: A prospective patient cohort study. *Cancer Sci.* **2020**, *111*, 2558–2569. [CrossRef] [PubMed]
15. Yang, Y.J.; Nam, S.J.; Kong, G.; Kim, M.K. A case-control study on seaweed consumption and the risk of breast cancer. *Br. J. Nutr.* **2010**, *103*, 1345–1353. [CrossRef] [PubMed]
16. Aisa, Y.; Miyakawa, Y.; Nakazato, T.; Shibata, H.; Saito, K.; Ikeda, Y.; Kizaki, M. Fucoidan induces apoptosis of human HS-sultan cells accompanied by activation of caspase-3 and down-regulation of ERK Pathways. *Am. J. Hematol.* **2005**, *78*, 7–14. [CrossRef]
17. Ale, M.T.; Maruyama, H.; Tamauchi, H.; Mikkelsen, J.D.; Meyer, A.S. Fucoidan from *Sargassum* sp. and *Fucus vesiculosus* reduces cell viability of lung carcinoma and melanoma cells in vitro and activates natural killer cells in mice in vivo. *Int. J. Biol. Macromol.* **2011**, *49*, 331–336. [CrossRef] [PubMed]
18. Kim, E.J.; Park, S.Y.; Lee, J.Y.; Park, J.H. Fucoidan present in brown algae induces apoptosis of human colon cancer cells. *BMC Gastroenterol.* **2010**, *10*, 96. [CrossRef]
19. Ha, S.; Lee, S.; Lee, J.; Kim, H.; Ko, H.-J.; Kim, K.; Choi, I.-G. Crystal structure of a key enzyme in the agarolytic pathway, α-neoagarobiose hydrolase from *Saccharophagus degradans* 2-40. *Biochem. Biophys. Res. Commun.* **2011**, *412*, 238–244. [CrossRef] [PubMed]
20. Kim, H.T.; Lee, S.; Lee, D.; Kim, H.S.; Bang, W.G.; Kim, K.H.; Choi, I.-G. Overexpression and molecular characterization of Aga50D from *Saccharophagus degradans* 2-40: An exo-type β-agarase producing neoagarobiose. *Appl. Microbiol. Biotechnol.* **2010**, *86*, 227–234. [CrossRef]
21. Kim, J.H.; Yun, E.J.; Seo, N.; Yu, S.; Kim, D.H.; Cho, K.M.; An, H.J.; Kim, J.H.; Choi, I.-G.; Kim, K.H. Enzymatic liquefaction of agarose above the sol-gel transition temperature using a thermostable endo-type β-agarase, Aga16B. *Appl. Microbiol. Biotechnol.* **2017**, *101*, 1111–1120. [CrossRef]
22. Underwood, M.A.; German, J.B.; Lebrilla, C.B.; Mills, D.A. *Bifidobacterium longum* subspecies *infantis*: Champion colonizer of the infant gut. *Pediatr. Res.* **2015**, *77*, 229–235. [CrossRef] [PubMed]
23. Yoshida, E.; Sakurama, H.; Kiyohara, M.; Nakajima, M.; Kitaoka, M.; Ashida, H.; Hirose, J.; Katayama, T.; Yamamoto, K.; Kumagai, H. *Bifidobacterium longum* subsp. *infantis* uses two different β-galactosidases for selectively degrading type-1 and type-2 human milk oligosaccharides. *Glycobiology* **2011**, *22*, 361–368. [CrossRef]
24. Garrido, D.; Ruiz-Moyano, S.; Lemay, D.G.; Sela, D.A.; German, J.B.; Mills, D.A. Comparative transcriptomics reveals key differences in the response to milk oligosaccharides of infant gut-associated bifidobacteria. *Sci. Rep.* **2015**, *5*, 13517. [CrossRef] [PubMed]
25. James, K.; Bottacini, F.; Contreras, J.I.S.; Vigoureux, M.; Egan, M.; Motherway, M.O.; Holmes, E.; van Sinderen, D. Metabolism of the predominant human milk oligosaccharide fucosyllactose by an infant gut commensal. *Sci. Rep.* **2019**, *9*, 15427. [CrossRef]
26. Kitaoka, M. Bifidobacterial enzymes involved in the metabolism of human milk oligosaccharides. *Adv. Nutr.* **2012**, *3*, 422S–429S. [CrossRef] [PubMed]
27. Yun, E.J.; Liu, J.-J.; Lee, J.W.; Kwak, S.; Yu, S.; Kim, K.H.; Jin, Y.-S. Biosynthetic routes for producing various fucosyl-oligosaccharides. *ACS Synth. Biol.* **2019**, *8*, 415–424. [CrossRef] [PubMed]
28. Yang, B.; Yu, G.; Zhao, X.; Jiao, G.; Ren, S.; Chai, W. Mechanism of mild acid hydrolysis of galactan polysaccharides with highly ordered disaccharide repeats leading to a complete series of exclusively odd-numbered oligosaccharides. *FEBS J.* **2009**, *276*, 2125–2137. [CrossRef] [PubMed]
29. Pluvinage, B.; Grondin, J.M.; Amundsen, C.; Klassen, L.; Moote, P.E.; Xiao, Y.; Thomas, D.; Pudlo, N.A.; Anele, A.; Martens, E.C.; et al. Molecular basis of an agarose metabolic pathway acquired by a human intestinal symbiont. *Nat. Commun.* **2018**, *9*, 1043. [CrossRef]
30. Yu, S.; Yun, E.J.; Kim, D.H.; Park, S.Y.; Kim, K.H. Dual agarolytic pathways in a marine bacterium, *Vibrio* sp. strain EJY3: Molecular and enzymatic verification. *Appl. Environ. Microbiol.* **2020**, *86*, e02724-19. [CrossRef]

31. Elmore, S. Apoptosis: A review of programmed cell death. *Toxicol. Pathol.* **2007**, *35*, 495–516. [CrossRef] [PubMed]
32. Barrangou, R.; Altermann, E.; Hutkins, R.; Cano, R.; Klaenhammer, T.R. Functional and comparative genomic analyses of an operon involved in fructooligosaccharide utilization by *Lactobacillus acidophilus*. *Proc. Natl. Acad. Sci. USA* **2003**, *100*, 8957–8962. [CrossRef]
33. Wefers, D.; Dong, J.; Abdel-Hamid, A.M.; Paul, H.M.; Pereira, G.V.; Han, Y.; Dodd, D.; Baskaran, R.; Mayer, B.; Mackie, R.I.; et al. Enzymatic mechanism for arabinan degradation and transport in the thermophilic bacterium *Caldanaerobius polysaccharolyticus*. *Appl. Environ. Microbiol.* **2017**, *83*, e00794-17. [CrossRef] [PubMed]
34. Freimoser, F.M.; Jakob, C.A.; Aebi, M.; Tuor, U. The MTT [3-(4,5-dimethylthiazol-2-yl)-2,5-diphenyltetrazolium bromide] assay is a fast and reliable method for colorimetric determination of fungal cell densities. *Appl. Environ. Microbiol.* **1999**, *65*, 3727–3729. [CrossRef]

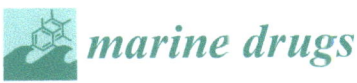

Article

On the Health Benefits vs. Risks of Seaweeds and Their Constituents: The Curious Case of the Polymer Paradigm

João Cotas [1,2], Diana Pacheco [1,2], Glacio Souza Araujo [3], Ana Valado [2,4], Alan T. Critchley [5,*] and Leonel Pereira [1,2]

1. Department of Life Sciences, University of Coimbra, 3000-456 Coimbra, Portugal; jcotas@uc.pt (J.C.); diana.pacheco@uc.pt (D.P.); leonel.pereira@uc.pt (L.P.)
2. Marine and Environmental Sciences Centre (MARE), Faculty of Sciences and Technology, University of Coimbra, 3001-456 Coimbra, Portugal; valado@estescoimbra.pt
3. Federal Institute of Education, Science and Technology of Ceará—IFCE, Campus Aracati, CE 040, km 137,1, Aracati 62800-000, Ceara, Brazil; glacio@ifce.edu.br
4. Department of Biomedical Laboratory Sciences, Polytechnic Institute of Coimbra, ESTeSC-Coimbra Health School, Rua 5 de Outubro, S. Martinho do Bispo, Apartamento 7006, 3046-854 Coimbra, Portugal
5. Verschuren Centre for Sustainability in Energy and the Environment, Sydney, NS B1P 6L2, Canada
* Correspondence: alan.critchley2016@gmail.com

Abstract: To exploit the nutraceutical and biomedical potential of selected seaweed-derived polymers in an economically viable way, it is necessary to analyze and understand their quality and yield fluctuations throughout the seasons. In this study, the seasonal polysaccharide yield and respective quality were evaluated in three selected seaweeds, namely the agarophyte *Gracilaria gracilis*, the carrageenophyte *Calliblepharis jubata* (both red seaweeds) and the alginophyte *Sargassum muticum* (brown seaweed). It was found that the agar synthesis of *G. gracilis* did not significantly differ with the seasons (27.04% seaweed dry weight (DW)). In contrast, the carrageenan content in *C. jubata* varied seasonally, being synthesized in higher concentrations during the summer (18.73% DW). Meanwhile, the alginate synthesis of *S. muticum* exhibited a higher concentration (36.88% DW) during the winter. Therefore, there is a need to assess the threshold at which seaweed-derived polymers may have positive effects or negative impacts on human nutrition. Furthermore, this study highlights the three polymers, along with their known thresholds, at which they can have positive and/or negative health impacts. Such knowledge is key to recognizing the paradigm governing their successful deployment and related beneficial applications in humans.

Keywords: polysaccharides; health benefits; health risks; biomedical; polymer seasonal variation

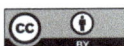

1. Introduction

The growing demand for seaweed feedstock is noteworthy, particularly since 1990, reaching its peak in 2018, when 31.5 million tons fresh weight (FW) of seaweeds were sustainably cultivated (this is the latest year for which reliable data are available), while around 1 million tons FW of seaweeds were exploited from wild stocks [1]. Seaweeds' rich nutritional profile (including phenolic compounds (e.g., phlorotannins), protein (e.g., phycobiliproteins), carbohydrates (e.g., alginates, fucoidans, ulvans, agars, and carrageenans), lipids (especially, ω-3 fatty acids), vitamins (in particular, A, B, C, D, E, and K and their precursors) and essential minerals (e.g., calcium, iron, iodine, magnesium, and potassium)) has led to their incorporation in the daily diet of several Asian and European countries [2–8]. Furthermore, a significant amount of the total annual seaweeds feedstock is used by the global phycocolloid industry [1]. The main phycocolloids (i.e., algal-derived) or polysaccharides for these industries are agars and carrageenans (i.e., extracted from red seaweeds) and alginates (i.e., extracted from brown seaweeds) [7,9,10]. Polysaccharides (sugars) are highly valuable macronutrients, which are indeed abundant in seaweeds, as they act as structural components of the varied morphologies of the thalli. In fact, these molecules can represent up to half of thallus dry weight [11–13]. Seaweeds are a polyphyletic group, and across the >12,000 species, a wide range of polysaccharides are synthesized, differing within species (even at the level of alternation of generations (i.e., n vs. 2n) of the same species) and may vary due to biotic and abiotic stimuli [12–16]. Moreover, the selection of the methods of extraction and purification may also directly affect their yield and purity [17].

Such biomolecules are receiving a high degree of economic interest from several industries, including the feed, food, cosmetics and pharmaceuticals industries, due to their rheological (i.e., gelling/thickening) and increasingly wide range of biological activities. In particular, interest has blossomed in the food and pharmaceutical industries, because of many research studies on their bioactive properties, which include: antitumor [18], anticoagulant [19,20], anti-thrombotic [21,22], antiviral [23–25], immunomodulatory [26,27] and anti-fungal [28,29] activities, presented collectively and/or individually by these phycocolloids [30].

Currently, many seaweed polysaccharides are widely used in the food industry as stabilizers or emulsifiers for their gelling properties [31]. In fact, agar (E 406) [32,33], carrageenan (E 407), processed carrageenan (E 407a) [34,35] and alginate (E 401) [36,37] are authorized food additives and are generally recognized as safe (GRAS) for human consumption. Therefore, when food products with these seaweed polysaccharides (as additives) are ingested, they present properties similar to a dietary fiber, not least since humans do not have the required enzymes to break the glycosidic bonds of the long-chain carbohydrates [38]. Indubitably, humans need to metabolize sugars in order to fuel the body and the nervous system [39]. Hence, the inclusion of polysaccharides such as agar, carrageenan and alginate play important roles in human nutrition, since they promote satiety and intestinal function regulation, and enhance intestinal flora, consequently achieving higher nutrient absorption rates [11,16,40–42]. The consumption of algal polysaccharides provides several additional health benefits, such as regulation of glycemic index values and reduction of low-density lipoprotein (LDL) cholesterol [11,41,43,44].

Despite the many health benefits that seaweeds and their compounds provide, there are some concerns hampering some consumers from including them in their daily diet. Among these are iodine, metals, pesticides, antibiotics and or other noxious compounds (e.g., radionuclides), which some seaweeds may accumulate from coastal seawater [45–47]. Thus, the European Food Safety Authority (EFSA) and the competent North American authorities, e.g., the Food and Drug Administration (FDA), have established a threshold for the consumption of certain seaweeds and their components, through several health risk assessment studies [48–50]. It is key to note that only specific seaweeds are on these lists, while other species that are not in those lists are considered "novel food" and require a considerable amount of generational data and clinical trial evidence before being allowed in food supply chains.

The carrageenophyte *Calliblepharis jubata* is widely distributed through the European coastline, while the agarophyte *Gracilaria gracilis* and the alginophyte *Sargassum muticum* are widespread throughout the globe, and all are considered edible seaweeds [2]. All the forementioned species are perennial species in Portugal, meaning that they are present throughout the year [51]. Thus, they are species with potential for industrial exploitation.

Herein, this study aimed to analyze the seasonal variation of the polysaccharide content of three different seaweed species of agarophyte, carrageenophyte and alginophyte. It was further assessed whether the polysaccharide content met the threshold established by the competent authorities, thereby guaranteeing the safety for human consumption of the wild seaweeds. Additionally, the literature was reviewed in order to understand the positive and potentially negative effects of seaweed polysaccharides on human health.

2. Results

Throughout the seasons evaluated, the carrageenophyte *Callibepharis jubata* (Figure 1a) produced the lowest polysaccharide content, as compared to the agarophyte *Gracilaria gracilis* (Figure 1b) and the alginophyte *Sargassum muticum* (Figure 1c). Furthermore, different seasonal patterns were observed with respect to their polysaccharide profiles.

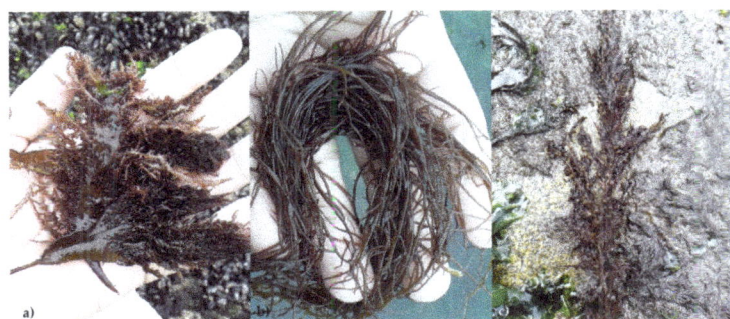

Figure 1. Three seaweeds studied at the collection site (Figueira da Foz, Portugal): (**a**) *Calliblepharis jubata* (Rhodophyta—carrageenan-bearing); (**b**) *Gracilaria gracilis* (Rhodophyta—agar bearing); (**c**) *Sargassum muticum* (Phaeophyta—alginate-bearing).

2.1. Red Seaweed Polymers

2.1.1. Carrageenan Content and Identification

Regarding the red seaweed *C. jubata* (Figure 2), this species presented the lowest content during the autumn, with a concentration of 10.37 ± 0.416% DW. However, during the summer it was possible to extract 18.73 ± 2.382% DW carrageenan, which was the highest value during the observation period.

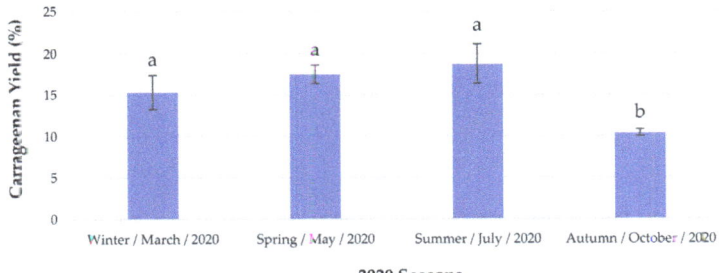

Figure 2. Carrageenan content analyzed seasonally. The extraction yields are expressed as mean ± standard deviation (n = 3). ^{a,b} The same letters indicate no significant differences at the p-value < 0.05 level.

The FTIR-ATR spectrum (Figure 3) of the phycocolloids extracted from *C. jubata* showed bands at approximately 930 and 845 cm^{-1}. However, an additional well-defined feature was visible at around 805 cm^{-1}, indicating the presence of two sulfate ester groups on the anhydro-D-galactose residues, a characteristic band of the iota-carrageenan (Table 1) [52,53].

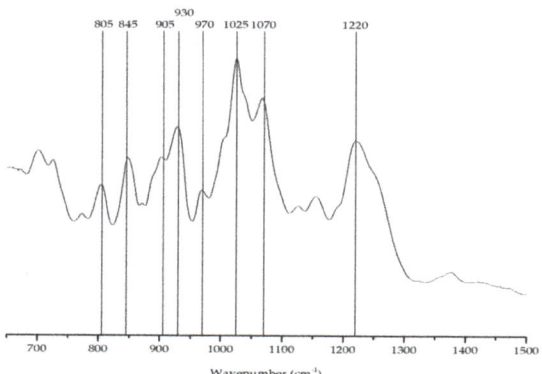

Figure 3. FTIR-ATR spectrum of the carrageenan extracted from *Callblepharis jubata*.

Table 1. FTIR-ATR band identification and characterization of the red seaweed *Callblepharis jubata* polysaccharides (carrageenan), based on the literature [53,54].

Wave Number (cm^{-1})	Chemical Group	Letter Code
805	C–O–SO$_3$ on C2 of 3,6-anhydrogalactose	DA2S
845	D-galactose-4-sulfate	G4S
905	C–O–SO$_3$ on C2 of 3,6-anhydrogalactose	DA2S
930	C–O of 3,6-anhydrogalactose (agar/carrageenan)	(DA)
970–975	Galactose	G/D
1025	Sulfate esters	S=O
1070	C–O of 3,6-anhydrogalactose	DA
1240–1260	Sulfate esters	S=O

2.1.2. Agar Content and Identification

The red seaweed *G. gracilis* produced the highest agar concentration (Figure 4) during the autumn, with 27.04 ± 2.684% DW. However, this did not differ greatly seasonally. Thus, its production was not statistically significantly different over the study period.

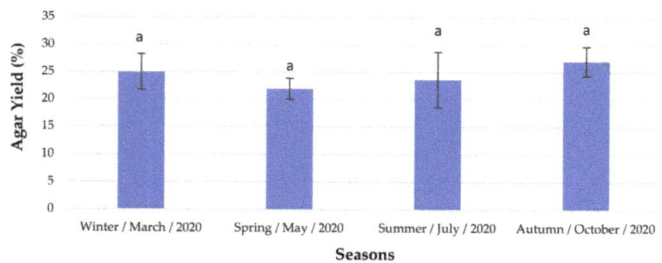

Figure 4. Agar content analyzed seasonally. The extraction yield results are expressed as mean ± standard deviation (n = 3). ^{a} The letters indicate no significant differences at the p-value < 0.05 level.

Agars differ from carrageenans, as they have an L-configuration for the 4-linked galactose residue; nevertheless, they have some structural similarities with carrageenans (Table 2). The characteristic broad band of sulfate esters, generally between 1210 and 1260 cm^{-1} (Figure 5), was much stronger in carrageenans than agars [54].

Table 2. FTIR-ATR band identification and characterization of the red seaweed *Gracilaria gracilis* polysaccharides (agar), based on [53,54].

Wave Number (cm^{-1})	Chemical Group	Letter Code
690	3,6-anhydro-L-galactose (agar)	Agar
741	C-S/C-O-C bending mode in glycosidic linkages of agars	Agar
790	Characteristic of agar-type in second derivative spectra	Agar
805	C–O–SO$_3$ on C2 of 3,6-anhydrogalactose	DA2S
845	D-galactose-4-sulfate	G4S
890–900	Unsulfated b-D-galactose	G/D
930	C–O of 3,6-anhydrogalactose (agar/carrageenan)	(DA)
1012	Sulfate esters	S=O
1070	C–O of 3,6-anhydrogalactose	DA
1100	Sulfate esters	S=O
1240–1260	Sulfate esters	S=O

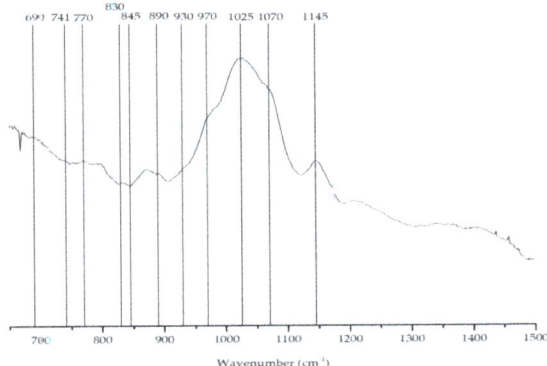

Figure 5. FTIR-ATR spectrum of the agar extracted from *Gracilaria gracilis*.

2.2. Brown Seaweed Polymers

Alginate Content and Identification

Regarding the non-indigenous seaweed *S. muticum* (Figure 6), the highest alginate concentration was observed during winter (e.g., 36.88 ± 2.953% DW).

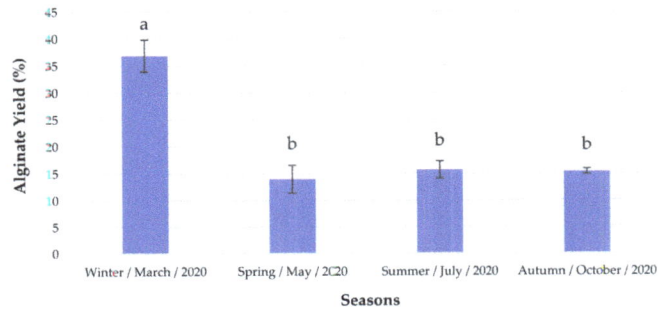

Figure 6. Alginate content analyzed seasonally. The extraction yields are expressed as mean ± standard deviation ($n = 3$). ^{a,b} Similar letters indicate no significant differences at the *p*-value < 0.05 level.

The main polysaccharide found in the brown alga (*S. muticum*) was alginic acid, a linear copolymer of mannuronic (M) and guluronic acid (G). Different types of alginic acid present different proportions and/or alternating patterns of different guluronic (G) and mannuronic (M) units. The presence of these acids can be identified from their characteristic bands in the vibrational spectrum (Figure 7). The extracted colloid showed two characteristic bands: 806 cm^{-1}, assigned to M units, and 788 cm^{-1}, assigned to G units, suggesting the presence of similar amounts of mannuronate and guluronate residues (Table 3) [54,55].

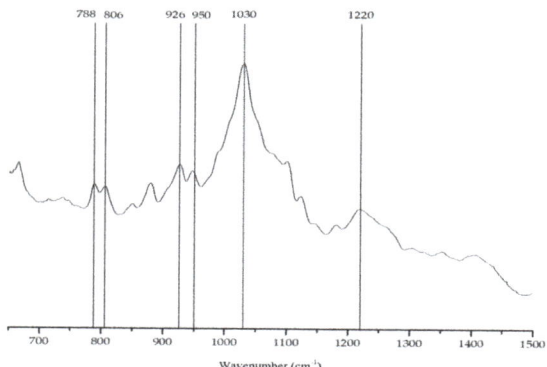

Figure 7. FTIR-ATR spectrum of the alginate extracted from *Sargassum muticum*.

Table 3. FTIR-ATR band identification and characterization of the brown seaweed *Sargassum muticum* polysaccharides (alginate), based on [54].

Wave Number (cm^{-1})	Chemical Group
788	Mannuronic acids residues
806	Guluronic acids residues
1020	Alginic acid
1232	Fucoidan
930–950	C-O stretching vibration of uronic acids

3. Discussion

Seasonal variation in the concentration of different polysaccharides such as carrageenan, agar and alginate was investigated in order to better understand the impact of the season on the polysaccharide yield and quality, due to their economic value and applications. From an industrial management point of view, it is pivotal to assess the extraction yield and the costs associated with the production of these seaweed polysaccharides. The FTIR-ATR is a known method for characterizing and evaluating the overall quality and composition of the seaweed polymers, mainly on the basis of the concentration or modifications in the sulfate esters groups, which are among those groups that can vary seasonally [56–59]. The results of FTIR-ATR evaluation demonstrated similar spectra between seasons, thus revealing that the quality of the polysaccharide extracted differed only in terms of their yield in the *C. jubata* and *S. muticum*.

With respect to the carrageenophyte *C. jubata*, the optimum season to harvest this seaweed for the highest yield of carrageenan was mid-spring to the beginning of the summer. This red seaweed synthesizes lower carrageenan concentrations during the autumn and winter [59]. This observation was supported by other reports assessing seasonal yield variation in carrageenan on the Normandy (France) and Portuguese coasts [59,60]. It was found that in Normandy, carrageenan yields fluctuated from 15% (in winter) to 45% DW (at the end of the spring/beginning of the summer) [60]. On the Portuguese coast, the lowest carrageenan content was found during winter (i.e., 4% DW), but with a maximum yield during the spring (i.e., 40.4% DW, a 10 fold increase) [59]. Previous research has shown that *C. jubata* collected during spring 2020, at the same sampling site as the present study, produced a carrageenan yield of 23% DW [61]. The FTIR-ATR analysis of carrageenan from *C. jubata* was in concordance with the analysis of Pereira et al. [53], which detected iota-carrageenan with a low/residual content of kappa-carrageenan.

The increased accumulation of this biological reserve by *C. jubata* could be explained by the fact that the seaweed is typically from cold-temperate waters, so the increase of the surface seawater temperatures (SST) during the summer could be a stressor enhancing carrageenan biosynthesis [60].

The agarophyte *G. gracilis* is an opportunistic seaweed that is present in temperate-warm waters, and is already an important commercial source of agar, of which there is currently a global supply shortage [62–64]. Previous research has highlighted seasonal differences in the yield of agar from this species [65–67]. In agreement with the results of this study, *G. gracilis* collected on the Patagonian coast (Argentina) recorded the highest agar production during the summer and spring seasons (i.e., 41 and 30% DW, respectively) [65,66]. Using materials collected from the Venice Lagoon (Italy), an average agar yield of 25% DW was reported [67]. The lower agar yield during the spring/summer, can be attributed to the increased nutrient concentrations and lower turbidity and planktonic blooms that often characterize these seasons [67]. The FTIR-ATR analysis of the agar from *G. gracilis* demonstrated the presence of typical bonds for agar, with sulfate esters being evident. The observations are similar to the results obtained by Pereira et al. [54] with other agarophyte species (e.g., *Gelidium* spp.).

The alginophyte *S. muticum* is a brown seaweed introduced and well established in European and North American waters [62,68–71]. This seaweed can be used as a feedstock for alginate extraction, e.g., *S. muticum* harvested in Morocco produced a 25.6% DW yield at the beginning of spring [55,72]. The FTIR-ATR spectra of the alginate from *S. muticum* presented alginate peaks, but sulfate esters were also revealed, which could have been derived from sulfated polysaccharides such as fucoidan and laminarin [54].

The FTIR-ATR spectra were very similar between the seasons, demonstrating that the main factor was the quantity and not the quality. These results are in concordance with literature reports [54,59,64].

Seaweed polysaccharides, with a high molecular weight, are generally considered to be good dietary fibers. Specific applications of these are recognized as key players in human health and disease prevention [73]. These benefits are especially enhanced because there is an interplay with the gut microbiome at intestinal, as well as systemic, levels, resulting in homeostasis between the host and the microflora. Food intake can modify the microflora equilibrium positively or negatively, resulting in immunological, physiological, metabolic and even psychological effects. Consequently, the human diet can modulate health status: indubitably, we are what we eat [74–76].

In addition to their biological properties, seaweed polysaccharides also have innate properties that are very important for intestinal health; these include mainly the viscosity and the high potential for water-binding activity, which adjusts the transit time of food through the gut. Such properties are demonstrated to promote satiety and weight loss; additionally, they delay gastric emptying, thereby promoting glycemic control (i.e., reducing the incidence of diabetes). In the intestinal tract, all seaweed-derived polysaccharides are reported to enhance gut transit, maintaining regular stool bulking, and promoting beneficial alterations to the composition of the microbiome. Taken together, these benefits result in improved metabolization of volatile fatty acids (VFAs), which are also considered to be short chain fatty acids (SCFAs) by members of the microflora, promoting positive impacts in the gastrointestinal system, and thus resulting in the improved status of cardiometabolic, immune, bone, and mental health conditions [3,77–80].

It is now clear that various seaweeds have an interesting dietary fiber content, which can have a positive impact on the health status of production and companion animals, as well as on the health status of humans. Furthermore, this source is natural and uniquely different from crop and fruit plants. However, from this study and others, it is patently clear that not all seaweed polymers are "the same". They have a structural function in the seaweed thalli and can be expected to vary seasonally. Hence, there is considerable need to quantify them, in order to ensure good intake without passing the intake limits. It has been shown that excessive consumption of dietary fiber can lead to negative impacts on human (and animal) health, e.g., recurrent symptoms of soft stools or diarrhea [3,77–79,81,82]. All good things should be taken in moderation. For instance, the study of Calvante et al. [83] demonstrated that a commercial powder of *Crassiphycus birdiae* at a low dosage, which is the recommend dosage intake of seaweed dried biomass supplement daily (5%) can induce reproductive toxicity and cellular damage when ingested with other chemicals. Thus, the full analysis of seaweed is required to fully understand the impact of seaweed compounds in the food industry and, more importantly, in the seaweed for direct intake [84,85], mainly with respect to metals (arsenic, cadmium, mercury, and lead) and other contaminants. In our study, the polymers were seasonally stable and the major differences in *C. jubata* and *S. muticum* were related to the yield.

The diversity of seaweed polysaccharides (and particularly their lower-molecular-weight oligomers) needs to be quantified, due to the negative effects that can arise if their cumulative dosage exceeds the limit of 25 g/day [82,86]. In this case, the consumption of wild harvested seaweeds would need to be limited according to their season of harvest (Table 1). Taking just three examples in the present study, *C. jubata* had the highest values in autumn; *G. gracilis* was the seaweed with the most consistent levels across the seasons; and *S. muticum* had the highest polymer levels during the winter. These observations are important in order to maximize the benefits of ingestion of particular types of seaweeds. This is because if the seaweed intake exceeds the recommended levels, the constituent polysaccharides, such as dietary fibers, can de-regulate the intestinal system, inducing bloating, abdominal pain, flatulence, loose stools or diarrhea, etc., as well as a reduction of blood glycemic values, which for diabetic patients, in particular, is a serious health risk [87].

However, due to the considerable diversity of seaweeds and their composition, the recommended daily intake for a generic "seaweed" is normally only 5 g DW/day, due to its high mineral/metal content; this was demonstrated by Milinovic et al. [88] as a result of the iodine content in seaweeds collected at Figueira da Foz, Portugal, which is a limiting factor in the seaweed intake. Due to the advice presented in the Recommended Dietary Allowance [89,90], it is necessary to standardize of the analyses applied to seaweed, especially for applications in the food industry [91]. Considering the examples in this study, the three species represent between 2 and 7% of the recommended daily intake (Table 4) [82,86].

Table 4. Thresholds of daily consumption of seaweeds based on their polysaccharide content.

Season	*C. jubata* (g of Dried Seaweed for 25 g of Dietary Fiber)	*C. jubata* (g of Dietary Fiber for 5 g of Dried Seaweed)	*G. gracilis* (g of Dried Seaweed for 25 g of Dietary Fiber)	*G. gracilis* (g of Dietary Fiber for 5 g of Dried Seaweed)	*S. muticum* (g of Dried Seaweed for 25 g of Dietary Fiber)	*S. muticum* (g of Dietary Fiber for 5 g of Dried Seaweed)
Winter	163.04	0.77	100.11	1.25	67.79	1.84
Spring	142.93	0.86	114.07	1.10	179.14	0.70
Summer	133.48	0.94	105.70	1.18	159.57	0.78
Autumn	241.15	0.52	92.45	1.35	163.29	0.77

Table 4 demonstrates that, overall, each of the seaweeds analyzed had a good dietary fiber content, which could be exploited commercially. In particular, *G. gracilis* did not exhibit a great deal of seasonal variability. However, *C. jubata* and *S. muticum* showed significant, although different, seasonal variations. From a commercial point of view, for the greatest benefit to the consumer, the seaweed raw materials need to be harvested in specific seasons in order that the level of polysaccharide content does not exceed the threshold of consumption. However, there is the need for a complete biochemical profile if the specific seaweed is to be consumed whole [90]. In particular, the macro- and trace elements present in the seaweeds need to be known due to their potential accumulation from the surrounding environment [88,92]. However, the effects due to the intake of whole seaweeds appear to be less when compared with the purified seaweed polysaccharide associated with water, milk, or prepared in a juice [93–95]. Consequently, ongoing research in this area is targeting applications of seaweed polysaccharides in novel foods with nutraceutical properties [6,96,97].

Anti-obesity effects have been described as being among the most beneficial attributes of seaweed polysaccharides for human consumption due to their fermentation in the intestinal tract, thereby reducing the microfloral/bile salt hydrolase activity, which is one theory behind this observed effect [96,98–101]. In this case, the microbiome composition was found to change to an augmented state, including populations of *Bifidobacterium*, *Bacteroides, Lactobacillus, Roseburia, Parasutterella, Fusicatenibacter, Coprococcus*, and *Fecalibacterium* colonies in in vitro experiments [96,98–101]. The nutritional values of the targeted seaweeds demonstrate a general fluctuation on the basis of the location at which the seaweed was collected, as demonstrated by Pacheco et al. [69]. Thus, the harvest site greatly influences the nutritional value, with carbohydrate yield being one of the principal variations (see Table 5). There is a lack of studies regarding the nutritional profile of *C. jubata*; however, there is a study by Araújo et al. [61] that characterizes its carbohydrate and lipidic profile.

Table 5. Range of nutritional values of selected seaweeds analyzed around the world (% DW).

Seaweed Species	Protein	Lipid	Carbohydrate	Ash	Ref.
G. gracilis	5.83–20.2	low	9.52–68.13	6.78–24.78	[102–105]
S. muticum	4.64–22	0.12–3.2	27.9–69	13.2–26.4	[69]

However, as a food supplement, the safety of the dietary inclusion of seaweeds also needs to have various biochemical constituents checked before the alga can be made commercially available for regular human consumption [6,106]. Studies thus far have demonstrated that some wild harvested seaweeds, without thorough analysis of their nutrient and metal concentrations, can provoke negative impacts on health. However, there is little information available on this, relative to the more adverse pathologies (i.e., compared to those described above). This important topic is well described in the reviews of Cherry et al. [96] and Weiner [81], as well as Wierner and McKim [107], who demonstrated that within the daily recommend intake, there are indeed relatively low health risks to consumption. Nonetheless, major concerns have been expressed over seaweed polysaccharides present at low molecular weights, and poligeenan in particular. This has also been referred to as "degraded carrageenan", and is not the natural chemical structure of the polysaccharide. Indeed, it can provoke harmful impacts, such as the powerful induction of inflammation. Intake of degraded carrageenan can happen when the legislation regarding polysaccharide preparation and usage in the food industry is not followed. Because of this, seaweed polysaccharide applications in the food industry are regulated, in order to guarantee the safety of the final product [6,32,34,36,81]. Aside from the general considerations regarding the safety of seaweed polysaccharides, there is ongoing debate arising from several in vitro and in vivo assay reports [108–115]. Unfortunately, there is still a lack of standard methods, and there are only a few in vivo assays with fully characterized seaweed polysaccharides [3,96]. This was demonstrated by Kumar and Sharma [116], where several deaths and illnesses that had been attributed to consumption of seaweeds were found to be mainly due to wild harvesting at unsuitable (polluted) sites, unreasonably high consumption, and the noted presence of highly potent secondary metabolites/toxins (some microalgal bloom related).

However, despite these negative reports, which occur only rarely, judicial (i.e., in moderation) consumption of seaweed polysaccharides have overall positive effects on several aspects of human health. These polymers work as nutraceutical compounds, thereby promoting human welfare and health. Indeed cautious and responsible consumption of seaweeds is no different from that of other terrestrial and marine food sources [117]. Taken alone, isolated seaweed polysaccharides have demonstrated numerous interesting properties for use in pharmaceutical and medical applications. In this regard, several specific seaweeds and their components are already in use commercially, while others are still in the research and development stage [117]. As commercial examples, the use of alginate in wound dressings, carrageenans in antiviral solutions, and agar in encapsulation of pharmacological drugs are all impressive [118–122]. In experimental development, selected seaweed polymers are being targeted mainly for the development of new hydrogel-based models for various human conditions, such as tumor or cardiovascular diseases, in order to provide more comprehensive models with which to understand drug and human cell interactions without using in vivo animal models, thereby providing more accurate/predictable responses [123]. This approach also enhances the development of new hydrogels for tissue engineering, where seaweed polymers have demonstrated good results in the early stage of development [124–126].

Seaweed polysaccharides can be applied as cosmetic ingredients, being used as gelling agents, thickeners, protective colloid emulsifier and stabilizer agents in hand lotions and liquid soap, deodorants, makeup, exfoliant, cleanser, shaving cream, facial moisturizer/lotion or in creams for acne and anti-aging care [127]. Similarly polysaccharide formulations can also be used in skin protection cosmetics to combat dermatitis, psoriasis, eczema, and dryness [128].

Carrageenans are one of the most bioactive polysaccharides from seaweeds; their chemical structure allows the formation of hydrogels, thereby allowing them to be used in anti-viral and anti-bacterial ingredients in various formulae [128,129]. There are compelling reasons for the use of these compounds, given the high levels of safety, efficacy and biocompatibility reported, in addition to their being biodegradable and non-toxic [118,130]. Furthermore, ancient records show that carrageenan has been used as a traditional medicine to ameliorate coughs and the common cold. These "old wives' tales" have been supported more recently by *in vitro* and *in vivo* assays using animal models. This functionality is mainly derived from the actions of carrageenans in inhibiting the aggregation of blood platelets (i.e., anticoagulant activity) [74,131]. Various carrageenans have other demonstrable bioactivities such as anti-tumor, anti-viral and immunomodulation activities [116,132], which are already being exploited commercially. The anti-viral mechanism is based on blocking the entrance of viral particles into the cell. Good results have been demonstrated against the herpes simplex virus type 1 and type 2, HIV-1, and the human rhinovirus [133,134]. These anti-viral activities have mainly been observed in iota-carrageenan (which is the carrageenan type produced by *C. jubata*) [53,59,133]. However, in pharmacodynamics, carrageenans that are harmful for human consumption (specifically, in the form of oligo-carrageenans or poligeenans) are regularly used as a pro-inflammatory factor in diverse *in vitro* and *in vivo* assays, due to the high inherent bioactivity when degraded to a low molecular weight [117]. Oligo-carrageenans can also be used to induce pleurisy, paw edema and ulceration in animal models, and as such, they are used as tools for medical research [135].

In contrast to carrageenans, agars and alginates are not recognized as bioactive molecules—instead they are seen as excellent polymers with reduced bioactivities (i.e., they are biologically inert) that can be inserted and used as a barrier/encapsulation to stabilize active ingredients and develop new biomedical and pharmaceutical methods and techniques [129,136]. Agar is used in pharmaceutical products such as a bulking and suspension ingredients for medical solutions, anti-coagulant agents, and laxatives in capsules and tablets [132,137]. Alginates are perhaps the most used seaweed polysaccharides in medical and pharmaceutical products already on the market, namely in wound and battle dressings, and also in wound-healing products in the form of hydrogels [34]. Alginates, when used in the biomedical and pharmaceutical areas, are linked to cations, such calcium, sodium or magnesium, to produce a biopolymer with no bioactivity and low toxicity that is easy to manipulate so as to permit the development of hydrogels for tissue regeneration, as well as application in other areas such as in burn or diabetic wound-healing dressings [118].

However, seaweed polysaccharides have been further explored in drug delivery systems, where the polymers have demonstrated features such as natural biocompatibility, variation of viscosity and gelation conditions, low toxicity, low-cost polymers, and biodegradability, with easy adaptation and manipulation for the assembly of polymer-derivatives with new physical characteristics [117,118,138]. Seaweed-derived polysaccharides have adaptable swelling properties that respond to temperature modifications, which is important for on-demand and time-dependent modulation of drug release [139]. In the post-rheology, pharmaceutical and medical arenas, seaweed polysaccharides must have a high level of purity in order to reduce the impact of potential inclusion of impurities in the application of polymers in products and solutions, permitting clean application without any associated health risks or hazards [140].

4. Materials and Methods

4.1. Reagents

The reagents used for carrageenan extraction, i.e., methanol, acetone, ethanol and sodium hydroxide, were acquired from the suppliers José Manuel Gomes dos Santos, Lda., Odivelas, Portugal; Ceamed, Lda., Funchal, Portugal; Valente e Ribeiro. Lda., Belas, Portugal and Sigma-Aldrich GmbH, Steinheim, Germany, respectively.

The reagents used for alginate extraction, i.e., sodium carbonate and hydrochloric acid, were purchased from Fisher Chemical, Leicestershire, United Kingdom.

4.2. Seaweed Collection

Seaweeds belonging to the Rhodophyta, i.e., *Gracilaria gracilis* (Stackhouse) Steentoft, L.M Irvine & Farnham 1995, and *Calliblepharis jubata* (Goodenough & Woodward) Kützing 1843 and the Ochrophyta, i.e., *Sargassum muticum* (Yendo) Fensholt, were collected during low-low tide the intertidal of Buarcos Bay, located in Figueira da Foz, Portugal (40°10'18.6'' N, 8°53'44.4'' W), Portugal. The seasonal sampling was conducted during 2020 (see Table 6) from sites with well-established seaweed populations without epiphytes or degradation visible to the eye. The specimens were collected from three different tidal pools at the same height on the shore. Approximately 100 g FW of *C. jubata*, 300 g FW of *G. gracilis*, 200 g FW of *S. muticum* were collected. After harvesting, each species was kept separately in plastic bags, inside a cool box, and transported to the laboratory (50 min from the harvest location). Firstly, the thalli were washed with filtered seawater to remove sand and other detritus. Thereafter, the samples were washed with distilled water, aiming for the removal of excess salts caused by the previous washing process and then placed on plastic trays and placed into an air-forced oven (Raypa DAF-135, R. Espinar S.L., Barcelona, Spain) at 60 °C, for 48 h. The dried algae were finely ground to make uniform ($\leq$1 mm) samples with a commercial mill (Taurus aromatic, Oliana, Spain) and then stored in a box with silica gel to reduce humidity, in the dark, at room temperature ($\pm$24 °C).

Table 6. Seaweed collection data.

Season	Date	Water Temperature (°C)	pH	Salinity (ppm)	Conductivity (µS/cm)	ORP (mV)	O$_2$ (%)
Winter	9 March 2020	14.13 $\pm$ 0.08	7.8 $\pm$ 0.09	35.12 $\pm$ 0.17	42146 $\pm$ 130.07	111.07 $\pm$ 5.27	113.2 $\pm$ 6.12
Spring	27 May 2020	17.15 $\pm$ 0.07	8.55 $\pm$ 0.06	35.60 $\pm$ 0.10	44149 $\pm$ 53.68	53.68 $\pm$ 27.33	94.775 $\pm$ 6.41
Summer	20 July 2020	17.94 $\pm$ 0.62	8.24 $\pm$ 0.19	36.20 $\pm$ 0.05	54595 $\pm$ 184.33	184.33 $\pm$ 16.87	35.16 $\pm$ 3.68
Autumn	19 October 2020	14.49 $\pm$ 0.08	8.06 $\pm$ 0.10	35.78 $\pm$ 0.12	54065 $\pm$ 83.56	83.56 $\pm$ 7.62	88.77 $\pm$ 4.00

4.3. Polysaccharide Extraction

4.3.1. Agar

Agar extraction was based on the technique reported by Li et al. [141], with adaptations. The extraction was performed in triplicate, using 20 g of dried seaweed and 600 mL of distilled water. Afterwards, the solution was placed in an electric pressure cooker

(Aigostar 300008IAU, Aigostar, Madrid, Spain) at a temperature of 115 °C with an air pressure of 80 Kpa, for 2 h. The solution was hot filtered, under vacuum, in a Buchner funnel, through a cloth filter. The extract was then vacuum filtered with a Goosh funnel (porosity G2). At room temperature, the filtrate was allowed to gel, frozen overnight and thawed. The thawed gel was finally dried (60 °C, 48 h) in an air-forced oven (Raypa DAF-135, R. Espinar S.L., Barcelona, Spain).

4.3.2. Carrageenan

The extraction of carrageenan was carried out in triplicate, according to the method defined by Pereira and van de Velde [142]. To remove the organic-soluble fraction, 1 g of milled seaweed was pre-treated with an acetone:methanol (1:1) solution at a final concentration of 1% (m/v) for 16 h, at 4 °C. The liquid solution was decanted, and the seaweed residues were collected and dried at 60 °C in an air-forced oven (Raypa DAF-135, R. Espinar S.L., Barcelona, Spain).

Dried samples were immersed in 150 mL of NaOH (1 M) in a hot water bath (GFL 1003, GFL, Burgwedel, Germany), at 85–90 °C, for 3 h. The solutions were hot filtered, under vacuum, in a Buchner funnel with a cloth filter. The extract was vacuum filtered with a Goosh funnel (porosity G2). Under vacuum, the extract was evaporated (rotary evaporator model: 2600000, Witeg, Germany) to one-third of the initial volume. The carrageenan was precipitated by adding twice the final volume of 96% ethanol. The polysaccharide was washed with 96% ethanol for 48 h at 4 °C and dried in an air forced oven (60 °C, 48 h).

4.3.3. Alginate

The extraction of alginic acid was performed in triplicate, employing the adjusted method of Sivagnanavelmurugan et al. [143]. Milled seaweed was added to a solution of HCl at 1.23% (1:30 v:v) and kept at room temperature for 48 h. The solution was filtered under vacuum with a Goosh funnel (porosity G2). The residue was rinsed with distilled water two to three times. The residue was submitted to an alkali extraction in 2% sodium carbonate for 48 h. The solution was filtered under vacuum through a cloth filter supported in a Goosh funnel (porosity G2), to remove any residues from the alginate solution. This process was followed by the addition of a solution of 37% HCl to the filtrate, producing the alginic acid precipitation (1 mL of 37% of HCl: 30 mL of the final solution). The precipitate was separated by centrifugation (4000 rpm, for 15 min) and then dried in an air forced oven (60 °C, 48 h).

4.4. Carbohydrate Characterization

Polysaccharide Analysis

For Fourier-Transform Infrared Spectroscopy–Attenuated Total Reflection (FTIR-ATR) analyses, the dried polysaccharides were powdered using a commercial mill, and then subjected to direct analysis. FTIR-ATR spectra were recorded on a Perkin Elmer Spectrum 400 spectrometer (Waltham, MA, USA), with no need for sample preparation, since these assays only require dried samples [52–54]. All spectra presented are the average of two independent measurements from 650–1500 cm^{-1} with 128 scans, each at a resolution of 2 cm^{-1}. The FTIR-ATR spectra in the manuscript were performed with the polymers extracted in the autumn.

4.5. Statistical Analyses

The statistical analyses were performed using Sigma Plot v.14. This included an ANOVA analysis to assess statistically differences between the extraction yields. Holms-Sidak multiple comparison analysis was used after the rejection of the ANOVA null hypothesis, to discriminate any differences. The analyses were considered statistically different when p-value < 0.05. Error bars are the standard deviation of the mean.

5. Conclusions

The seaweeds analyzed in this study demonstrated that wild harvested materials can indeed vary in terms of polysaccharide yield. Such variance could significantly change the nutritional value/properties on a seasonal basis. Therefore, the direct intake of seaweeds should be carefully analyzed.

Seaweed-derived polymers (polysaccharides) as food sources/ingredients are compared to dietary fiber due to their high molecular weight and because algal polysaccharides are not digestible compounds, being an important nutraceutical for good gastrointestinal functioning. However, if the polysaccharide is degraded (by over hydrolysis), the low-molecular-weight fractions can have negative impacts on human health. Likewise, over-dosage/consumption may be an issue, and thus moderation in all things is a key.

However, for the commodity food sector, there is a need to guarantee similar nutritional values in all supplies, independent of the season. In this context, seaweed cultivation can present a solution for controlling seaweed food safety; this is something in which Asian countries are already well practiced [144–148], and which Western countries need to learn and adapt to.

In the future, long-term assays should be conducted in different years to understand any fluctuations that may occur. Thus, seaweed cultivation (on land or in the sea) may provide more homogenous raw materials. In the nutraceutical/biomedical field, there is a need to understand the digestive part of the polymers in order to provide greater security for the consumption of seaweed polymers. As demonstrated, there is a need to understand the ecological factors affecting seaweed biomass in order to obtain safe and high-quality polymers to support their many applications in the food industry.

Author Contributions: Conceptualization, J.C., D.P., G.S.A., A.V., A.T.C. and L.P.; Seaweed laboratory work, J.C., D.P., G.S.A.; writing—original draft preparation, J.C., D.P., G.S.A.; writing—review and editing, J.C., D.P., A.V., A.T.C. and L.P.; supervision, A.V., A.T.C. and L.P. All authors have read and agreed to the published version of the manuscript.

Funding: This research received no external funding.

Institutional Review Board Statement: Not applicable.

Data Availability Statement: Data available from authors.

Acknowledgments: This work was financed by national funds through FCT (Foundation for Science and Technology), I.P., within the scope of the projects UIDB/04292/2020 (MARE, Marine and Environmental Sciences Centre). Diana Pacheco thanks to PTDC/BIA-CBI/31144/2017-POCI-01 project -0145-FEDER-031144-MARINE INVADERS, co-financed by the ERDF through POCI (Operational Program Competitiveness and Internationalization) and by the Foundation for Science and Technology (FCT, IP). João Cotas thanks to the European Regional Development Fund through the Interreg Atlantic Area Program, under the project NASPA (EAPA_451/2016).

Conflicts of Interest: The authors declare no conflict of interest.

References

1. FAO. *The State of World Fisheries and Aquaculture 2020 Sustainability in Action*; FAO: Rome, Italy, 2020; ISBN 978-92-5-132692-3.
2. Pereira, L. *Edible Seaweeds of the World*; CRC Press: Boca Raton, FL, USA, 2016.
3. Cherry, P.; O'Hara, C.; Magee, P.J.; McSorley, E.M.; Allsopp, P.J. Risks and benefits of consuming edible seaweeds. *Nutr. Rev.* **2019**, *77*, 307–329. [CrossRef] [PubMed]
4. Rajapakse, N.; Kim, S.K. *Nutritional and Digestive Health Benefits of Seaweed*, 1st ed.; Elsevier Inc.: Amsterdam, The Netherlands, 2011; Volume 64, ISBN 9780123876690.
5. Mišurcová, L.; Machů, L.; Orsavová, J. Seaweed minerals as nutraceuticals. *Adv. Food Nutr. Res.* **2011**, *64*, 371–390. [CrossRef]
6. Leandro, A.; Pacheco, D.; Cotas, J.; Marques, J.C.; Pereira, L.; Gonçalves, A.M.M. Seaweed's Bioactive Candidate Compounds to Food Industry and Global Food Security. *Life* **2020**, *10*, 140. [CrossRef] [PubMed]
7. Shannon, E.; Abu-Ghannam, N. Seaweeds as nutraceuticals for health and nutrition. *Phycologia* **2019**, *58*, 563–577. [CrossRef]
8. Cotas, J.; Leandro, A.; Monteiro, P.; Pacheco, D.; Figueirinha, A.; Gonçalves, A.M.M.; da Silva, G.J.; Pereira, L. Seaweed Phenolics: From Extraction to Applications. *Mar. Drugs* **2020**, *18*, 384. [CrossRef]
9. McHugh, D.J. *A Guide to the Seaweed Industry*; FAO: Rome, Italy, 2003.

10. Ferrara, L. Seaweeds: A Food for Our Future. *J. Food Chem. Nanotechnol.* **2020**, *6*, 56–64. [CrossRef]
11. Pereira, L. A review of the nutrient composition of selected edible seaweeds. In *Seaweed: Ecology, Nutrient Composition and Medicinal Uses*; Pomin, V.H., Ed.; Nova Science Publishers, Inc: New York, USA, 2011; pp. 15–33, ISBN 9781614708780.
12. Catarino, M.; Silva, A.; Cardoso, S. Phycochemical Constituents and Biological Activities of *Fucus* spp. *Mar. Drugs* **2018**, *16*, 249. [CrossRef]
13. Lahaye, M.; Robic, A. Structure and Functional Properties of Ulvan, a Polysaccharide from Green Seaweeds. *Biomacromolecules* **2007**, *8*, 1765–1774. [CrossRef]
14. Wijesinghe, W.A.J.P.; Jeon, Y.-J. Enzyme-assistant extraction (EAE) of bioactive components: A useful approach for recovery of industrially important metabolites from seaweeds: A review. *Fitoterapia* **2012**, *83*, 6–12. [CrossRef]
15. Charoensiddhi, S.; Lorbeer, A.J.; Lahnstein, J.; Bulone, V.; Franco, C.M.M.; Zhang, W. Enzyme-assisted extraction of carbohydrates from the brown alga *Ecklonia radiata*: Effect of enzyme type, pH and buffer on sugar yield and molecular weight profiles. *Process. Biochem.* **2016**, *51*, 1503–1510. [CrossRef]
16. Devillé, C.; Gharbi, M.; Dandrifosse, G.; Peulen, O. Study on the effects of laminarin, a polysaccharide from seaweed, on gut characteristics. *J. Sci. Food Agric.* **2007**, *87*, 1717–1725. [CrossRef]
17. Yaich, H.; Garna, H.; Besbes, S.; Paquot, M.; Blecker, C.; Attia, H. Effect of extraction conditions on the yield and purity of ulvan extracted from *Ulva lactuca*. *Food Hydrocoll.* **2013**. [CrossRef]
18. Khotimchenko, M.; Tiasto, V.; Kalitnik, A.; Begun, M.; Khotimchenko, R.; Leonteva, E.; Bryukhovetskiy, I.; Khotimchenko, Y. Antitumor potential of carrageenans from marine red algae. *Carbohydr. Polym.* **2020**, *246*, 116568. [CrossRef] [PubMed]
19. Barros Gomes Camara, R.; Silva Costa, L.; Pereira Fidelis, G.; Duarte Barreto Nobre, L.T.; Dantas-Santos, N.; Lima Cordeiro, S.; Santana Santos Pereira Costa, M.; Guimaraes Alves, L.; Oliveira Rocha, H.A. Heterofucans from the Brown Seaweed *Canistrocarpus cervicornis* with Anticoagulant and Antioxidant Activities. *Mar. Drugs* **2011**, *9*, 124–138. [CrossRef]
20. Yu, X.; Zhang, Q.; Cui, W.; Zeng, Z.; Yang, W.; Zhang, C.; Zhao, H.; Gao, W.; Wang, X.; Luo, D. Low Molecular Weight Fucoidan Alleviates Cardiac Dysfunction in Diabetic Goto-Kakizaki Rats by Reducing Oxidative Stress and Cardiomyocyte Apoptosis. *J. Diabetes Res.* **2014**, *2014*, 1–13. [CrossRef]
21. Reis, S.E.; Andrade, R.G.C.; Accardo, C.M.; Maia, L.F.; Oliveira, L.F.C.; Nader, H.B.; Aguiar, J.A.K.; Medeiros, V.P. Influence of sulfated polysaccharides from *Ulva lactuca* L. upon Xa and IIa coagulation factors and on venous blood clot formation. *Algal Res.* **2020**, *45*, 101750. [CrossRef]
22. Cui, K.; Tai, W.; Shan, X.; Hao, J.; Li, G.; Yu, G. Structural characterization and anti-thrombotic properties of fucoidan from *Nemacystus decipiens*. *Int. J. Biol. Macromol.* **2018**, *120*, 1817–1822. [CrossRef] [PubMed]
23. Pereira, L.; Critchley, A.T. The COVID 19 novel coronavirus pandemic 2020: Seaweeds to the rescue? Why does substantial, supporting research about the antiviral properties of seaweed polysaccharides seem to go unrecognized by the pharmaceutical community in these desperate times? *J. Appl. Phycol.* **2020**, *32*, 1875–1877. [CrossRef]
24. Sun, Q.-L.; Li, Y.; Ni, L.-Q.; Li, Y.-X.; Cui, Y.-S.; Jiang, S.-L.; Xie, E.-Y.; Du, J.; Deng, F.; Dong, C.-X. Structural characterization and antiviral activity of two fucoidans from the brown algae *Sargassum henslowianum*. *Carbohydr. Polym.* **2020**, *229*, 115487. [CrossRef]
25. Richards, C.; Williams, N.A.; Fitton, J.H.; Stringer, D.N.; Karpiniec, S.S.; Park, A.Y. Oral Fucoidan Attenuates Lung Pathology and Clinical Signs in a Severe Influenza A Mouse Model. *Mar. Drugs* **2020**, *18*, 246. [CrossRef] [PubMed]
26. Ponce, M.; Zuasti, E.; Anguís, V.; Fernández-Díaz, C. Effects of the sulfated polysaccharide ulvan from *Ulva ohnoi* on the modulation of the immune response in Senegalese sole (*Solea senegalensis*). *Fish Shellfish Immunol.* **2020**, *100*, 27–40. [CrossRef]
27. Li, Y.; Huo, Y.; Wang, F.; Wang, C.; Zhu, Q.; Wang, Y.; Fu, L.; Zhou, T. Improved antioxidant and immunomodulatory activities of enzymatically degraded *Porphyra haitanensis* polysaccharides. *J. Food Biochem.* **2020**, *44*. [CrossRef]
28. Tyśkiewicz, K.; Tyśkiewicz, R.; Konkol, M.; Rój, E.; Jaroszuk-Ściseł, J.; Skalicka-Woźniak, K. Antifungal Properties of *Fucus vesiculosus* L. Supercritical Fluid Extract Against *Fusarium culmorum* and *Fusarium oxysporum*. *Molecules* **2019**, *24*, 3518. [CrossRef] [PubMed]
29. Souza, R.B.; Frota, A.F.; Silva, J.; Alves, C.; Neugebauer, A.Z.; Pinteus, S.; Rodrigues, J.A.G.; Cordeiro, E.M.S.; de Almeida, R.R.; Pedrosa, R.; et al. In vitro activities of kappa-carrageenan isolated from red marine alga *Hypnea musciformis*: Antimicrobial, anticancer and neuroprotective potential. *Int. J. Biol. Macromol.* **2018**, *112*, 1248–1256. [CrossRef]
30. Biris-Dorhoi, E.-S.; Michiu, D.; Pop, C.R.; Rotar, A.M.; Tofana, M.; Pop, O.L.; Socaci, S.A.; Farcas, A.C. Macroalgae—A Sustainable Source of Chemical Compounds with Biological Activities. *Nutrients* **2020**, *12*, 3085. [CrossRef] [PubMed]
31. MacArtain, P.; Gill, C.I.R.; Brooks, M.; Campbell, R.; Rowland, I.R. Nutritional Value of Edible Seaweeds. *Nutr. Rev.* **2008**, *65*, 535–543. [CrossRef]
32. Mortensen, A.; Aguilar, F.; Crebelli, R.; Di Domenico, A.; Frutos, M.J.; Galtier, P.; Gott, D.; Gundert-Remy, U.; Lambré, C.; Leblanc, J.; et al. Re-evaluation of agar (E 406) as a food additive. *EFSA J.* **2016**, *14*. [CrossRef]
33. Food and Drug Administration Sec. 184.1115 of the Federal Food and Drug Administration Act (21CFR184.1115). In *Code of Federal Regulations Title 21 Food and Drugs*; FDA: Silver Spring, ML, USA, 2020.
34. Younes, M.; Aggett, P.; Aguilar, F.; Crebelli, R.; Filipič, M.; Frutos, M.J.; Galtier, P.; Gott, D.; Gundert-Remy, U.; Kuhnle, G.G.; et al. Re-evaluation of carrageenan (E 407) and processed Eucheuma seaweed (E 407a) as food additives. *EFSA J.* **2018**, *16*. [CrossRef]
35. Food and Drug Administration Sec. 172.620 of the Federal Food and Drug Admnistration Act (21CFR172.620). In *Code of Federal Regulations Title 21 Food and Drugs*; FDA: Silver Spring, ML, USA, 2020.

36. Younes, M.; Aggett, P.; Aguilar, F.; Crebelli, R.; Filipič, M.; Frutos, M.J.; Galtier, P.; Gott, D.; Gundert-Remy, U.; Kuhnle, G.G.; et al. Re-evaluation of alginic acid and its sodium, potassium, ammonium and calcium salts (E 400–E 404) as food additives. *EFSA J.* **2017**, *15*. [CrossRef]
37. Food and Drug Administration Sec. 184.1724 of the Federal Food and Drug Admnistration Act (21CFR184.1724). In *Code of Federal Regululations Title 21 Food and Drugs*; FDA: Silver Spring, ML, USA, 2020.
38. Lunn, J.; Buttriss, J.L. Carbohydrates and dietary fibre. *Nutr. Bull.* **2007**, *32*, 21–64. [CrossRef]
39. Sun, S.Z.; Empie, M.W. Fructose metabolism in humans—What isotopic tracer studies tell us. *Nutr. Metab.* **2012**, *9*, 89. [CrossRef] [PubMed]
40. Chen, L.; Xu, W.; Chen, D.; Chen, G.; Liu, J.; Zeng, X.; Shao, R.; Zhu, H. Digestibility of sulfated polysaccharide from the brown seaweed *Ascophyllum nodosum* and its effect on the human gut microbiota in vitro. *Int. J. Biol. Macromol.* **2018**, *112*, 1055–1061. [CrossRef]
41. Li, Y.O.; Komarek, A.R. Dietary fibre basics: Health, nutrition, analysis, and applications. *Food Qual. Saf.* **2017**, *1*, 47–59. [CrossRef]
42. Cherry, P.; Yadav, S.; O'Callaghan, C.; Popper, Z.A.; Ross, R.P.; McSorley, E.M.; Allsopp, P.J.; Stanton, C. In-vitro fermentation of whole seaweed and a polysaccharide-rich extract derived from the edible red seaweed *Palmaria palmata*. *Proc. Nutr. Soc.* **2016**, *75*, E57. [CrossRef]
43. Valado, A.; Pereira, M.; Caseiro, A.; Figueiredo, J.P.; Loureiro, H.; Almeida, C.; Cotas, J.; Pereira, L. Effect of Carrageenans on Vegetable Jelly in Humans with Hypercholesterolemia. *Mar. Drugs* **2019**, *18*, 19. [CrossRef]
44. Lattimer, J.M.; Haub, M.D. Effects of Dietary Fiber and Its Components on Metabolic Health. *Nutrients* **2010**, *2*, 1266–1289. [CrossRef]
45. Sundhar, S.; Shakila, R.J.; Jeyasekaran, G.; Aanand, S.; Shalini, R.; Arisekar, U.; Surya, T.; Malini, N.A.H.; Boda, S. Risk assessment of organochlorine pesticides in seaweeds along the Gulf of Mannar, Southeast India. *Mar. Pollut. Bull.* **2020**, *161*, 111709. [CrossRef]
46. Ahmed, D.A.E.A.; Gheda, S.F.; Ismail, G.A. Efficacy of two seaweeds dry mass in bioremediation of heavy metal polluted soil and growth of radish (*Raphanus sativus* L.) plant. *Environ. Sci. Pollut. Res.* **2020**. [CrossRef]
47. Costa, M.; Henriques, B.; Pinto, J.; Fabre, E.; Dias, M.; Soares, J.; Carvalho, L.; Vale, C.; Pinheiro-Torres, J.; Pereira, E. Influence of toxic elements on the simultaneous uptake of rare earth elements from contaminated waters by estuarine macroalgae. *Chemosphere* **2020**, *252*. [CrossRef] [PubMed]
48. Delcour, J.A.; Aman, P.; Courtin, C.M.; Hamaker, B.R.; Verbeke, K. Prebiotics, Fermentable Dietary Fiber, and Health Claims. *Adv. Nutr.* **2016**, *7*, 1–4. [CrossRef]
49. Sá Monteiro, M.; Sloth, J.; Holdt, S.; Hansen, M. Analysis and Risk Assessment of Seaweed. *EFSA J.* **2019**, *17*. [CrossRef]
50. Food and Drug Administration. *CFR—Code of Federal Regulations. Title 21: Food and Drugs. Electronic Code Federal Regulation*; FDA: Silver Spring, MD, USA, 2014.
51. APA—Agência Portuguesa do Ambiente. *Sistema de Classificação ele Macroalgas em Águas Costeiras*; APA: Lisbon, Portugal, 2007.
52. Pereira, L.; Mesquita, J.F. Carrageenophytes of occidental Portuguese coast: 1-spectroscopic analysis in eight carrageenophytes from Buarcos bay. *Biomol. Eng.* **2003**, *20*, 217–222. [CrossRef]
53. Pereira, L.; Critchley, A.T.; Amado, A.M.; Ribeiro-Claro, P.J.A. A comparative analysis of phycocolloids produced by underutilized versus industrially utilized carrageenophytes (Gigartinales, Rhodophyta). *J. Appl. Phycol.* **2009**, *21*, 599–605. [CrossRef]
54. Pereira, L.; Gheda, S.F.; Ribeiro-claro, P.J. a Analysis by Vibrational Spectroscopy of Seaweed Polysaccharides with Potential Use in Food, Pharmaceutical, and Cosmetic Industries. *Int. J. Carbohydr. Chem.* **2013**, 1–7. [CrossRef]
55. El Atouani, S.; Bentiss, F.; Reani, A.; Zrid, R.; Belattmania, Z.; Pereira, L.; Mortadi, A.; Cherkaoui, O.; Sabour, B. The invasive brown seaweed *Sargassum muticum* as new resource for alginate in Morocco: Spectroscopic and rheological characterization. *Phycol. Res.* **2016**, *64*, 185–193. [CrossRef]
56. Gómez-Ordóñez, E.; Rupérez, P. FTIR-ATR spectroscopy as a tool for polysaccharide identification in edible brown and red seaweeds. *Food Hydrocoll.* **2011**, *25*, 1514–1520. [CrossRef]
57. Pereira, L.; Amado, A.M.; Critchley, A.T.; van de Velde, F.; Ribeiro-Claro, P.J.A. Identification of selected seaweed polysaccharides (phycocolloids) by vibrational spectroscopy (FTIR-ATR and FT-Raman). *Food Hydrocoll.* **2009**, *23*, 1903–1909. [CrossRef]
58. Cotas, J.; Figueirinha, A.; Pereira, L.; Batista, T. The effect of salinity on *Fucus ceranoides* (Ochrophyta, Phaeophyceae) in the Mondego River (Portugal). *J. Oceanol. Limnol.* **2019**, *37*, 881–891. [CrossRef]
59. Pereira, L. Estudos em Macroalgas Carragenófitas (Gigartinales, Rhodophyceae) da Costa Portuguesa—Aspectos Ecológicos, Bioquímicos e Citológicos. Ph.D. Thesis, University of Coimbra, Coimbra, Portugal, 2004.
60. Zinoun, M.; Cosson, J. Seasonal variation in growth and carrageenan content of *Callibepharis jubata* (Rhodophyceae, Gigartinales) from the Normandy coast, France. *J. Appl. Phycol.* **1996**, *8*, 29–34. [CrossRef]
61. Araujo, G.S.; Cotas, J.; Morais, T.; Leandro, A.; García-Poza, S.; Gonçalves, A.M.M.; Pereira, L. *Callibepharis jubata* Cultivation Potential—A Comparative Study between Controlled and Semi-Controlled Aquaculture. *Appl. Sci.* **2020**, *10*, 7553. [CrossRef]
62. Guiry, M.; Guiry, G. Algaebase. Available online: https://www.algaebase.org/ (accessed on 28 December 2020).
63. Gioele, C.; Marilena, S.; Valbona, A.; Nunziacarla, S.; Andrea, S.; Antonio, M. *Gracilaria gracilis*, Source of Agar: A Short Review. *Curr. Org. Chem.* **2017**, *21*, 380–386. [CrossRef]
64. Pereira, L.; Sousa, A.; Coelho, H.; Amado, A.M.; Ribeiro-Claro, P.J.A. Use of FTIR, FT-Raman and 13C-NMR spectroscopy for identification of some seaweed phycocolloids. *Biomol. Eng.* **2003**, *20*, 223–228. [CrossRef]

65. Martín, L.A.; Rodríguez, M.C.; Matulewicz, M.C.; Fissore, E.N.; Gerschenson, L.N.; Leonardi, P.I. Seasonal variation in agar composition and properties from *Gracilaria gracilis* (Gracilariales, Rhodophyta) of the Patagonian coast of Argentina. *Phycol. Res.* **2013**, *61*, 163–171. [CrossRef]
66. Rodríguez, M.C.; Matulewicz, M.C.; Noseda, M.D.; Ducatti, D.R.B.; Leonardi, P.I. Agar from *Gracilaria gracilis* (Gracilariales, Rhodophyta) of the Patagonic coast of Argentina—Content, structure and physical properties. *Bioresour. Technol.* **2009**, *100*, 1435–1441. [CrossRef] [PubMed]
67. Sfriso, A.A.; Gallo, M.; Baldi, F. Seasonal variation and yield of sulfated polysaccharides in seaweeds from the Venice Lagoon. *Bot. Mar.* **2017**, *60*. [CrossRef]
68. Kraan, S. Sargassum muticum (Yendo) Fensholt in Ireland: An invasive species on the move. In *Nineteenth International Seaweed Symposium*; Springer: Dordrecht, The Netherlands, 2008; pp. 375–382.
69. Pacheco, D.; Araújo, G.S.; Cotas, J.; Gaspar, R.; Neto, J.M.; Pereira, L. Invasive Seaweeds in the Iberian Peninsula: A Contribution for Food Supply. *Mar. Drugs* **2020**, *18*, 560. [CrossRef] [PubMed]
70. Monteiro, C.; Engelen, A.H.; Serrão, E.A.; Santos, R. Habitat differences in the timing of reproduction of the invasive alga *Sargassum muticum* (Phaeophyta, Sargassaceae) over tidal and lunar cycles. *J. Phycol.* **2009**, *45*, 1–7. [CrossRef] [PubMed]
71. Incera, M.; Olabarria, C.; Cacabelos, E.; César, J.; Troncoso, J.S. Distribution of *Sargassum muticum* on the North West coast of Spain: Relationships with urbanization and community diversity. *Cont. Shelf. Res.* **2011**, *31*, 488–495. [CrossRef]
72. Belattmania, Z.; Kaidi, S.; El Atouani, S.; Katif, C.; Bentiss, F.; Jama, C.; Reani, A.; Sabour, B.; Vasconcelos, V. Isolation and FTIR-ATR and 1H NMR characterization of alginates from the main alginophyte species of the atlantic coast of Morocco. *Molecules* **2020**, *25*, 4335. [CrossRef]
73. Tuohy, K.M.; Probert, H.M.; Smejkal, C.W.; Gibson, G.R. Using probiotics and prebiotics to improve gut health. *Drug Discov. Today* **2003**, *8*, 692–700. [CrossRef]
74. Brown, E.M.; Allsopp, P.J.; Magee, P.J.; Gill, C.I.; Nitecki, S.; Strain, C.R.; McSorley, E.M. Seaweed and human health. *Nutr. Rev.* **2014**, *72*, 205–216. [CrossRef] [PubMed]
75. Rastall, R.A.; Gibson, G.R.; Gill, H.S.; Guarner, F.; Klaenhammer, T.R.; Pot, B.; Reid, G.; Rowland, I.R.; Sanders, M.E. Modulation of the microbial ecology of the human colon by probiotics, prebiotics and synbiotics to enhance human health: An overview of enabling science and potential applications. *FEMS Microbiol. Ecol.* **2005**, *52*, 145–152. [CrossRef] [PubMed]
76. Rowland, I. Optimal nutrition: Fibre and phytochemicals. *Proc. Nutr. Soc.* **1999**, *58*, 415–419. [CrossRef] [PubMed]
77. EFSA. Panel on Dietetic Products Scientific Opinion on the substantiation of health claims related to dietary fibre (ID 744, 745, 746, 748, 749, 753, 803, 810, 855, 1415, 1416, 4308, 4330) pursuant to Article 13(1) of Regulation (EC) No 1924/2006. *EFSA J.* **2010**, *8*, 1735. [CrossRef]
78. EFSA. Panel on Dietetic Products Scientific Opinion on the substantiation of health claims related to the replacement of mixtures of saturated fatty acids (SFAs) as present in foods or diets with mixtures of monounsaturated fatty acids (MUFAs) and/or mixtures of polyunsaturated fatty aci. *EFSA J.* **2011**, *9*, 2069. [CrossRef]
79. Clark, M.J.; Slavin, J.L. The Effect of Fiber on Satiety and Food Intake: A Systematic Review. *J. Am. Coll. Nutr.* **2013**, *32*, 200–211. [CrossRef]
80. Gibson, G.R.; Hutkins, R.; Sanders, M.E.; Prescott, S.L.; Reimer, R.A.; Salminen, S.J.; Scott, K.; Stanton, C.; Swanson, K.S.; Cani, P.D.; et al. Expert consensus document: The International Scientific Association for Probiotics and Prebiotics (ISAPP) consensus statement on the definition and scope of prebiotics. *Nat. Rev. Gastroenterol. Hepatol.* **2017**, *14*, 491–502. [CrossRef]
81. Weiner, M.L. Food additive carrageenan: Part II: A critical review of carrageenan *in vivo* safety studies. *Crit. Rev. Toxicol.* **2014**, *44*, 244–269. [CrossRef]
82. EFSA. Panel on Dietetic Products Scientific Opinion on Dietary Reference Values for carbohydrates and dietary fibre. *EFSA J.* **2010**, *8*. [CrossRef]
83. Cavalcante, D.; Garcia, M.; Aranha, M.; Almeida, A.; Merey, F.M.; do Amaral Crispim, B.; Barufatti, A.; Pisani, L.; Fonseca, G.; Braga, A.R.C.; et al. The controversial effects of dehydrated powder of *Gracilaria birdiae* as a food supplement to juvenile male rats. *J. Appl. Phycol.* **2021**. [CrossRef]
84. Kejžar, J.; Jagodic Hudobivnik, M.; Nečemer, M.; Ogrinc, N.; Masten Rutar, J.; Poklar Ulrih, N. Characterization of Algae Dietary Supplements Using Antioxidative Potential, Elemental Composition, and Stable Isotopes Approach. *Front. Nutr.* **2021**, *7*. [CrossRef] [PubMed]
85. Darias-Rosales, J.; Rubio, C.; Gutiérrez, Á.J.; Paz, S.; Hardisson, A. Risk assessment of iodine intake from the consumption of red seaweeds (*Palmaria palmata* and *Chondrus crispus*). *Environ. Sci. Pollut. Res.* **2020**, *27*, 45737–45741. [CrossRef] [PubMed]
86. Teas, J. *Dietary Seaweed and Breast Cancer: A Randomized Trial*; Clinical Trials.gov: Columbia, SC, USA, 2005.
87. Bliss, D.Z.; Savik, K.; Jung, H.-J.G.; Whitebird, R.; Lowry, A. Symptoms Associated With Dietary Fiber Supplementation Over Time in Individuals With Fecal Incontinence. *Nurs. Res.* **2011**, *60*, S58–S67. [CrossRef]
88. Milinovic, J.; Rodrigues, C.; Diniz, M.; Noronha, J.P. Determination of total iodine content in edible seaweeds: Application of inductively coupled plasma-atomic emission spectroscopy. *Algal Res.* **2021**, *53*, 102149. [CrossRef]
89. Krela-Kaźmierczak, I.; Czarnywojtek, A.; Skoracka, K.; Rychter, A.M.; Ratajczak, A.E.; Szymczak-Tomczak, A.; Ruchała, M.; Dobrowolska, A. Is There an Ideal Diet to Protect against Iodine Deficiency? *Nutrients* **2021**, *13*, 513. [CrossRef] [PubMed]
90. CEVA-Centre d'Étude & de Valorisation des Algues. *Edible Seaweed and Microalgae-Regulatory Status in France and Europe*; CEVA: Pleubian, France, 2019; Volume 11.

91. Sloth, J.J.; Holdt, S.L. Setting the standards for seaweed analysis. In *New Food*; Russell Publishing Ltd.: Kent, UK, 2021.
92. Paz, S.; Rubio, C.; Frías, I.; Luis-González, G.; Gutiérrez, Á.J.; González-Weller, D.; Hardisson, A. Human exposure assessment to macro- and trace elements in the most consumed edible seaweeds in Europe. *Environ. Sci. Pollut. Res.* **2019**, *26*, 36478–36485. [CrossRef]
93. Brownlee, I.A.; Allen, A.; Pearson, J.P.; Dettmar, P.W.; Havler, M.E.; Atherton, M.R.; Onsøyen, E. Alginate as a Source of Dietary Fiber. *Crit. Rev. Food Sci. Nutr.* **2005**, *45*, 497–510. [CrossRef] [PubMed]
94. Chater, P.I.; Wilcox, M.; Cherry, P.; Herford, A.; Mustar, S.; Wheater, H.; Brownlee, I.; Seal, C.; Pearson, J. Inhibitory activity of extracts of Hebridean brown seaweeds on lipase activity. *J. Appl. Phycol.* **2016**, *28*, 1303–1313. [CrossRef] [PubMed]
95. El Khoury, D.; Goff, H.D.; Anderson, G.H. The Role of Alginates in Regulation of Food Intake and Glycemia: A Gastroenterological Perspective. *Crit. Rev. Food Sci. Nutr.* **2015**, *55*, 1406–1424. [CrossRef] [PubMed]
96. Cherry, P.; Yadav, S.; Strain, C.R.; Allsopp, P.J.; Mcsorley, E.M.; Ross, R.P.; Stanton, C. Prebiotics from seaweeds: An ocean of opportunity? *Mar. Drugs* **2019**, *17*, 327. [CrossRef]
97. *Bioactive Seaweeds for Food Applications*; Qin, Y., Ed.; Elsevier: Amsterdam, The Netherlands, 2018; ISBN 9780128133125.
98. Liu, J.; Kandasamy, S.; Zhang, J.; Kirby, C.W.; Karakach, T.; Hafting, J.; Critchley, A.T.; Evans, F.; Prithiviraj, B. Prebiotic effects of diet supplemented with the cultivated red seaweed *Chondrus crispus* or with fructo-oligo-saccharide on host immunity, colonic microbiota and gut microbial metabolites. *BMC Complement. Altern. Med.* **2015**, *15*, 279. [CrossRef]
99. Huebbe, P.; Nikolai, S.; Schloesser, A.; Herebian, D.; Campbell, G.; Glüer, C.-C.; Zeyner, A.; Demetrowitsch, T.; Schwarz, K.; Metges, C.C.; et al. An extract from the Atlantic brown algae *Saccorhiza polyschides* counteracts diet-induced obesity in mice via a gut related multi-factorial mechanisms. *Oncotarget* **2017**, *8*, 73501–73515. [CrossRef]
100. Fu, X.; Cao, C.; Ren, B.; Zhang, B.; Huang, Q.; Li, C. Structural characterization and in vitro fermentation of a novel polysaccharide from *Sargassum thunbergii* and its impact on gut microbiota. *Carbohydr. Polym.* **2018**, *183*, 230–239. [CrossRef] [PubMed]
101. Charoensiddhi, S.; Conlon, M.A.; Vuaran, M.S.; Franco, C.M.M.; Zhang, W. Polysaccharide and phlorotannin-enriched extracts of the brown seaweed *Ecklonia radiata* influence human gut microbiota and fermentation in vitro. *J. Appl. Phycol.* **2017**, *29*, 2407–2416. [CrossRef]
102. Rioux, L.; Turgeon, S.L. Seaweed carbohydrates. In *Seaweed Sustainability: Food and Non-Food Applications*; Tiwari, B.K., Troy, D.J., Eds.; Academic Press: Cambridge, MA, USA, 2015; pp. 141–192, ISBN 9780124186972.
103. Padam, B.S.; Chye, F.Y. *Seaweed Components, Properties, and Applications*; Elsevier Inc.: Amsterdam, The Netherlands, 2020; ISBN 9780128179437.
104. Rasyid, A.; Ardiansyah, A.; Pangestuti, R. Nutrient Composition of Dried Seaweed *Gracilaria gracilis*. *ILMU Kelaut. Indones. J. Mar. Sci.* **2019**, *24*, 1. [CrossRef]
105. Rodrigues, D.; Freitas, A.C.; Pereira, L.; Rocha-Santos, T.A.P.; Vasconcelos, M.W.; Roriz, M.; Rodríguez-Alcalá, L.M.; Gomes, A.M.P.; Duarte, A.C. Chemical composition of red, brown and green macroalgae from Buarcos bay in Central West Coast of Portugal. *Food Chem.* **2015**, *183*, 197–207. [CrossRef]
106. Wells, M.L.; Potin, P.; Craigie, J.S.; Raven, J.A.; Merchant, S.S.; Helliwell, K.E.; Smith, A.G.; Camire, M.E.; Brawley, S.H. Algae as nutritional and functional food sources: Revisiting our understanding. *J. Appl. Phycol.* **2017**, *29*, 949–982. [CrossRef] [PubMed]
107. Weiner, M.L.; McKim, J.M. Comment on "Revisiting the carrageenan controversy: Do we really understand the digestive fate and safety of carrageenan in our foods?" by S. David, C.S. Levi, L. Fahoum, Y. Ungar, E.G. Meyron-Holtz, A. Shpigelman and U. Lesmes, *Food Funct.*, **2018**, *9*, 1344–1352. *Food Funct.* **2019**, *10*, 1760–1762. [CrossRef]
108. Tobacman, J.K. Review of harmful gastrointestinal effects of carrageenan in animal experiments. *Environ. Health Perspect.* **2001**, *109*, 983–994. [CrossRef] [PubMed]
109. Bixler, H.J. The carrageenan controversy. *J. Appl. Phycol.* **2017**, *29*, 2201–2207. [CrossRef]
110. Bhattacharyya, S.; Liu, H.; Zhang, Z.; Jam, M.; Dudeja, P.K.; Michel, G.; Linhardt, R.J.; Tobacman, J.K. Carrageenan-induced innate immune response is modified by enzymes that hydrolyze distinct galactosidic bonds. *J. Nutr. Biochem.* **2010**, *21*, 906–913. [CrossRef] [PubMed]
111. McKim, J.M. Food additive carrageenan: Part I: A critical review of carrageenan in vitro studies, potential pitfalls, and implications for human health and safety. *Crit. Rev. Toxicol.* **2014**, *44*, 211–243. [CrossRef] [PubMed]
112. Weiner, M.L. Parameters and pitfalls to consider in the conduct of food additive research, Carrageenan as a case study. *Food Chem. Toxicol.* **2016**, *87*, 31–44. [CrossRef]
113. Sokolova, E.V.; Bogdanovich, L.N.; Ivanova, T.B.; Byankina, A.O.; Kryzhanovskiy, S.P.; Yermak, I.M. Effect of carrageenan food supplement on patients with cardiovascular disease results in normalization of lipid profile and moderate modulation of immunity system markers. *PharmaNutrition* **2014**, *2*, 33–37. [CrossRef]
114. David, S.; Shani Levi, C.; Fahoum, L.; Ungar, Y.; Meyron-Holtz, E.G.; Shpigelman, A.; Lesmes, U. Revisiting the carrageenan controversy: Do we really understand the digestive fate and safety of carrageenan in our foods? *Food Funct.* **2018**, *9*, 1344–1352. [CrossRef]
115. McKim, J.M.; Willoughby, J.A.; Blakemore, W.R.; Weiner, M.L. Clarifying the confusion between poligeenan, degraded carrageenan, and carrageenan: A review of the chemistry, nomenclature, and in vivo toxicology by the oral route. *Crit. Rev. Food Sci. Nutr.* **2019**, *59*, 3054–3073. [CrossRef] [PubMed]
116. Kumar, M.S.; Sharma S.A. Toxicological effects of marine seaweeds: A cautious insight for human consumption. *Crit. Rev. Food Sci. Nutr.* **2021**, *61*, 500–521. [CrossRef]

117. Tanna, B.; Mishra, A. Nutraceutical Potential of Seaweed Polysaccharides: Structure, Bioactivity, Safety, and Toxicity. *Compr. Rev. Food Sci. Food Saf.* **2019**, *18*, 817–831. [CrossRef] [PubMed]
118. Pereira, L.; Cotas, J. Introductory Chapter: Alginates—A General Overview. In *Alginates—Recent Uses of This Natural Polymer*; IntechOpen: London, UK, 2020.
119. Aswathy, S.H.; Narendrakumar, U.; Manjubala, I. Commercial hydrogels for biomedical applications. *Heliyon* **2020**, *6*, e03719. [CrossRef] [PubMed]
120. Argudo, P.G.; Guzmán, E.; Lucia, A.; Rubio, R.G.; Ortega, F. Preparation and Application in Drug Storage and Delivery of Agarose Nanoparticles. *Int. J. Polym. Sci.* **2018**, *2018*, 1–9. [CrossRef]
121. Koenighofer, M.; Lion, T.; Bodenteich, A.; Prieschl-Grassauer, E.; Grassauer, A.; Unger, H.; Mueller, C.A.; Fazekas, T. Carrageenan nasal spray in virus confirmed common cold: Individual patient data analysis of two randomized controlled trials. *Multidiscip. Respir. Med.* **2014**, *9*, 57. [CrossRef]
122. Marais, D.; Gawarecki, D.; Allan, B.; Ahmed, K.; Altini, L.; Cassim, N.; Gopolang, F.; Hoffman, M.; Ramjee, G.; Williamson, A.-L. The effectiveness of Carraguard, a vaginal microbicide, in protecting women against high-risk human papillomavirus infection. *Antivir. Ther.* **2011**, *16*, 1219–1226. [CrossRef]
123. Sepantafar, M.; Maheronnaghsh, R.; Mohammadi, H.; Radmanesh, F.; Hasani-sadrabadi, M.M.; Ebrahimi, M.; Baharvand, H. Engineered Hydrogels in Cancer Therapy and Diagnosis. *Trends Biotechnol.* **2017**, *35*, 1074–1087. [CrossRef]
124. Popa, E.G.; Reis, R.L.; Gomes, M.E. Seaweed polysaccharide-based hydrogels used for the regeneration of articular cartilage. *Crit. Rev. Biotechnol.* **2015**, *35*, 410–424. [CrossRef] [PubMed]
125. Bilal, M.; Iqbal, H.M.N. Marine Seaweed Polysaccharides-Based Engineered Cues for the Modern Biomedical Sector. *Mar. Drugs* **2019**, *18*, 7. [CrossRef]
126. Carvalho, D.N.; Inácio, A.R.; Sousa, R.O.; Reis, R.L.; Silva, T.H. Seaweed polysaccharides as sustainable building blocks for biomaterials in tissue engineering. In *Sustainable Seaweed Technologies*; Elsevier: Amsterdam, The Netherlands, 2020; pp. 543–587.
127. Pereira, L. Seaweeds as Source of Bioactive Substances and Skin Care Therapy—Cosmeceuticals, Algotheraphy, and Thalassotherapy. *Cosmetics* **2018**, *5*, 68. [CrossRef]
128. Morais, T.; Cotas, J.; Pacheco, D.; Pereira, L. Seaweeds Compounds: An Ecosustainable Source of Cosmetic Ingredients? *Cosmetics* **2021**, *8*, 8. [CrossRef]
129. Beaumont, M.; Tran, R.; Vera, G.; Niedrist, D.; Rousset, A.; Pierre, R.; Shastri, V.P.; Forget, A. Hydrogel-Forming Algae Polysaccharides: From Seaweed to Biomedical Applications. *Biomacromolecules* **2021**, *22*, 1027–1052. [CrossRef]
130. Pacheco-Quito, E.-M.; Ruiz-Caro, R.; Veiga, M.-D. Carrageenan: Drug Delivery Systems and Other Biomedical Applications. *Mar. Drugs* **2020**, *18*, 583. [CrossRef] [PubMed]
131. Liu, L.; Heinrich, M.; Myers, S.; Dworjanyn, S.A. Towards a better understanding of medicinal uses of the brown seaweed *Sargassum* in Traditional Chinese Medicine: A phytochemical and pharmacological review. *J. Ethnopharmacol.* **2012**, *142*, 591–619. [CrossRef] [PubMed]
132. Pal, A.; Kamthania, M.C.; Kumar, A. Bioactive Compounds and Properties of Seaweeds—A Review. *OALib* **2014**, *01*, 1–17. [CrossRef]
133. Grassauer, A.; Weinmuellner, R.; Meier, C.; Pretsch, A.; Prieschl-Grassauer, E.; Unger, H. Iota-Carrageenan is a potent inhibitor of rhinovirus infection. *Virol. J.* **2008**, *5*, 107. [CrossRef] [PubMed]
134. Peñuela, A.; Bourgougnon, N.; Bedoux, G.; Robledo, D.; Madera-Santana, T.; Freile-Pelegrín, Y. Anti-Herpes simplex virus (HSV-1) activity and antioxidant capacity of carrageenan-rich enzymatic extracts from *Solieria filiformis* (Gigartinales, Rhodophyta). *Int. J. Biol. Macromol.* **2021**, *168*, 322–330. [CrossRef]
135. Wijesekara, I.; Pangestuti, R.; Kim, S.-K. Biological activities and potential health benefits of sulfated polysaccharides derived from marine algae. *Carbohydr. Polym.* **2011**, *84*, 14–21. [CrossRef]
136. Silva, T.H.; Alves, A.; Ferreira, B.M.; Oliveira, J.M.; Reys, L.L.; Ferreira, R.J.F.; Sousa, R.A.; Silva, S.S.; Mano, J.F.; Reis, R.L. Materials of marine origin: A review on polymers and ceramics of biomedical interest. *Int. Mater. Rev.* **2012**, *57*, 276–306. [CrossRef]
137. Pereira, L. Biological and therapeutic properties of the seaweed polysaccharides. *Int. Biol. Rev.* **2018**, *2*. [CrossRef]
138. Zhong, H.; Gao, X.; Cheng, C.; Liu, C.; Wang, Q.; Han, X. The Structural Characteristics of Seaweed Polysaccharides and Their Application in Gel Drug Delivery Systems. *Mar. Drugs* **2020**, *18*, 658. [CrossRef]
139. Roy, D.; Cambre, J.N.; Sumerlin, B.S. Future perspectives and recent advances in stimuli-responsive materials. *Prog. Polym. Sci.* **2010**, *35*, 278–301. [CrossRef]
140. Lee, K.Y.; Mooney, D.J. Alginate: Properties and biomedical applications. *Prog. Polym. Sci.* **2012**, *37*, 106–126. [CrossRef]
141. Li, H.; Yu, X.; Jin, Y.; Zhang, W.; Liu, Y. Development of an eco-friendly agar extraction technique from the red seaweed *Gracilaria lemaneiformis*. *Bioresour. Technol.* **2008**, *99*, 3301–3305. [CrossRef] [PubMed]
142. Pereira, L.; Van De Velde, F. Portuguese carrageenophytes: Carrageenan composition and geographic distribution of eight species (Gigartinales, Rhodophyta). *Carbohydr. Polym.* **2011**, *84*, 614–623. [CrossRef]
143. Sivagnanavelmurugan, M.; Radhakrishnan, S.; Palavesam, A.; Arul, V.; Immanuel, G. Characterization of alginic acid extracted from *Sargassum wightii* and determination of its anti-viral activity of shrimp *Penaeus monodon* post larvae against white spot syndrome virus. *Int. J. Curr. Res. Life Sci.* **2018**, *7*, 1863–1872.

144. García-Poza, S.; Leandro, A.; Cotas, C.; Cotas, J.; Marques, J.C.; Pereira, L.; Gonçalves, A.M.M. The Evolution Road of Seaweed Aquaculture: Cultivation Technologies and the Industry 4.0. *Int. J. Environ. Res. Public Health* **2020**, *17*, 6528. [CrossRef] [PubMed]
145. Hwang, E.K.; Yotsukura, N.; Pang, S.J.; Su, L.; Shan, T.F. Seaweed breeding programs and progress in eastern Asian countries. *Phycologia* **2019**, *58*, 484–495. [CrossRef]
146. Kim, J.K.; Yarish, C.; Hwang, E.K.; Park, M.; Kim, Y. Seaweed aquaculture: Cultivation technologies, challenges and its ecosystem services. *ALGAE* **2017**, *32*, 1–13. [CrossRef]
147. Hwang, E.K.; Park, C.S. Seaweed cultivation and utilization of Korea. *ALGAE* **2020**, *35*, 107–121. [CrossRef]
148. Abbott, D.W.; Aasen, I.M.; Beauchemin, K.A.; Grondahl, F.; Gruninger, R.; Hayes, M.; Huws, S.; Kenny, D.A.; Krizsan, S.J.; Kirwan, S.F.; et al. Seaweed and Seaweed Bioactives for Mitigation of Enteric Methane: Challenges and Opportunities. *Animals* **2020**, *10*, 2432. [CrossRef] [PubMed]

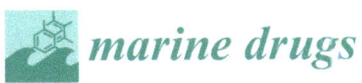

Review

Microalgal Peloids for Cosmetic and Wellness Uses

M. Lourdes Mourelle *, Carmen P. Gómez and José L. Legido

FA2 Research Group, Applied Physics Department, University of Vigo, 36310 Vigo, Spain; carmengomez@uvigo.es (C.P.G.); xllegido@uvigo.es (J.L.L.)
* Correspondence: lmourelle@uvigo.es; Tel.: +34-696413531

Abstract: Peloids have been used for therapeutic purposes since time immemorial, mainly in the treatment of locomotor system pathologies and dermatology. Their effects are attributed to their components, i.e., to the properties and action of mineral waters, clays, and their biological fraction, which may be made up of microalgae, cyanobacteria, and other organisms present in water and clays. There are many studies on the therapeutic use of peloids made with microalgae/cyanobacteria, but very little research has been done on dermocosmetic applications. Such research demonstrates their potential as soothing, regenerating, antioxidant, anti-inflammatory, and antimicrobial agents. In this work, a method for the manufacture of a dermocosmetic peloid is presented based on the experience of the authors and existing publications, with indications for its characterization and study of its efficacy.

Keywords: peloids; microalgae; cyanobacteria; cosmetics; dermocosmetics; mineral water; seawater

1. Introduction

Peloids are therapeutic agents used in spas and thalassotherapy centers since time immemorial, mainly for treatment of osteo-articular and dermatological disorders, sports injuries, and generally in rehabilitation programs. Their use in cosmetics also dates back a long time, especially the ones made from clays, which are used in wellness programs and thermal spa centres nowadays [1].

Peloids are comprised of a solid fraction that includes various sediments, clays and peat, and a liquid fraction that can be either mineral-medicinal water (mineral water), seawater, or salt/brackish lake water. A biological fraction, consisting of microbiota present in mineral-medicinal water, clays, peat or sediments, and the microorganisms that thrive in the mixture during the peloid maturation processes, can also be present [2]. It is precisely during this maturation process (prolonged contact between solid substrate and liquid) that the different biological action compounds, partly responsible for the therapeutic actions, are formed [3].

Peloids either form "in situ" through contact between the mineral-medicinal water and the sediments surrounding it or are prepared artificially by mixing the above components [4]. When preparing peloids artificially, the biological fraction (microalgae and cyanobacteria) is usually from the natural mineral-medicinal water, while in the case of marine silt peloids, it is from cultivated microalgae; maturation times vary from 1–18 months but usually do not exceed 3 months [5]. According to Gomes et al. (2013), peloids can be classified regarding their origin, composition, and applications into "natural peloid" or "peloid *sensu strictu*"; "inorganic," "organic," or "mixed peloids"; and "medical" or "cosmetic" peloids (Figure 1) [4]. During the 3rd Symposium on Thermal Mud, held in 2004 in Dax, it was agreed to distinguish between the two main types of peloids: (i) muds or clays that are just mixed with mineral water with no maturation process—the extemporaneous or prepared *ad hoc* peloids—and (ii) muds or clays mixed with mineral water, including naturally or artificially matured peloids. Figures 2–5 show two different types of natural-maturation and artificial-maturation peloids [4].

In order to evaluate peloid suitability for therapeutic and cosmetic purposes, the thermal properties of the mixtures like density, specific heat, thermal conductivity, and retention capacity are studied, as well as other properties related to applicability such as viscosity and pH [6].

Applicability, spreadability, user, and efficacy tests should be performed when used in dermocosmetics and/or wellness programs in thermal spas and thalassotherapy centres. Marketing of cosmetic peloids must comply with national legislation, which usually includes safety reports, user and efficacy tests, etc.

Thermal spas and wellness centers seldom use microalgae peloids in dermocosmetics, which is why this study reviewed such peloids and proposed a method for their manufacture. Therefore, the intention was to encourage spas to manufacture their own products for use in cosmetic and wellness applications through the required research and experience.

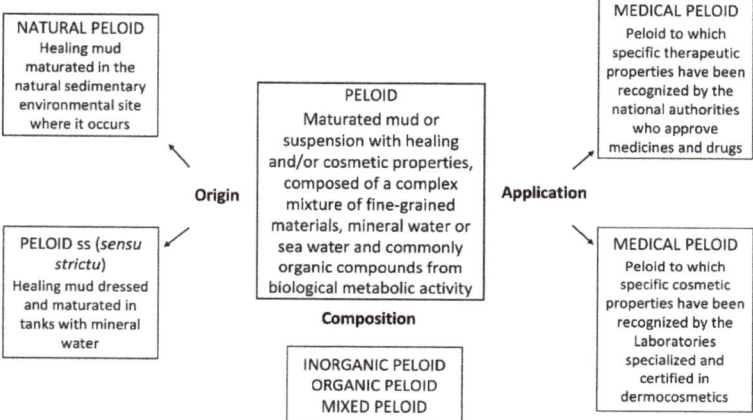

Figure 1. Peloid classification with regard to origin, composition, and applications (from Gomes et al. 2013).

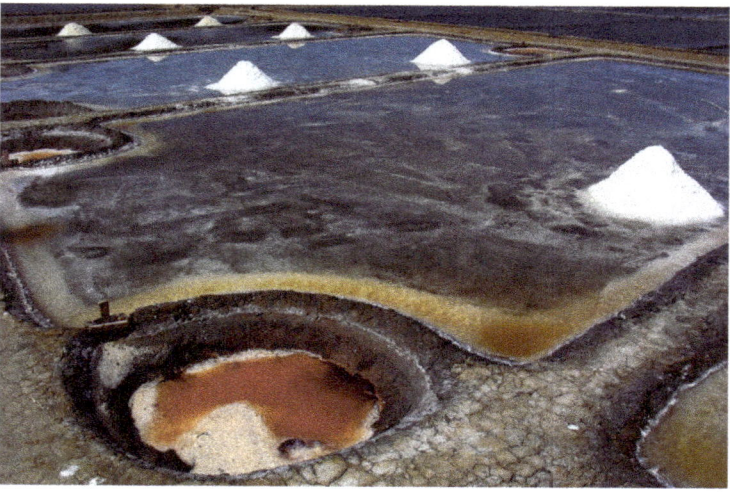

Figure 2. Natural maturation peloid (saline mud from Sečovlje salt pans, Sečovlje Nature Park, Slovenia).

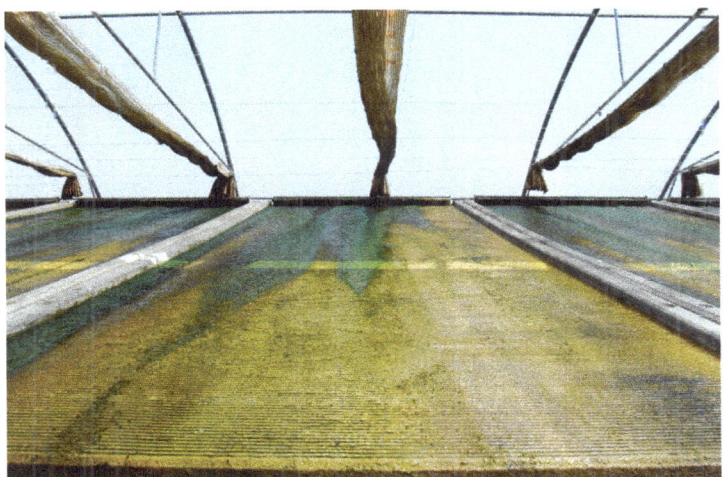

Figure 3. Cyanobacteria cultivation for peloid preparation (Dax, France).

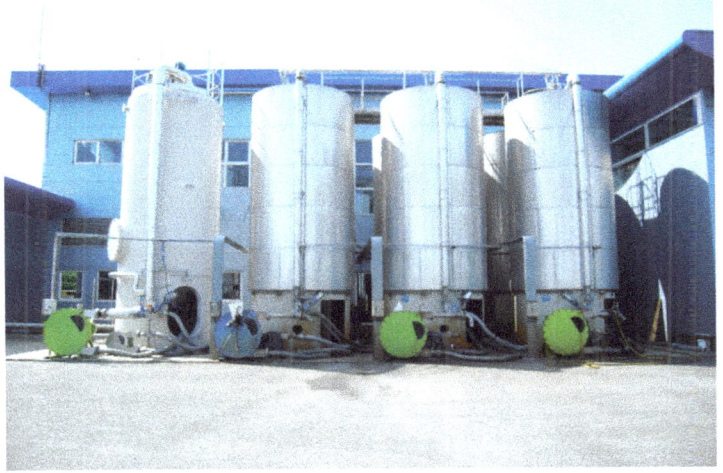

Figure 4. Tanks for artificial peloid maturation (Dax, France).

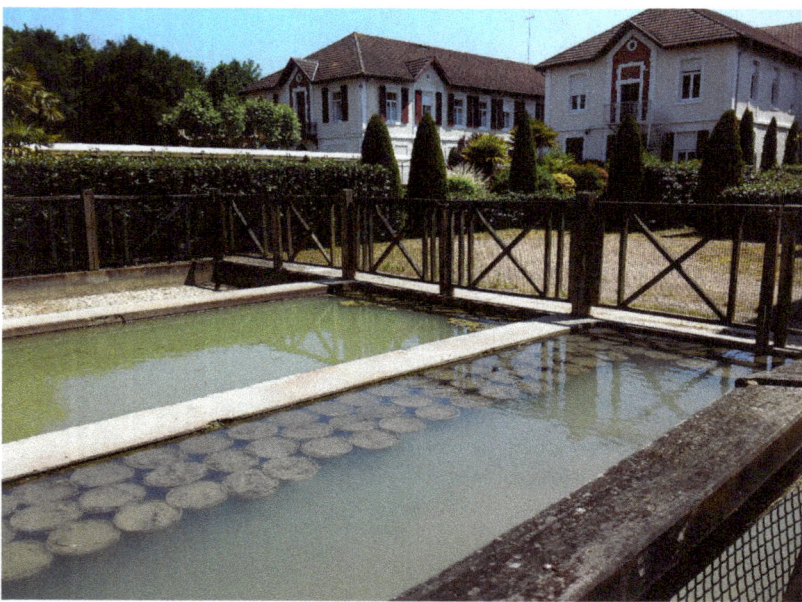

Figure 5. Thermal mud maturation (Dax, France).

2. Peloids for Dermocosmetics and Wellness

For this review, SciFinder, Pubmed, Web of Science, and Scopus databases were reviewed up to September 2021. Search terms included "pelotherapy," "mud therapy," "peloids and skin," "thermal mud," "microalgae and thermal water," "cyanobacteria and thermal water," mud and cosmetics," "mud and dermocosmetics," "mineral water and skin," and "seawater and skin".

Although frequently used empirically, peloids have important cosmetic actions, which are linked to the improvement of skin hydration, the removal of flaking cells, and the prevention of aging [7–9]. Traditionally, the types of peloids most used in cosmetics are volcanic, sulphurous, and chlorinated bromo-iodics, but this also includes peat due to its content of fulvic and ulmic acids [7].

There is also evidence of their action in treating dermatological diseases such as psoriasis and other skin disorders, an example being that of Dead Sea peloids [10], in which it has been observed to reduce all skin symptoms of this disease (PASI index) [11] when combined with Dead Sea water and phototherapy. This water is furthermore observed to have antimicrobial action [12], an aspect of interest in the treatment of related dermatological alterations such as dermatitis. Other studies have shown that these muds can improve wound healing [13]. The effects of biogleas in thermal muds from Guardia Piemontese-Acquappesa were studied and found to significantly reduce desquamation, erythema, and itching in psoriasis [14].

Similar muds used in skin disorder applications are the Peruíbe muds [15] for psoriasis, dermatitis, acne, and seborrhoea. Peloids from Balaruc-les-Bains have been recently used for their anti-inflammatory, antioxidant, and healing properties [16]. Additionally, Spilioti et al. (2017) investigated the anti-inflammatory properties of 13 mud samples from Greek spa resorts by assessing their effect on the expression of the adhesion molecules ICAM-1 and VCAM-1 by endothelial cells as well as their effects on monocyte adhesion to activated endothelial cells. Most of the mud extracts used in the study inhibited TNF-a-induced expression of VCAM-1 by endothelial cells but showed little alteration on ICAM1 expression. Interestingly, the majority of the examined mud extracts markedly reduced monocyte adhesion to activated endothelial cells indicating a potent anti-inflammatory activity [17].

In terms of peloid composition for cosmetic and welfare purposes, many studies attribute their curative properties to their clay (less frequently peat or sapropels), mineral and trace elements content, and to the presence of microalgae and cyanobacteria.

2.1. Clays and Dermocosmetic Peloids

The use of clays in the preparation of peloids and dermocosmetic products have been studied by a great number of authors [1,3,18–27]. The main phyllosilicates present in most peloids are smectites, kaolinite, illite, illite–smectite mixed layers, and chlorite in different proportions [21].

Although there are fewer studies published on the composition of sapropels from Lake Techirghiol in Romania [28] and from lakes in Latvia, there are some studies that evaluate their potential medicinal and cosmetic use [29].

A comparative physico-chemical composition study of muds from different areas in the Homogeneous Euganean Hills Hydromineral Basin (B.I.O.C.E.) (Italy) reported the composition of peloids as "clayey-silt" (65.42% silt and 24.62% clay) and "silty-clay" (64.37% clay and 34.41% silt). Their heavy metal content was studied by comparison with commercial cosmetic mud and was found to be higher than in commercial mud; however, no allergic reactions were detected. A proposal to establish a protocol for effective control of these types of natural products has been put forward [30].

2.2. Minerals and Trace Elements in Dermocosmetic Peloids

Peloids for dermocosmetic and wellness applications are characterised by their varied composition in minerals and trace elements. The moisturising, soothing, and regenerating properties of the Dead Sea mud are attributed to a high magnesium content [31], which is well known for its anti-inflammatory and antiphlogistic effects and for its capacity to inhibit the polyamines involved in psoriasis pathogenesis [7]. Dead Sea mud also exhibits antimicrobial action, which is attributed to the high salt and sulphide concentrations plus its low pH, and it is therefore used in the treatment of acne [31].

In the case of the above-mentioned Peruíbe peloids, Da Silva-Cardosc et al. (2015) noted that the mud is enriched with Br, Cr, Sb, SE, and Zn ions during the maturation process and that these may be responsible for their anti-inflammatory properties [15,32].

2.3. Microalgae and Cyanobacteria in Dermocosmetic Peloids

One of the most outstanding and studied characteristics of peloids is their content in microalgae and cyanobacteria, which seem to exert a great influence on their cosmetic properties, since they have been proven to generate biologically active substances (especially during the maturation process), which in turn are responsible for the beneficial effects and actions on the skin [33].

There is abundant recent scientific literature on the biological fraction of peloids, and worth highlighting among them are studies on Euganea basin muds in the Spa area of Abano Terme (Italy). Thus, Ceschi-Berrini et al. in 2004 [34] described the presence of the genus *Phormidium* in thermal waters of the Euganea basin and subsequently identified the presence of acylglycerolipids produced by the aforementioned cyanobacteria, which appeared to confer therapeutic and cosmetic properties to the mud [35]. In a study of microbial diversity in the same area, Moro et al. (2007) [36] described a new species of Cyanoprokaryote called *Cyanobacterium aponinum* in the microbial mats of Euganean thermal springs. Subsequently, Poli et al. (2009) [37] described a thermophilic bacterium in the mud from this thermal basin that they called *Anoxybacillus thermarum*, which provides an idea of the special characteristics of the biological composition of these muds. Additional studies by Moro et al. (2010) expanded the biodiversity of these muds to species of the genus *Leptolyngbya* and *Spirulina* (now *Arthrospira*), suggesting that the cyanobacterial composition of phototrophic mats in the rather unusual environment of the Euganean

Thermal District is variable, depending on the physico-chemical features of the different thermal spa waters. In fact, surveys carried out on 90 thermal spas suggest that the cyanobacterial diversity might be related to thermal mud processing in the different maturation tanks with thermal waters at different temperatures [38].

Research on the biological composition and organic matter present in the different maturation stages of Abano muds showed the presence of saturated and unsaturated fatty acids, hydroxyl acids, dicarboxylic acids, ketoacids, and alcohols and an increase in the lipid profile during the maturation process that peaked at six months. The presence of diatoms from clays was observed at the start of maturation; however, cyanobacteria belonging to the Oscillatoriales subsection progressively colonized the mud throughout maturation [39].

Centini et al. [40] recently analyzed the composition and antioxidant capacity of biogleas present in the Satunia Terme mud and confirmed earlier findings on the increased lipid profile during the maturation process and analyzed the hydrophilic fraction. Studies on antioxidant power revealed that bottom mud extracts are more active than surface extracts and that hydrophilic extracts are more active than lipid extracts.

A comprehensive study using more than 650 mud samples from 29 places in the Abano area compared mineralogical and geological parameter variations with chlorophyll A in sludge during the mud maturation and recycling process. The conclusion was that chlorophyll A is converted into its derivatives and generates molecules that pass to the matured mud. Such a decrease in the chlorophyll A amount warrants maturation to take place in open tanks in order to maintain the photosynthetic process and to ensure that the amount of chlorophyll A and its derivatives continue to be sensitive to the supply of fresh mud [41]. Subsequent research by Gris et al. (2020) on the same muds (Euganean Thermal Muds) confirmed that the predominant species is *Phormidium* sp. and that diversity is greater when the temperature is 37–47 °C. At lower and higher temperatures, populations lose stability, thus exhibiting a significant change in species composition, low biodiversity, and low cyanobacterial abundance [42]. Zampieri et al. (2020) likewise noted the anti-inflammatory activity of exopolyssacharides from *Phormidium* sp present in the Abano muds [43].

Studies carried out on mud from Pausilya Therme di Donn'Anna (Italy) revealed antimicrobial capacity and identified seven taxa of green algae, two taxa of cyanobacteria, and even diatom taxa. In terms of the microalgae community, mud samples ripened for 6 months (6-month mud) presented a higher biodiversity compared to mud allowed to ripen for 1 month (1-month mud). The most abundant benthic microalgae taxa, identified in both samples and isolated exclusively from ripened mud, are *Chlorella* sp., *Coccomyxa* sp., *Scenedesmus* sp., *Leptolyngbya* sp., *Anabaena* sp., *Cocconeis placentula*, *Rhoicosphenia abbreviata* and *Navicula cincta*. *Nostoc* sp., *Scenedesmus* sp., *Chlamydomonas* sp., *Pseudococcomyxa simplex*, *Monodus* sp., *Gomphonema acuminatum*, *Amphora ovalis*, and *Nitzschia palea* [44].

In a like manner, the microbiological diversity of waters and muds from Sirmione Terme was characterised (using next-generation sequencing technology) by studying the different mud maturation stages: young (2-month old), intermediate (4-month old), and mature (6-month old). The results showed that three genera predominate: *Pelobacter*, *Desulfomonile*, and *Thiobacillus* and that *Pelobacter* levels increase during maturation while those of *Desulfomonile* and *Thiobacillus* decrease. The increase in phospholipid and sulpho- glycolipid fraction of mature muds reported by other authors [45] was attributed to *Pelobacter* by these authors.

Muds from Balaruc-les-Bains (France) have also been analyzed to study the molecules responsible for their antioxidant, anti-inflammatory, and healing properties. Nine strains were analyzed and although no antioxidant activity was detected, a strong anti-inflammatory potential was observed for *Planktothricoides raciborskii*, *Nostoc* sp., and *Pseudo-chroococcus couteii*, and a slight wound-healing function was detected in extracts from *Aliinostoc* sp. [46], which is an activity of great interest in dermocosmetic and well-being treatments. Recent studies using morphological, ultrastructural, and molecular methods clearly identified the nine cyanobacterial isolates from the Thermes de Balaruc-Les-Bains muds as belonging to the orders Chroococcales: *Pseudochroococcus coutei*; Synechococcales: *Leptolyngbya boryana*; Oscillatoriales: *Planktothricoides raciborskii, Laspinema* sp., *Microcoleus vaginatus*, and *Lyngbya martensiana*; and Nostocales: *Nostoc* sp., *Aliinostoc* sp., and *Dulcicalothrix* sp. [47,48].

Dead Sea muds are well known for their use in the treatment of psoriasis [49]. They are high-salinity muds in which nine extremely halotolerant Bacillus species have been identified, one of them being *B. Paralicheniformis*, which confer a high antimicrobial action [50]. Subsequent studies have confirmed the antimicrobial property of *Bacillus persicusi* against different Gram+ and Gram− pathogens [51].

Organic fractions of mud from other environments have also been studied. Dolmaa et al. (2017) studied silty mud containing sulphide from Noggon Lake (Mongolia) and found that soluble organic matter contains a high percentage of hydrocarbons and their derivatives (33.68%) and that the lipid group contains fat-soluble vitamins including vitamins A, D, E, and their derivatives, plus steroids, which the authors relate to therapeutic and cosmetic properties [52].

Bigovic et al. (2019) examined the organic composition of Igalo Bay peloids (Montenegro), and they found them to mostly contain (saturated and unsaturated) fatty acids as well as essential amino acids, many of which have significant physiological, medical, and pharmaceutical properties [53].

Research carried out on the mineral peloids from Mariánské Lázne (Czech Republic) reported a new species of the genus *Aquitalea* (previously identified in humic lakes and peat marshes), which they called *Aquitalea pelogenes* ("derived or generated from mud"). They also found a profile of quinones and fatty acids upon analyzing the dry biomass. The polar lipids detected were diphosphatidylglycerol, phosphatidylethanolamine, phosphatidylglycerol, two unidentified phospholipids, and one unidentified aminophospholipid, to which the authors attributed the therapeutic properties [54].

Other studies reported changes in the microbial community composition of the peloid throughout maturation, wherein main changes take place in the early stages, with there being hardly any change between 3 and 6 months [55].

2.4. Safety of Peloids for Application in Dermocosmetics

Given that peloids are applied topically and in many cases on skin with dermatological disorders, their safety must be monitored for the possible presence of trace toxic metals and pathogenic microorganisms.

Ma'or et al. (2015) studied the safety of Dead Sea muds used in cosmetics, by evaluating traces of nickel and chrome, and concluded that nickel and chrome concentrations measured in the mud are safe for human health insofar as systemic toxicity is concerned. They also observed that skin exposure to nickel and chrome is much lower since both metals mainly attach to the clay components in mud and are not easily released into the aquatic solution. The use of Dead Sea mud is not recommended for Ni^-- or Cr^--sensitive persons [56].

Recently, Pavlovska et al. (2017) recommended testing in natural peloids (to be used as a raw material for pharmaceutical applications) not only heavy metals but also pesticides such as chlororganics, which are widely used as effective help to combat unwanted plant pests and pathogens and which have bioaccumulation and bioconcentration capabilities [29].

To ensure the quality and safety of the peloids, some properties should be determined; the most common are granulometry, plasticity, CEC and exchangeable cations, water content, pH, specific surface area, swelling power and swelling index, abrasiveness, density, rheological properties (viscosity), and thermal properties such as: specific heat capacity, thermal conductivity, thermal diffusivity, and thermal retentivity. For cosmetic uses could be also of interest to determine the parameters of hardness, springiness, adhesiveness, and cohesiveness, which are related to their visco-elastic properties [3]. From the microbiological quality and hygiene perspective, microbiological analyses such as total viable count (TVC), total coliforms, *E. coli*, enterococci, *S. aureus*, *P. aeruginosa*, and sulfite-reducing clostridia and dermatophytes fungi, must also be carried out [57].

3. Proposal for a Procedure to Manufacture Microalgae Peloids

This work puts forward a method that uses clays, microalgae/cyanobacteria, and mineral-medicinal water or seawater to manufacture peloids for use in cosmetics and in health and wellness programs at wellness centers.

Such peloids can be manufactured in the thermal spa itself for use with patients on the premises. Some examples of use in Europe are Abano Terme and Montecatini Terme (Italy), Dax Thermes, Eugenie-les-Bains or Barèges (France), Bad Bayersoien (Germany), and the thermal spas of Archena, Bohí, and El Raposo in Spain, these being mainly used to treat rheumatology and locomotor system disorders. Worth highlighting in Spain are the spas at Isla de la Toja and Balneario de Compostela that manufacture their own peloids for use in dermatology and dermocosmetics, with interesting results in psoriasis and dermatitis [58,59]. In such cases, the peloid is considered as a spa product derived from mineral-medicinal water and is governed by the spa legislation of each country. An example is shown in Figure 6.

However, if the product is destined for marketing as a cosmetic product, it is governed by cosmetic regulations. REGULATION (EC) No 1223/2009 OF THE EUROPEAN PARLIAMENT AND OF THE COUNCIL of 30 November 2009 on cosmetic products (https://eur-lex.europa.eu/legal-content/EN/TXT/?uri=CELEX:02009R1223-20190813 accessed on 21 October 2021) defines the stages involved in the manufacture and marketing of a cosmetic product in Europe, including the lifecycle of a cosmetic product, from its conception in R&D laboratories to the monitoring of its effects and effectiveness after marketing.

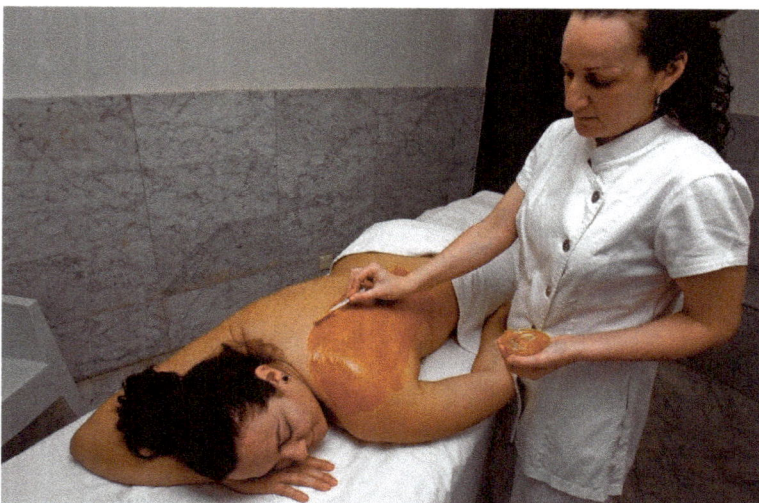

Figure 6. Manufactured peloid; application for psoriasis and dermatological conditions (La Toja thermal spa, Pontevedra, Spain).

3.1. Composition of a Peloid

A peloid is comprised of a solid fraction or substrate made of clays, sediments, or peat and a liquid fraction made of mineral-medicinal water, seawater, or brackish/salt-lake water, and it may contain a biological fraction from the water or the solid substrate [2,8]. When manufacturing peloids for dermocosmetic purposes, one should use high-quality clays to guarantee safety and effectiveness on skins, which in many cases are damaged. Their composition is shown in Figure 7.

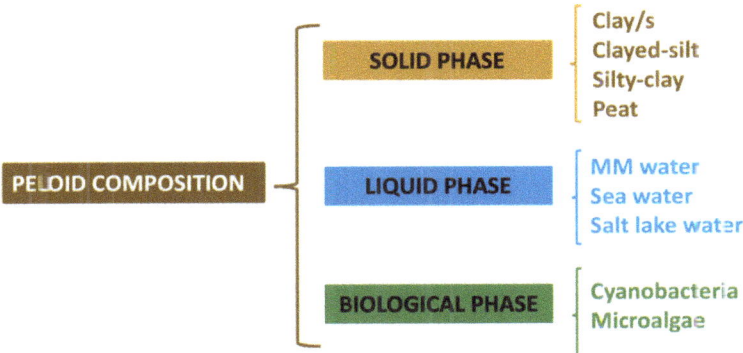

Figure 7. Composition of a peloid (MM: mineral-medicinal).

3.1.1. Solid Substrate: Clays

As indicated earlier, the solid component of a peloid can be diverse. In order to achieve good thermo-physical characteristics and applicability, we propose the use of clays containing smectite (bentonite) and kaolinite, since the former have very good plastic properties [21] and the latter help regulate skin secretions and the final pH of the mixtures [8].

3.1.2. Solid Substrate: Mineral-Medicinal Water and Seawater

Each mineral-medicinal water is unique and thus the first step is gaining knowledge of its chemical composition, including the majority and trace elements, as well as physico-chemical characteristics such as pH, electrical conductivity, and the possible presence of dissolved gases.

All mineral-medicinal waters must be analyzed periodically to guarantee quality before and during their application in spas, as provided for in the legislation of the different countries. This is why all of them are analyzed and quality is guaranteed. However, given that often only the major elements are analyzed, it is of utmost importance to analyze the trace elements when developing peloids for cosmetic us since their dermocosmetic potential lies in them [60]. Table 1 summarizes the principal majority and trace elements in mineral-medicinal waters of interest for the manufacture of cosmetic products.

Table 1. Majority and trace elements in mineral-medicinal waters that have an effect on the skin (Mourelle & Gómez, 2015).

Chemical Element	Effect on the Skin
Calcium	Effect on proteins that regulate cell divisions: calmodulin and cellular retinoic-acid-binding protein (CRAB) Catalysing action of differentiation enzymes: transglutaminase, protease, and phospholipases Indispensable for regulating permeability of cell membranes Regulation of proliferation and differentiation of keratinocytes
Sulphur	Cell regenerator, keratolytic/keratoplastic (dose-dependent) Antibacterial, antifungal
Magnesium	Inhibits synthesis of some polyamines involved in psoriasis pathogenesis at concentrations of 5×10^{-4}, and its reduction by magnesium improves disease condition Anti-inflammatory, antiphlogistic Catalyses synthesis of nucleic acids and proteins Catalyses ATP production Produces sedation in the central nervous system
Chloride	Fluid balance of tissues
Sodium	Fluid balance of tissues

Table 1. *Cont.*

Copper	Anti-inflammatory, immune system maintenance
Chromium	Enzymatic activator
Fluorine	Energy supply in keratinocytes
Manganese	Immune system modulator
Nickel	Stimulates cell development in tissues
Zinc	Antioxidant; prevents ageing; healing and regeneration of skin tissues
Silicon	Involved in collagen and elastin synthesis and cell metabolism Present in colloidal silica form in many mineral waters used in dermatology Has a dermoabrasive and emollient effect on psoriatic plaques

3.1.3. Microalgae and Cyanobacteria

They are one of the differential components in a peloid; and given that each mineral-medicinal water is unique, one needs to study the type of microalgae/cyanobacteria present therein. The plankton composition in seawater differs through latitudes unlike the composition of seawater, which is similar at all latitudes, and hence one needs to study the type of microalgae present in a particular environment.

We therefore propose that microalgae/cyanobacteria cultures be sourced from the mineral-medicinal waters or seawater, by means of a process adapted to the characteristics of each species or genus predominant therein. The culture process includes growth in an appropriate medium (mineral-medicinal or seawater) with the necessary nutrients and light stimulation depending on the type of species (Figure 8).

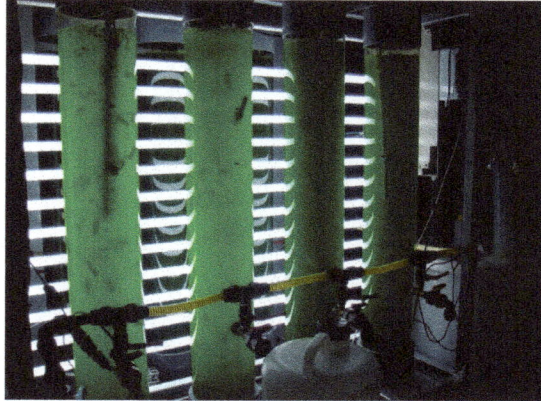

Figure 8. Photobioreactor with microalgae (cultivation at FA2 lab; Applied Physics Department; University of Vigo).

3.2. Preparation of a Dermocosmetic Peloid with Microalgae

The process of preparing a peloid with microalgae or cyanobacteria involves a few prior stages in which raw materials are first studied before carrying out tests on the mixtures. The stages are summarised in Figure 9 and in the following subsections: (i) selection of raw materials (clays, thermal waters, and microalgae cyanobacteria); (ii) characterization of raw materials (different test and determinations to asess its suitability and optimal properties); (iii) preparation and testing mixtures (using different proportions of the raw materials); (iv) characterization of the peloid sample (including maturation process if necessary); and (v) use and effectiveness test.

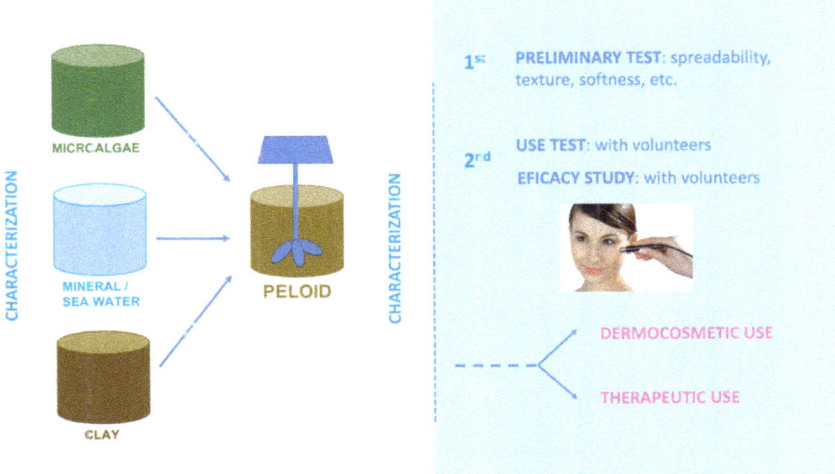

Figure 9. Peloid manufacture: procedure and test.

3.2.1. Selection of Raw Materials

Raw materials or initial materials (clays, microalgae, and waters) are selected for the intended purposes. Given that the peloid is intended for dermocosmetic and/or welfare uses the clays selected must be of a high quality and have an affinity for the skin (kaolinites, bentonites, etc.). The water used is the one present at the spa: mineral-medicinal water (or seawater), and the microalgae/cyanobacteria can either be those present at the thermal spa or the thalassotherapy center, but others acquired lyophilized or frozen can also be used.

3.2.2. Characterization of Raw Materials

All raw materials must be properly characterised. The most frequent tests performed on clays are mineralogical analysis; chemical composition; granulometry; SEM study; swelling; cation exchange capacity and exchangeable cations; percentage of water, solids, and ash; and differential thermal analysis and thermogravimetry [6,21,61–63].

The spa water or seawater must also be analyzed to study the majority and trace elements, in addition to other physico-chemical analyses. The most important parameters are temperature, electrical conductivity, dry residue, turbidity, cations and anions, dissolved gases, radioactivity, hardness, and alkalinity. One also needs to study properties such as density, thermal conductivity, specific heat, viscosity, and thermal diffusivity [63–65].

It is furthermore important to characterize microalgae or cyanobacteria and undertake studies to isolate and obtain a mono-specific and clonal culture. The sample is characterized through a chemical analysis, determination of crystalline phases, and by studying its composition (proteins, lipids, carbohydrates, vitamins, etc.) [66].

3.2.3. Preparation and Testing of Mixtures

Mixtures are prepared using different proportions of the three raw materials and tested for texture, spreadability, ease of application, etc.

The mixtures are then selected, characterized, and subject to use and efficacy tests.

3.2.4. Characterization of the Peloid Sample

The most common analyses carried out on the sample of the selected peloid or mixture are density, thermal conductivity, specific heat, viscosity, rheological behavior, and thermal diffusivity [62,65,67,68]. For a peloid to be suitable for pelotherapy uses, it should have several properties, such as a low cooling rate, a high absorption capacity, a high cationic exchange capacity, good adhesiveness, handling easiness, and a pleasant feeling when applied to the skin. Among all the above properties, the cooling rate is one of the most critical ones, since the heat contributed by the peloid also plays a role as a therapeutic agent. In many therapeutic applications, therefore, the peloid must be kept at a higher temperature than that of the patient's body during application [6].

If peloids need maturing, then one must also establish the temperature, light, agitation, etc. conditions. In any case, the characterization analyses are the same, and samples need to be taken after 15 days, 1 month, 2 months, etc. until the maturation process is complete and no further changes in the physico-chemical parameters are observed [39,55,61,69,70].

3.2.5. Use and Effectiveness Tests

Different analyses and tests are carried out on volunteers to evaluate user acceptance of the peloid and its effectiveness. Inclusion and exclusion criteria for both tests must be established, taking into account that these preliminary studies are carried out on healthy persons. Additional controlled clinical trials must be done if the peloid is finally destined to treat skin conditions such as psoriasis, dermatitis, etc.

The use test consists of a set of questions related to texture, ease of application, sensations during and after application, skin condition after product removal, etc. In Figure 10, an example of a microalgal peloid is shown.

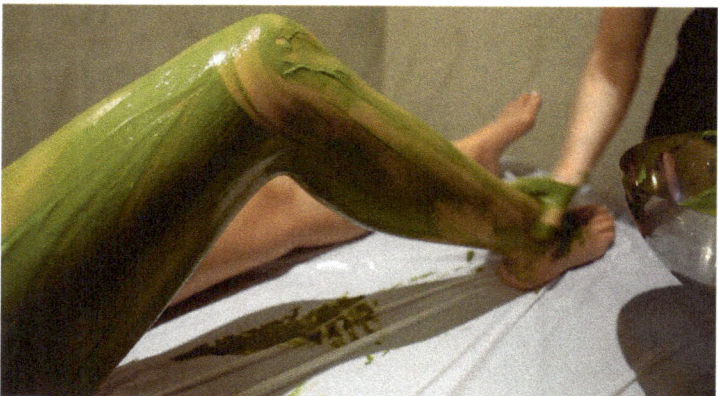

Figure 10. Application of microalgal peloid (Talaso Atlántico, Baiona, Pontevedra, Spain).

Efficacy studies are usually objective determinations done through skin biometrology techniques, such as hydration (by corneometry), grade of sebum (with sebumeter), skin elasticity (cutometry or elastometry), and, sometimes, transepidermal water loss [71–73].

4. Conclusions

Peloids have been used for therapeutic purposes since time immemorial, mainly in the treatment of locomotor-system pathologies and dermatology. Their effects are attributed to their components, i.e., to the properties and action of mineral waters, clays, and their biological fraction, which may be made up of microalgae, cyanobacteria, and other organisms present in water and clays. Different studies show that the biological fraction and the maturation process (in which components remain in contact for a certain length of time) contribute to the formation of biologically active compounds.

Even though there are many studies on the therapeutic use of peloids made with microalgae/cyanobacteria, very little research has been done on dermocosmetic applications. Such research demonstrates their potential as soothing, regenerating, antioxidant, anti-inflammatory, and antimicrobial agents. Their effect is related to the presence of unsaturated fatty acids, acylglycerolipids, sulfoglucolipids, vitamins, alcohols, phenols, etc., as well as sulphur derivatives, minerals (Ca, Mg, etc.), and trace elements (Zn, Se, Si, etc.).

Each thermal spa has a unique natural mineral water with specific physico-chemical characteristics, which are the basis of their therapeutic actions (along with other mechanisms related to the application technique). Moreover, specific microbiota consisting mainly of microalgae and/or cyanobacteria are often found in it. This is why thermal spas, thalassotherapy centres, and wellness centres in general should progress towards making their own dermocosmetic products using their natural mineral water or seawater; a solid substrate, preferably clay; and the microalgae/cyanobacteria. Hence, a method for the manufacture of a dermocosmetic peloid was presented based on the experience of the authors and existing publications, with indications for its characterization and efficacy study.

Author Contributions: Writing—original draft preparation, M.L.M.; writing—review and editing, M.L.M.; C.P.G., and J.L.L. All authors have read and agreed to the published version of the manuscript.

Funding: This research received no external funding.

Conflicts of Interest: The authors declare no conflict of interest.

References

1. Silva, P.S.C.; Oliveira, S.M.B.; Farias, F.; Fávaro, D.I.I.; Mazzilli, B.P. Chemical and radiological characterization of clay minerals used in pharmaceutics and cosmetics. *Appl. Clay Sci.* **2011**, *52*, 145–149. [CrossRef]
2. Maraver, F.; Fernández-Torán, M.A.; Corvillo, I.; Morer, C.; Vázquez, I.; Aguilera, L.; Armijo, F. Pelotherapy, a review. *Med. Nat.* **2015**, *9*, 38–46.
3. Carretero, M.I. Clays in pelotherapy. A review. Part II: Organic compounds, microbiology and medical applications. *Appl. Clay Sci.* **2020**, *189*, 105531. [CrossRef]
4. Gomes, C.; Carretero, M.I.; Pozo, M.; Maraver, F.; Cantista, P.; Armijo, F.; Legido, J.L.; Teixeira, F.; Rautureau, M.; Delgado, R. Peloids and pelotherapy: Historical evolution, classification and glossary. *Appl. Clay Sci.* **2013**, *75*, 28–38. [CrossRef]
5. Veniale, F.; Barberis, E.; Carcangiu, G.; Morandi, N.; Setti, M.; Tamanini, M.; Tessier, D. Formulation of muds for pelotherapy: Effects of "maturation" by different mineral waters. *Int. J. Biometeorol.* **2004**, *25*, 135–148. [CrossRef]
6. Legido, J.; Medina, C.; Mourelle, M.L.; Carretero, M.; Pozo, M. Comparative study of the cooling rates of bentonite, sepiolite and common clays for their use in pelotherapy. *Appl. Clay Sci.* **2007**, *36*, 148–160. [CrossRef]
7. Meijide, R.; Mourelle, M.L. Afecciones dermatológicas y cosmética dermotermal. In *Técnicas y Tecnologías en Hidrología Médica e Hidroterapia. Agencia de Evaluación de Tecnologías Sanitarias*; Hernández Torres, A., Ed.; Instituto Carlos III: Madrid, Spain, 2006; pp. 175–194. (In Spanish)
8. Mourelle, M.L. Caracterización Termofísica de Peloides para Aplicaciones Termoterapéuticas en Centros Termales Ph.D. Thesis, Universidade de Vigo, Galicia, Spain, 2006. (In Spanish).
9. Carbajo, J.M.; Corvillo, I.; Aguilera, A.; Meijide, R.; Diestro, P.; Crespo, V.; Maraver, F. Biophysical skin effects of peloids according to their maturity time. *Balnea* **2012**, *6*, 169–170.
10. Halevy, S.; Sukenik, S. Different Modalities of Spa Therapy for Skin Diseases at the Dead Sea Area. *Arch. Dermatol.* **1998**, *134*, 1416–1420. [CrossRef]
11. Emmanuel, T.; Lybæk, D.; Johansen, C.; Iversen, L. Effect of Dead Sea Climatotherapy on Psoriasis; A Prospective Cohort Study. *Front. Med.* **2020**, *7*, 83. [CrossRef]
12. Ma'or, Z.; Henis, Y.; Alon, Y.; Orlov, E.; Sørensen, K.; & Oren, A. Antimicrobial properties of Dead Sea black mineral mud. *Int. J. Dermatol.* **2006**, *45*, 504–511. [CrossRef]
13. Abu-al-Basal, M.A. Histological evaluation of the healing properties of Dead Sea black mud on full-thickness excision cutaneous wounds in BALB/c mice. *Pak. J. Biol. Sci.* **2012**, *15*, 306–315. [CrossRef] [PubMed]
14. Mazzulla, S.; Chimenti, R.; Sesti, S.; De Stefano, S.; Morrone, M.; Martino, G. Effetto delle Bioglee solfuree su lesioni psoriasiche. *Clin. Ter.* **2004**, *155*, 499–504. (In Italian)
15. Da Silva, P.S.C.; Torrecilha, J.K.; Gouvea, P.F.D.M.; Máduar, M.F.; de Oliveira, S.M.B.; Scapin, M.A. Chemical and radiological characterization of Peruíbe Black Mud. *Appl. Clay Sci.* **2015**, *118*, 221–230. [CrossRef]
16. Shoieb, S.M.; Esmat, A.; Khalifa, A.E.; Abdel-Naim, A.B. Chrysin attenuates testosterone-induced benign prostate hyperplasia in rats. *Food Chem. Toxicol.* **2018**, *111*, 650–659. [CrossRef]
17. Spilioti, E.; Vargiami, M.; Letsiou, S.; Gardikis, K.; Sygouni, V.; Koutsoukos, P.; Chinou, I.; Kasi, E.; Moutsatsou, P. Biological properties of mud extracts derived from various spa resorts. *Environ. Geochem. Health* **2017**, *39*, 821–833. [CrossRef] [PubMed]
18. Zague, V.; de Almeida Silva, D.; Eaby, A.R.; Kaneko, T.M.; Velasco, M.V. Clay facial masks: Physicochemical stability at different storage temperatures. *J. Cosmet. Sci.* **2007**, *58*, 45–51. [CrossRef]

19. Carretero, M.I.; Pozo, M. Clay and non-clay minerals in the pharmaceutical industry: Part I. Excipients and medical applications. *Appl. Clay Sci.* **2009**, *4*, 73–80. [CrossRef]
20. Carretero, M.I.; Pozo, M. Clay and non-clay minerals in the pharmaceutical and cosmetic industries Part II. Active ingredients. *Appl. Clay Sci.* **2010**, *47*, 171–1801. [CrossRef]
21. Carretero, M.I. Clays in pelotherapy. A review. Part I: Mineralogy, chemistry, physical and physicochemical properties. *Appl. Clay Sci.* **2020**, *189*, 105526. [CrossRef]
22. Kamitsou, M.D.; Sygouni, V.; Kanellopoulou, D.G.; Gardikis, K.; Koutsoukos, P.G. Physicochemical characterization of sterilized muds for pharmaceutics/cosmetics applications. *Environ. Geochem. Health* **2018**, *40*, 1449–1464. [CrossRef]
23. Silva-Valenzuela, M.; Chambi-Peralta, M.M.; Sayeg, I.J.; Carvalho, F.; Wang, S.; Valenzuela-Díaz, F. Enrichment of clay from Vitoria da Conquista (Brazil) for applications in cosmetics. *Appl. Clay Sci.* **2018**, *155*, 111–119. [CrossRef]
24. Khiari, I.; Mefteh, S.; Sánchez-Espejo, R.; Aguzzi, C.; López-Galindo, A.; Jamoussi, F.; Iborra, C. Study of traditional Tunisian medina clays used in therapeutic and cosmetic mud-packs. *Appl. Clay Sci.* **2014**, *101*, 141–148. [CrossRef]
25. Viseras, C.; Carazo, E.; Borrego-Sánchez, A.; García-Villén, F.; Sánchez-Espejo, R.; Cerezo, P.; Aguzzi, C. Clay Minerals in Skin Drug Delivery. *Clays Clay Miner.* **2019**, *67*, 59–71. [CrossRef]
26. García-Villén, F.; Sánchez-Espejo, R.; Borrego-Sánchez, A.; Cerezo, P.; Perioli, L.; Viseras, C. Safety of Nanoclay/Spring Water Hydrogels: Assessment and Mobility of Hazardous Elements. *Pharmaceutics* **2020**, *12*, 764. [CrossRef]
27. Katona, G.; Vojvodić, S.; Kalić, M.; Sarač, M.S.; Klimó, A.; Jovanović Lješković, N. The effect of Kanjiža peloid on skin hydration and skin barrier function. *Maced. Pharm. Bull.* **2020**, *66*, 105–106. [CrossRef]
28. Hoteteu, M.; Munteanu, C.; Ionescu, E.; Almășan, R.; Balnear, T.; Sanatorium, R. Bioactive substances of the Techirghiol therapeutic mud. *Balneo Res. J.* **2018**, *9*, 5–10. [CrossRef]
29. Pavlovska, I.; Klaviņa, J.; Auce, A.; Vanadziņš, I.; Silova, A.; Komarovska, L.; Silamiķele, B.; Dobkeviča, L.; Paegle, L. Assessment of sapropel use for pharmaceutical products according to legislation, pollution parameters, and concentration of biologically active substances. *Sci. Rep.* **2020**, *10*, 21527. [CrossRef]
30. Bergamaschi, B.; Marzola, L.; Radice, M.; Manfredini, S.; Baldini, E.; Vicentini, C.B.; Marrocchino, E.; Molesini, S.; Ziosi, P.; Vaccaro, C.; et al. Comparative Study of SPA Mud from "Bacino Idrominerario Omogeneo dei Colli Euganei (B.I.O.C.E.)-Italy" and Industrially Optimized Mud for Skin Applications. *Life* **2020**, *10*, 78. [CrossRef]
31. Bawab, A.A.; Bozeya, A.; Abu-Mallouh, S.; Irmaileh, B.A.; Daqour, I.; Abu-Zurayk, R. The Dead Sea Mud and Salt: A Review of Its Characterization, Contaminants, and Beneficial Effects. *IOP Conf. Ser. Mater. Sci. Eng.* **2018**, *305*, 012003. [CrossRef]
32. Britschka, Z.M.N.; Teodoro, W.R.; Velosa, A.P.P.; Mello, S.B.V. The efficacy of Brazilian black mud treatment in chronic experimental arthritis. *Rheumatol. Int.* **2007**, *28*, 39–45. [CrossRef]
33. Yarkent, Ç.; Gürlek, C.; Oncel, S.S. Potential of microalgal compounds in trending natural cosmetics: A review. *Sustain. Chem. Pharm.* **2020**, *17*, 100304. [CrossRef]
34. Ceschi-Berrini, C.; de Appolonia, F.; Dalla Valle, L.; Komárek, J.; Andreoli, C. Morphological and molecular characterization of a thermophilic cyanobacterium (Oscillatoriales) from Euganean Thermal Springs (Padua, Italy). *Arch. Hydrobiol. Algol. Stud.* **2004**, *113*, 73–85.
35. Marcolongo, G.; de Appolonia, F.; Venzo, A.; Berrie, C.P.; Carofiglio, T.; Ceschi Berrini, C. Diacylglycerolipids isolated from a thermophile cyanobacterium from the Euganean hot springs. *Nat. Prod. Res.* **2006**, *20*, 766–774. [CrossRef]
36. Moro, I.; Rascio, N.; La Rocca, N.; Di Bella, M.; Andreoli, C. Cyanobacterium aponinum, a new Cyanoprokaryote from the microbial mat of Euganean Thermal Springs (Padua, Italy). *Arch. Hydrobiol. Suppl. Algol. Stud.* **2007**, *123*, 1–15. [CrossRef]
37. Poli, A.; Romano, I.; Cordella, P.; Orlando, P.; Nicolaus, B.; Ceschi Berrini, C. *Anoxybacillus thermarum* sp. nov., a novel thermophilic bacterium isolated from thermal mud in Euganean hot springs, Abano Terme, Italy. *Extremophiles* **2009**, *13*, 867–874. [CrossRef] [PubMed]
38. Moro, I.; Rascio, N.; La Rocca, N.; Sciuto, K.; Albertano, P.; Bruno, L.; Andreoli, C. Polyphasic characterization of a thermo-tolerant filamentous cyanobacterium isolated from the Euganean thermal muds (Padua, Italy). *Eur. J. Phycol.* **2010**, *45*, 143–154. [CrossRef]
39. Centini, M.; Tredici, M.R.; Biondi, N.; Buonocore, A.; Maffei Facino, R.; Anselmi, C. Thermal mud maturation: Organic matter and biological activity. *Int. J. Cosmet. Sci.* **2015**, *37*, 339–347. [CrossRef] [PubMed]
40. Centini, M.; Roberto Tredici, M.; Biondi, N.; Buonocore, A.; Facino, R.M.; Anselmi, C. Bioglea as a Source of Bioactive Ingredients: Chemical and Biological Evaluation. *Cosmetics* **2020**, *7*, 81. [CrossRef]
41. Calderan, A.; Carraro, A.; Honisch, C.; Lalli, A.; Ruzza, P.; Tateo, F. Euganean therapeutic mud (NE Italy): Chlorophyll a variations over two years and relationships with mineralogy and geochemistry. *Appl. Clay Sci.* **2020**, *185*, 105361. [CrossRef]
42. Gris, B.; Treu, L.; Zampieri, R.M.; Caldara, F.; Romualdi, C.; Campanaro, S.; La Rocca, N. Microbiota of the Therapeutic Euganean Thermal Muds with a Focus on the Main Cyanobacteria Species. *Microorganisms* **2020**, *8*, 1590. [CrossRef]
43. Zampieri, R.M.; Adessi, A.; Caldara, F.; Codato, A.; Furlan, M.; Rampazzo, C.; De Philippis, R.; La Rocca, N.; Dalla Valle, L. Anti-Inflammatory Activity of Exopolysaccharides from *Phormidium* sp. ETS05, the Most Abundant Cyanobacterium of the Therapeutic Euganean Thermal Muds, Using the Zebrafish Model. *Biomolecules* **2020**, *10*, 582. [CrossRef]
44. Giorgio, A.; Carraturo, F.; Aliberti, F.; De Bonis, S.; Libralato, G.; Morra, M.; Guida, M. Characterization of microflora composition and antimicrobial activity of algal extracts from Italian thermal muds. *J. Nat. Sci. Biol. Med.* **2018**, *9*, 150–158.
45. Paduano, S.; Valeriani, F.; Romano-Spica, V.; Bargellini, A.; Borella, P.; Marchesi, I. Microbial biodiversity of thermal water and mud in an Italian spa by metagenomics: A pilot study. *Water Sci. Technol. Water Supply* **2017**, *18*, 1456–1465. [CrossRef]

46. Demay, J.; Halary, S.; Knittel-Obrecht, A.; Villa, P.; Duval, C.; Hamlaoui, S.; Roussel, T.; Yéprémian, C.; Reinhardt, A.; Bernard, C.; et al. Anti-Inflammatory, Antioxidant, and Wound-Healing Properties of Cyanobacteria from Thermal Mud of Balaruc-Les-Bains, France: A Multi-Approach Study. *Biomolecules* **2021**, *11*, 28. [CrossRef] [PubMed]
47. Duval, C.; Hamlaoui, S.; Piquet, B.; Toutirais, G.; Yéprémian, C.; Reinhardt, A.; Duperron, S.; Marie, B.; Demay, J.; Bernard, C. Characterization of cyanobacteria isolated from thermal muds of Balaruc-Les-Bains (France) and description of a new genus and species *Pseudo-chroococcus coutei*. *bioRxiv* **2020**. [CrossRef]
48. Duval, C.; Hamlaoui, S.; Piquet, B.; Toutirais, G.; Yéprémian, C.; Reinhardt, A.; Duperron, S.; Marie, B.; Demay, J.; Bernard, C. Diversity of cyanobacteria from thermal muds (Balaruc-Les-Bains, France) with the description of *Pseudochroococcus coutei* gen. nov., sp. nov. *FEMS Microbes* **2021**, *2*, xtab006. [CrossRef]
49. Halevy, S.; Giryes, H.; Friger, M.; Grossman, N.; Karpas, Z.; Sarov, B.; Sukenik, S. The role of trace elements in psoriatic patients undergoing balneotherapy with Dead Sea bath salt. *IMAJ* **2001**, *3*, 828–832. [PubMed]
50. Obeidat, M. Isolation and characterization of extremely halotolerant Bacillus species from Dead Sea black mud and determination of their antimicrobial and hydrolytic activities. *Afr. J. Microbiol. Res.* **2017**, *11*, 1303–1314.
51. Al-Karablieh, N. Antimicrobial Activity of *Bacillus Persicus* 24-DSM Isolated from Dead Sea Mud. *Open Microbiol. J.* **2017**, *11*, 372–383. [CrossRef]
52. Dolmaa, G.; Bayaraa, B.; Tserenkhand, B.; Nomintsetseg, B.; Ganzaya, G. Chemical investigation of medical mud from Lake Nogoon. *Proc. Mong. Acad. Sci.* **2018**, *57*, 15–23. [CrossRef]
53. Bigovic, M.; Pantovic, S.; Milašević, I.; Ivanović, L.; Djurović, D.; Slavić, V.; Popovic, M.; Vrvić, M.; Roganovic, M. Organic composition of Igalo Bay peloid (Montenegro). *IJTK* **2019**, *18*, 837–848.
54. Sedláček, I.; Kwon, S.W.; Švec, P.; Mašlaňová, I.; Kýrová, K.; Holochová, P.; Černohlávková, J.; Busse, H.J. *Aquitalea pelogenes* sp. nov., isolated from mineral peloid. *Int. J. Syst. Evol. Microbiol.* **2016**, *66*, 962–967. [CrossRef] [PubMed]
55. Pesciaroli, C.; Viseras, C.; Aguzzi, C.; Rodelas, B.; González-López, J. Study of bacterial community structure and diversity during the maturation process of a therapeutic peloid. *Appl. Clay Sci.* **2016**, *132–133*, 59–67. [CrossRef]
56. Ma'or, Z.; Halicz, L.; Portugal-Cohen, M.; Russo, M.; Robino, F.; Vanhaecke, T.; Rogiers, V. Safety evaluation of traces of nickel and chrome in cosmetics: The case of Dead Sea mud. *Regul. Toxicol. Pharmacol.* **2015**, *73*, 797–801. [CrossRef]
57. Baldovin, T.; Amoruso, I.; Caldara, F.; Buja, A.; Baldo, V.; Cocchio, S.; Bertoncello, C. Microbiological Hygiene Quality of Thermal Muds: A Pilot Study in Pelotherapy Facilities of the Euganean Thermal District (NE Italy). *Int. J. Environ. Res. Public Health* **2020**, *13*, 5040. [CrossRef]
58. Arribas, M.; Gómez, C.P.; Mourelle, M.L. Nuevos casos clínicos tratados con peloide La Toja. In Proceedings of the Libro de resúmenes del V Congreso Iberoamericano de peloides, Badajoz, Spain, 11–14 June 2017. (In Spanish).
59. Cabana, B.; Galiñares, M.; Mourelle, L. Estudio preliminar con peloides en paciente con psoriasis. In Proceedings of the Libro de resúmenes del V Congreso Iberoamericano de peloides, Badajoz, Spain, 11–14 June 2017. (In Spanish).
60. Mourelle, M.L.; Gómez, C.P.; Legido, J.L. Cosmética dermotermal: Valor añadido para los centros termales. In Proceedings of the I Congreso Internacional del Agua—Termalismo y Calidad de Vida, Ourense, Spain, 23–24 September 2015. (In Spanish).
61. Carretero, M.I.; Pozo, M.; Legido, J.L.; Fernández-González, M.V.; Delgado, R.; Gómez, I.; Armijo, F.; Maraver, F. Assessment of three Spanish clays for their use in pelotherapy. *Appl. Clay Sci.* **2017**, *99*, 131–143.
62. Glavaš, N.; Mourelle, M.L.; Gómez, C.P.; Legido, J.L.; Šmuc, N.R.; Dolenec, M.; Kovac, N. The mineralogical, geochemical, and thermophysical characterization of healing saline mud for use in pelotherapy. *Appl. Clay Sci.* **2017**, *135*, 119–128.
63. Maraver, F.; Vázquez, I.; Armijo, F. *Vademécum III de Aguas Mineromedicinales Españolas*; Ediciones Complutense: Madrid, Spain, 2020. (In Spanish)
64. Quattrini, S.; Pampaloni, B.; Brandi, M.L. Natural mineral waters: Chemical characteristics and health effects. *Clin. Cases Miner. Bone Metab.* **2016**, *13*, 173–180. [CrossRef] [PubMed]
65. Casas, L.M.; Pozo, M.; Gómez, C.P.; Pozo, E.; Bessieres, D.; Plantier, F.; Legido, J.L. Thermal behavior of mixtures of bentonitic clay and saline solutions. *Appl. Clay Sci.* **2013**, *72*, 18–25.
66. Dolganyuk, V.; Andreeva, A.; Budenkova, E.; Sukhikh, S.; Babich, O.; Ivanova, S.; Prosekov, A.; Ulrikh, E. Study of Morphological Features and Determination of the Fatty Acid Composition of the Microalgae Lipid Complex. *Biomolecules* **2020**, *10*, 1571. [CrossRef] [PubMed]
67. Casas, L.M.; Legido, J.L.; Pozo, M.; Mourelle, L.; Plantier, F.; Bessieres, D. Specific heat of mixtures of bentonitic clay with sea water or distilled water for their use in thermotherapy. *Thermochim. Acta* **2011**, *524*, 68–73. [CrossRef]
68. Mato, M.M.; Casas, L.M.; Legido, J.L.; Gómez, C.P.; Mourelle, L.; Bessieres, D.; Plantier, F. Specific heat of mixtures of kaolin with sea water or distilled water for their use in thermotherapy. *J. Therm. Anal. Calorim.* **2017**, *130*, 479–484. [CrossRef]
69. Sánchez-Espejo, R.; Cerezo, P.; Aguzzi, C.; López-Galindo, A.; Machado, J.; Viseras, C. Physicochemical and in vitro cation release relevance of therapeutic muds "maturation". *Appl. Clay Sci.* **2015**, *116–117*, 1–7. [CrossRef]
70. Carretero, M.I.; Pozo, M.; Sánchez, C.; García, F.J.; Medina, J.A.; Bernabé, J.M. Comparison of saponite and montmorillonite behaviour during static and stirring maturation with seawater for pelotherapy. *Appl. Clay Sci.* **2007**, *36*, 161–173. [CrossRef]
71. Constantin, M.M.; Bucur, S.; Serban, E.D.; Olteanu, R.; Bratu, O.G.; Constantin, T. Measurement of skin viscoelasticity: A non-invasive approach in allergic contact dermatitis. *Exp. Ther. Med.* **2020**, *20*, 184. [CrossRef] [PubMed]

72. Qassem, M.; Kyriacou, P.A. Review of Modern Techniques for the Assessment of Skin Hydration. *Cosmetics* **2019**, *6*, 19. [CrossRef]
73. Kim, M.A.; Kim, E.J.; Lee, H.K. Use of SkinFibrometer® to measure skin elasticity and its correlation with Cutometer® and DUB® Skinscanner. *Skin Res. Technol.* **2018**, *24*, 466–471. [CrossRef]

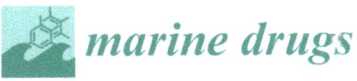

Review

Applying Seaweed Compounds in Cosmetics, Cosmeceuticals and Nutricosmetics

Lucía López-Hortas [1], Noelia Flórez-Fernández [1], Maria D. Torres [1], Tania Ferreira-Anta [1], María P. Casas [1], Elena M. Balboa [1], Elena Falqué [2] and Herminia Domínguez [1,*]

[1] Centro de Investigaciones Biomédicas (CINBIO), Departamento de Enxeñería Química, Universidade de Vigo (Campus Ourense), Edificio Politécnico, As Lagoas, 32004 Ourense, Spain; luclopez@uvigo.es (L.L.-H.); noelia.florez@uvigo.es (N.F.-F.); matorres@uvigo.es (M.D.T.); ta.ferreiraan@gmail.com (T.F.-A.); mariapc@uvigo.es (M.P.C.); elenamba@uvigo.es (E.M.B.)

[2] Departamento de Química Analítica, Universidade de Vigo (Campus Ourense), Edificio Politécnico, As Lagoas, 32004 Ourense, Spain; efalque@uvigo.es

* Correspondence: herminia@uvigo.es; Tel.: +34-988-387082

Abstract: The interest in seaweeds for cosmetic, cosmeceutics, and nutricosmetics is increasing based on the demand for natural ingredients. Seaweeds offer advantages in relation to their renewable character, wide distribution, and the richness and versatility of their valuable bioactive compounds, which can be used as ingredients, as additives, and as active agents in the formulation of skin care products. Bioactive compounds, such as polyphenols, polysaccharides, proteins peptides, amino acids, lipids, vitamins, and minerals, are responsible for the biological properties associated with seaweeds. Seaweed fractions can also offer technical features, such as thickening, gelling, emulsifying, texturizing, or moistening to develop cohesive matrices. Furthermore, the possibility of valorizing industrial waste streams and algal blooms makes them an attractive, low cost, raw and renewable material. This review presents an updated summary of the activities of different seaweed compounds and fractions based on scientific and patent literature.

Keywords: marine macroalgae; ingredients; additives; bioactives; nutricosmetics

1. Introduction

Consumer preferences towards green and eco-friendly products have increased in the last few years [1,2]. This trend is also found in cosmetics, which represent a competitive and rapidly changing global market demanding natural, safe, and efficient ingredients for the development of novel skin care products [3–5]. Other relatively new products are cosmeceuticals and nutricosmetics. The term cosmeceutical is used to define active and safe products developed and tested by the cosmetics industry to provide benefits to skin appearance and are effective for preventing and treating different dermatologic conditions [6] by offering a variety of functions [6–8]. A number of active ingredients, including vitamins, phytochemicals, enzymes, antioxidants, and essential oils, are also considered [9], and can be used for the formulation of creams, lotions, ointments, or masks. The use of cosmeceuticals has drastically risen in the last few years [10], in a market that also incorporates other less-traditional population segments, such as men and children [11–13]. Both cosmetics and cosmeceuticals have to be safe, efficient, and have good sensorial quality features [6,14]; nutricosmetics also require optimal characteristics. For the optimal development of these products, cooperation in areas such as biotechnology, chemistry, food technology, pharmaceutical technology, and toxicology is needed [15].

Marine resources represent a widely available and promising source of unique and active compounds with the potential to produce cosmetics, cosmeceuticals, and nutricosmetics. Among them, seaweeds represent a sustainable and renewable resource, gaining increasing attention for these applications [16,17]. Furthermore, valorization of waste seaweeds, such as beach-casts, which are disposed of in landfills without commercial value, could represent an attractive low-cost source for cosmeceutical industries [18]. Similarly, the valorization of invasive species could contribute to the creation of natural and eco-friendly ingredients for the cosmetic industry [19] while also contributing to the restoration of affected environments. Regardless the origin and type of seaweed, the development of environmentally-friendly sustainable extraction methods, allowing a low extraction time, minimum usage of solvents, higher extraction yields, and quality, are increasingly demanded [5,19–22].

The use of seaweed-derived ingredients in cosmetic products has increased in recent years as a result of the many scientific studies that have proved the potential skincare properties of seaweed bioactives [23,24]. Among those biologically active molecules, carotenoids, fatty acids, polysaccharides, phlorotannins, vitamins, sterols, tocopherol, phycobilins, and phycocyanins have attracted attention [9,25–29]. Such rich compositions have converted seaweed into potential ingredients in classical cosmetics, such as solid soaps, to replace sodium lauryl sulfate/sodium laureth sulfate [22], but many algal extracts have also been used in nutritional supplements, cosmetics, and alternative medicines recommended for skin-related diseases [30]. In this latter case, they are added as the active ingredient, because they can provide a variety of activities, including photoprotective, moisturizing, antioxidant, anti-melanogenic, anti-allergic, anti-inflammatory, anti-acne, anti-wrinkling, antimicrobial, antiaging, whitening, etc. [16,31–33]. Furthermore, they exhibit low cytotoxicity and low allergen contents [34].

Excellent comprehensive reviews on the subject have recently been published, including on the chemical diversity and unique properties of algal bioactive molecules or extracts for cosmetic uses [5,16,28,33,35–37] and the progress made in the application of bioactives from marine organisms as cosmeceuticals [27,38,39]. Most of these have emphasized the importance and scientific evidence of algae-derived compounds and their benefits, as well as current application in the cosmetic industry and their challenges and limitations in the development of cosmeceuticals [3,23,24,29,34,40]. Others have reported on particular components, such as carbohydrates [41,42], or the specific beneficial actions on hyperpigmentation, photoaging, and acne [2,23,24], as well as on perspectives for the development of greener extraction methods [35], particularly those using safe solvents [3].

The present review tries to update the advances in this field, presenting an initial section summarizing the activities of algal components of particular relevance for cosmetic and cosmeceutical formulations and then by trying to offer the multiple and faceted benefits and functions that these seaweed components can provide to products where they can be incorporated as ingredients and additives, conferring other textural, functional, and sensorial properties. The potential applications are presented based on information in the scientific literature, but also using patents claiming the use of algae and algal components.

2. Seaweed Components and Bioactivity
2.1. Polysaccharides

Seaweeds contain an important carbohydrate fraction forming part of their cell walls and these polysaccharides are specific to each type of algae: in brown alginate, laminaran and fucoidan; in green ulvan and in red agar, carrageenan is the most important. Polysaccharides are receiving increasing attention for their biofunctional and physicochemical characteristics [43]. Sulfated polysaccharides are highly interesting due to their health benefits and biological activities [32,44–50]. A key aspect of these polysaccharides is the close relationship between the activity and their composition and structure, particularly, their molecular weight. Therefore, depolymerization is usually proposed to enhance the activity [51], but other structural modifications can also be performed. Simple hydrophobization reactions, such as esterification, acylation, alkylation, amidation, or cross-linking reactions on native hydroxyl-, amine, or carboxylic acid functions can also enhance bioactivity [52]. Examples of these activities are summarized in Table 1.

Table 1. Some activities and properties of seaweeds polysaccharides of interest in cosmeceutical formulations.

Component	Properties/Activities	Seaweed	References
Agar	Thickener; antioxidant	Pterocladia, Pterocladiella, Gelidium amansii, Gracilaria	[23,46,53–55]
Alginate	High stability, thickening agent, gelling agent	Brown seaweeds	[34,56,57]
Carrageenans	Antioxidant, antitumor, antiaging, thickeners properties, radiation protection	Red seaweeds, Porphyra haitanensis, Gracilaria chouae, Gracilaria blodgettii	[16,49,58–62]
Fucoidans	Photoaging inhibition; minimized elastase activity; antioxidant, anti-inflammatory collagenase and elastase inhibition, skin-whitening	Fucoidan (Sigma), Ascophyllum nodosum, Chnoospora minima, Ecklonia maxima, Hizikia fusiforme, Saccharina japonica, Sargassum hemiphyllum, Sargassum horneri, Sargassum polycystum, Sargassum vachellianum	[2,23,24,43,44,46, 48,63–67]
Laminaran	Reconstructed dermis; skin cell anti-inflammation; antioxidant	Saccharina longicruris, Laminarin (Sigma)	[68,69]
Polysaccharides	Hydration	Saccharina japonica, Chondrus crispus, Codium tomentosum	[28]
Ulvan	Antiaging, antiherpetic	Ulva pertusa, Ulva sp.	[51,70]

Alginates composed of chains of D-mannuronic acid and L-guluronic acid are found in brown seaweeds. These compounds show other properties in relation to cosmetics and well-being products, particularly anti-allergic properties [32,71], an action that is also observed in formulations of hydrogels with alginate [72], and can also prevent obesity [73,74]. Laminarin does not form viscous solutions and has prebiotic [75,76], antioxidant [77–79], and anti-photoaging and regenerative [69] properties. Based on the wound healing [80] properties of laminarin sulfate, novel hydrogel systems have been developed [81–83]. In addition, promising outcomes have been exhibited in several biomedical applications, such as tissue engineering, cancer therapies, antioxidant, and anti-inflammatory properties [84]. Degradation by irradiation can enhance the radical scavenging capacity and inhibitory activity against melanin synthesis in melanoma cells [2,59].

Fucoidans are heteropolysaccharides with fucose and other monosaccharides, such as xylose, galactose, mannose, and glucuronic acid, as well as other components, mainly sulfate, uronic acids, and acetyl groups. Fucoidans offer promising potential as cosmetic ingredient [34,85,86] since they are non-toxic, biodegradable, and biocompatible [87,88], and they present a wide variety of biological properties [23,24,49,61,89–91]; they also reduce antioxidant and antiradical properties [23,24,34,67,92], depending on the molecular weight and sulfate content [93,94]. Fucoidans have shown confirmed benefits for preventing and treating skin photoaging and have in vitro inhibition of UVB-induced collagenase and gelatinase activities, ex vivo inhibition on elastase activity in human skin [2,64,66,95], inhibition of wrinkle-related enzymes and enhanced collagen synthesis in human dermal fibroblasts [67], and anti-inflammatory action in relation to extracellular matrix degradation by matrix metalloproteinases [27,32,42,65,96].

Sulfated polysaccharides from green algae (rhamnans, arabinogalactans, galactans and mannans) present variable compositions and structures and some properties are highly influenced by the molecular weight in terms of antiradical and chelating properties [97–100]. Ulvans are highly complex and variable sulfated polysaccharides from ulvales, composed mainly of rhamnose, xylose, glucose, glucuronic acid, iduronic acid, and sulfate [34,89,101,102]. Ulvans exhibit a variety of activities, including gelling [101,103], anti-aging [51], anti-hyperlipidemic and antiherpetic properties [71,104].

Agar is mainly composed of β-D-galactopyranose and 3,6-anhydro-α-L-galactopyranose units with variable amounts of sulfate, pyruvate, and uronate substituents. Agar has pharmaceutical and industrial cosmetic applications, including its use as a thickener and as an ingredient for tablets or capsules to carry and release drugs [105,106]. Carrageenans are generally recognized as safe (GRAS) and are approved for food applications, and are high-molecular-weight sulfated linear polysaccharides with a backbone of alternating 3- α-D-galactopyranose and 4-β-D-galactopyranose with anhydrogalactose residues [54,55,107,108]. Porphyran is a complex sulfated galactan found in Porphyra sp. with interesting therapeutic properties. These polysaccharides have uses as gelling agent, nutritional supplement, with antioxidants [109–112], and are antiallergic [32,113], show tyrosinase inhibitory activity [62], protection against ultraviolet B radiation [59], anti-inflammatory and antitumoral activity, and can promote the growth of beneficial bacteria in intestinal microbiota [76,113] without toxicity in mice models [114,115]. Agaro-oligosaccharides (AOS) and carrageenan-oligosaccharides (COS) present enhanced biological properties compared to native ones, in relation to prebiotic, antitumoral, and antioxidant actions, related to their chemical structure, molecular weight, degree of polymerization, and the flexibility of the glycosidic linkages [116].

2.2. Proteins, Peptides and Aminoacids

Some seaweeds are a rich source of proteins, their cultivation offers a higher protein yield per unit area (2.5–7.5 tons/Ha/year) compared to terrestrial crops, but their successful extraction is largely influenced by the presence of polysaccharides, such as alginates in brown seaweed or carrageenans in red seaweed [117]. Seasonal variations and habitat affect the proteins, peptides, and amino acids contents in seaweed; generally, red algae (Rhodophyceae) have higher contents (up to 47%) than green (Chlorophyceae) (between 9–26%), whereas brown (*Phaeophyceae*) have a lower concentration (3–15%) [73,118–120]. The proteins in the three groups of macroalgae contain all essential amino acids, and non-essential amino acids are also present [25,121–123]. Protein and bioactive peptides from seaweed show many health benefits and have high antioxidant properties, mainly in molecules with low molecular weights, which are also considered safer than synthetic molecules and have reduced side effects [3,124–127].

Bioactive peptides usually contain 3–20 amino acid residues and both their amino acid composition and the sequence influences their activities, such as antioxidant and antimicrobial activities, among others of pharmacological interest [128–131]. Carnosine, glutathione, and taurine are peptides with antioxidant and chelating properties [132]. Due to the lack of a carboxyl group, taurine is not a "true" amino acid but has a number of health-promoting properties, being accumulated in the thalli of several red algae, such as *Ahnfeltia plicata*, *Euthora cristata*, and *Ceramium virgatum* [133]. The peptide, PPY1, is composed of five amino acids and is obtained by enzymatic hydrolysis from *Pyropia yezoensis*, and it shows anti-inflammatory effects through the suppression of inflammatory cytokines [134]. The peptides, PYP1-5 and Porphyra 334, extracted from *Porphyra yezoensis* f. coreana Ueda showed an increase in elastin and collagen production and a decrease in the expression of matrix metalloproteinases (MMP) [135]. Ultrasound-assisted enzymatic hydrolysis has also been proposed for the successful extraction of iodinated amino acids from *Palmaria palmata* and *Porphyra umbilicalis* (red seaweeds) [136].

Mycosporine-like amino acids (MAAs) are secondary metabolites synthesized for protection against solar radiation [28,137,138]. They consist of cyclohexenone or cyclohex-enimine chromophore with various amino acids, mainly glycine or iminoalcohol groups, as substituents and show antioxidant and photoprotective properties [3,137,139–144]. Among the most abundant compounds, mainly in Rhodophyceae shinorine, porphyra-334, palythine, asterina-330, mycosporine-glycine, palythinol, and palythene have been described [145,146], and their contents are dependent on the geographic, seasonal and bathymetric conditions, increasing during summer and decreasing with water depth [147]. A multifunctional cosmetic liposome formulation containing UV filters, vitamins (A, C, and E), Ginkgo biloba extract (rich on quercetin), and Phorphyra umbilicalis extract (rich in proteins, vitamins, minerals and mainly in MAA's porphyra-334 and shinorine) was efficient against signs of aging [148] by increasing hydration and reducing wrinkles and skin roughness. Leandro et al. [149] incorporated an extract of *Asparagopsis armata* (ASPAR'AGE™) containing MAA molecules in lotions with anti-aging properties, a hydrolyzed extract Aosaine® (three-quarters of aosaine consists of amino acids that are very similar those responsible for skin elasticity) extracted from *Ulva lactuca*, which present anti-aging, anti-wrinkle and stimulation of collagen properties. An extract (rich in minerals, trace elements and amino acids) from *Gelidium corneum* improves skin softness and restores elasticity. Therefore, MAAs have different properties, such as serving as natural sunscreens, possess antioxidants, anti-inflammatory, and anti-aging, and are stimulators of skin renewal, activators of cells proliferation, etc., making them a promising and safe option for pharmaceutical and cosmetic industries [150] (Table 2).

Table 2. Some activities and properties of seaweeds protein, peptides, and amino acids of interest in the cosmeceutical formulations.

Extract/Compound	Activity	Seaweed	Reference
Eleven mycosporine-like amino acids	UV-protective effect, antioxidant	*Agarophyton chilense*, *Pyropia plicata* and *Champia novae-zelandiae*	[147]
Mycosporine-like amino acids extract (with porphyra-334 and shinorine in a ratio of 2:1)	Anti-aging	*Phorphyra umbilicalis*	[151]
Mycosporine-like amino acids extract (mainly palythine and asterina-330)	Antioxidant, UV-protective effect, anti-aging	*Curdieara covitzae*, *Iridaea cordata*	[152]
Mycosporine-like amino acids extract (mainly porphyra-334, shinorine, palythine and asterina-330)	Antioxidant; UV-protective effect	*Gracilaria vermiculophylla*	[153]
Mycosporine-like amino acids extract (mainly palythine, asterina-330, shinorine, palythinol, porphyra-334 and usujirene)	Antioxidant, antiproliferative	*Chondrus crispus*, *Mastocarpus stellatus*, *Palmaria palmata*	[154]
Mycosporine-like amino acids extract (mainly deoxygadusol, palythene and usujirene)	Antioxidant	*Rhodymenia pseudopalmata*	[155]
Aqueous extract from freshwater macroalga (mainly polysaccharides and amino acids)	Skin moisturizing effect	*Rhizoclonium hieroglyphicum*	[156]
Peptide PPY1	Anti-inflammatory	*Pyropia yezoensis*	[134]
Peptides PYP1-5 and porphyra 334	Increase production of elastin and collagen	*Porphyra yezoensis* f. *coreana* Ueda	[135]
Methanol extract rich in proteins, vitamins, minerals, porphyra-334 and shinorine	Hydration, skin protective, anti-wrinkle, anti-roughness	*Phorphyra umbilicalis*	[148]
Phycobiliproteins (R-phycoerythrin allophycocyanin and phycocyanin)	Antioxidant	*Gracilaria gracilis*	[157]
Hydrolyzed extract	Antitumor	*Porphyra haitanesis*	[158]
Algae extract	Decrease of progerin production, anti-elastase, anti-collagenase	*Alaria esculenta*	[159]

Due to the toxic effect of several synthetic dyes and the high consumer demand for natural colors in food, pharmaceuticals, cosmetics, and textile industries there has been increasing interest in the use of phycobiliproteins in the food (C-phycocyanin) and cosmetic fields (C-phycocyanin and R-phycoerythrin). Phycobiliproteins are a class of water-soluble compounds composed of proteins that are covalently bound to linear tetrapyrroles, known as phycobilins, with fluorescent properties and high molecular weights and can be used for reddish colorings [28,118,160–163]. B-phycoerythrin resists changes in pH, possesses antioxidant properties [164], and can be used as a pink or purple dye in cosmetics [165]. Phycobilins can be red (phycoerytrins) or blue (phycocyanins and allophycocyanins) and phycocyanin is usually the major pigment microalgae (*Spirulina* spp.), whereas the characteristic red color of Rhodophyta phyla is due to both the phycoerythrin and phycocyanin pigments. Phycobiliproteins (concretely, R-phycoerythrin, phycocyanin, and allophycocyanin) extracted from *Gracilaria gracilis* presented high antioxidant and radical scavenging activities, primarily when harvested in winter [157], and the extraction can yield up to 46.5% of R-phycoerythrin using an aqueous solution of ionic liquids (cholinium chloride) to remove it from fresh algal biomass [166]. Saluri et al. [167] studied *Furcellaria lumbricalis* and *Coccotylus truncatus* and found an exponential correlation between R-phycoerythrin and allophycocyanin concentrations and collection depth. The contents of phycoerythrin and phycocyanin were slightly higher and lower, respectively, for dried commercial *Porphyra* spp. extracts in comparison to *Spirulina* spp. [168].

2.3. Phenolics and Terpenoids

Phenolic compounds are secondary plant metabolites with a basic structure with one or more aromatic rings, presenting one or more attached -OH groups. They are synthesized as part of the defense mechanisms in plants. Phlorotannins are secondary metabolites of phloroglucinol (1,3,5-trihydroxybenzene), are structurally less complex than terrestrial tannins, and are found in polymerized structures with ether, phenyl or 1,4-dibenzodioxin linkages [169,170].

Phlorotanins are increasingly considered for cosmeceutical applications, based on their antioxidative [171–175], anti-allergic [27,176–179], anti-inflammatory [27,180,181], tyrosinase inhibitory [182–186], and antidiabetic [175] activities. Skin protection against UV irradiation was confirmed in mouse skin models [187,188]. Phlorotannins also attenuated the expression of MMP-1 (an interstitial collagenase mainly responsible for the degradation of dermal collagen in human skin aging process) [27,28,189]. Dioxinodehydroeckol from *Ecklonia cava* proved to be an effective repair agent for skin damage against UVB [190]. On the other hand, fucofuroeckol-A derived from the brown seaweed *Ecklonia stolonifera Okamura*, exhibited protective activity against UVB radiation [191]; other studies also exhibited similar results for eckol and dieckol [192,193]. A correlation between the antioxidant activity and the hyaluronidase inhibitory capacity with higher molecular weight phlorotannins was observed [172], a behavior that was also observed in other works [194–196]. Some properties of brown algal phlorotannins are summarized in Table 3.

Table 3. Examples of recent studies confirming the phlorotannin activities of interest for cosmeceutical products.

Compound	Activity	Seaweed	References
Dioxinodehydroeckol	Preventive activity against UVB-induced apoptosis	*Ecklonia cava*	[190]
Dieckol	Adipogenesis inhibitory effect	*Ecklonia cava*	[197]
Eckol	Anti-inflammatory, anti-tyrosinase	*Eisenia bicyclis, Ecklonia stolonifera*	[192,193,198]
Eckol, 6,6'-bieckol, 8,8'-bieckol, dieckol, and phlorofucofuroeckol-A	Antiallergic	*Ecklonia cava, E. stolonifera*	[179]
Fucofuroeckol-A	Protective against UVB	*Ecklonia stolonifera Okamura*	[191]
Fuhalol	Antioxidant	*Cystoseira compressa*	[175]
Fucophloroethol (isomer)	Antioxidant	*Fucus vesiculosus*	[199]
Eckstolonol	Antioxidant enzymatic activities of catalase and superoxide dismutase	*Ecklonia cava*	[200]
Octaphlorethol A	Antioxidative effects	*Ishige foliacea*	[201]
Phlorofucofuroeckol A	Hepatoprotective effect against oxidative stress	*Eisenia bicyclis*	[93]
	Tyrosinase inhibitory activity	*Ecklonia stolonifera*	[182]
2-phloroeckol and 2-O-(2,4,6-trihydroxyphenyl)-6,60-bieckol	Tyrosinase inhibitory activity	*Ecklonia cava*	[185]
Phlorofucofuroeckol B	Antiallergic	*Eisenia arborea*	[202]
Phlorotannins	Antioxidant, anticoagulant, antiinflammatory, antibacterial, antiviral, antitumor; antidiabetic, photoprotective	Brown algae, *Ascophyllum nodosum*, *Fucus serratus*, *Himanthalia elongata*, *Halidrys siliquosa*	[45,172,175,198,203,204]

Meroterpenoids exhibited antioxidant properties and can prevent skin photoaging without the risk of cytotoxicity [205]. Other meroterpenoid derivatives have also shown interesting properties in relation to protection from cell damage caused by UVA irradiation [206] and photodamage attenuation on irradiated cells [207]. In addition, the hypopigmenting effect of meroterpenoids has been associated with brown algae [208].

2.4. Lipids

Seaweed present a low lipidic content (usually under 5%), but they are highly unsaturated and the ω3:ω-6 fatty acids ratio is highly favorable [73,209,210]. Among the most abundant fatty acids are γ-linolenic acid, arachidonic acid, eicosapentanoic acid, and docosahexanoic acid, but other lipid types, such as sterols and phospholipids, are also found [211,212]. The main sterols found are fucosterol, isofucosterol, and clionasterol [213,214]. Several biological properties have been associated with lipids [211,215]. Polyunsaturated fatty acids (PUFA) can benefit skin barrier protection and other biological functions can be enhanced nutricosmetics could contribute an anti-obesity effect [211,216,217] and the regulation of inflammatory responses [25,218]. Being structural components of cell membranes, sterols regulate membrane fluidity and permeability and other properties, such as antioxidant, antiproliferative, and anti-photodamage, and anti-inflammatory effects have been reported for fucosterol [28,188,219–221] An effect against the malarial parasite *Plasmodium falciparum* has been exhibited [222]. The viability of human keratinocytes irradiated with UVB was not affected when cells were incubated with fucosterol, and a marked decrease in UV-irradiated MMPs and increased type-I procollagen production were observed [28,206]; other authors obtained results consistent with these observations [49,61]. Phospholipids, mainly made up of fatty acids containing a phosphate group and a simple organic molecule, have been reported to help with carotenoid absorption [223]; in other work, authors showed a reduction of body weight and fat mass in mice drinking water with lipid capsules prepared using phospholipids [224]. In addition, seaweed essential oil has been evaluated, and Rexliene and Sridhar reported the antimicrobial and anti-dandruff properties of red seaweed *Portieria hornemannii* essential oil [225]. Subsequently, an antibacterial film was created with a carrageenan biopolymer blended with extracted seaweed essential oil, showing adequate bio-physical, mechanical, and anti-microbial properties. Table 4 summarizes the biological activities associated with lipids.

Table 4. Activities of seaweed lipids of interest in the formulation of cosmeceuticals.

Compound	Activity	Seaweed	References
E-10-oxooctadec-8-enoic acid, E-9-oxooctadec-10- enoic acid	Anti-inflammatory	*Gracilaria verrucosa*	[226]
Essential oil (tetradeconoic acid, hexadecanoic acid, (9Z, 12Z)-9,12-octadecadienoic acid, (9Z)-hexadec-9-enoic acid)	Antibacterial activity against *Staphylococcus aureus* and *Bacillus cereus* Antioxidant: radical scavenging (DPPH, superoxide, ABTS)	*Laminaria japonica*	[227]
Fucosterol	Antioxidant: increased antioxidative enzymes (superoxide dismutase, catalase, glutathione peroxidase)	*Pelvetia siliquosa*	[219,228]
Fucosterol	Anti-photodamage: decreased UVB-induced MMPs and increased procollagen Anti-inflammatory	*Hizikia fusiformis*	[60,188]
Phytosterol	Antitumoral	Commercial (Sigma)	[229]
Lipidic profile	Antioxidant, enzyme inhibition	*Ulva rigida*, *Gracilaria* sp., *Fucus vesiculosus*, *Saccharina latissima*	[211]
Unsaturated fatty acids	Antioxidant	Brown algae	[230]
Fatty acid profiling	Bioindicator of chemical stress	*Pterocladia capillacea*, *Sargassum hornschuchii*, *Ulva lactuca*	[231]

2.5 Vitamins

Vitamins obtained from diet and through topical application are essential for many functions of human skin. Supplementation is considered for protection against dehydration and premature aging of the skin, cosmetic prevention of damage by sun exposure, regulation of the secretory activity of the sebaceous glands, and the preservation of the anatomical integrity of adnexial structures [232]. Vitamins are popular ingredients in many cosmeceuticals and skin care products. Vitamins A, C, E, K and vitamin complex B are the most important and clinically validated for skin photoaging prevention and treatment [233] and the common vitamins in algae are vitamins A, B, C, and E [3,16,25,234].

Vitamin A or the retinol form shows antioxidant and antiwrinkle capacity [37,235,236] and is topically used in cosmetics to reduce facial hyperpigmentation and fine wrinkles [237]. The concentration of vitamin complex B (B_1, B_2, B_3 or niacine, B_6, B_9 or folic acid, B_{12}) is generally higher in green and red seaweeds [3,238]. Vitamin B_3 active forms added to skin care products include: niacinamide, nicotinic acid nicotinate esters. Niacinamide is an antioxidant, reduces hyperpigmentation (also due to blue light-induced), and improves aspects of the epidermis by reducing the trans-epidermal water loss [7,239]. Red algae and other species are good sources of vitamin B_{12} for vegetarians; this vitamin shows anti-aging properties and is essential for hair and nail growth and health [25,240–242].

Vitamin C is used in the cosmeceutical industry as it is an L-ascorbic acid of which the biologically active form is most known [236]. The red algae *Ceramium rubrum* and *Porphyra leucosticta* show high vitamin C or ascorbate content. This vitamin, topically applied, has antioxidant, detoxifying, antiviral, anti-inflammatory, antimicrobial, and anti-stress effects, and can be used for enhancing tissue cell growth, repairing blood vessels, teeth, and bones [7,243]. Many studies reported skin improvements in fine lines and reduction of pigmentation and inflammation if present in an appropriate concentration in a cosmetic formula [7,244]. Several works confer tyrosinase inhibition to vitamin C due to it interacting with copper ions, which reduces melanogenesis [236].

Vitamin E (α, ã, ä tocopherol), the most abundant fat-soluble vitamin of non-saponifiable lipids in many algae, can be extracted from different green, red, or/and brown seaweeds [245], and is effective against UV damage, photoaging, and skin cancer when is in a high concentration and in a non-esterified form [209,246]. Cosmetic formulations usually include vitamin C since it regenerates oxidized vitamin E [7]. Vitamin K, found in high concentrations in some seaweeds, has well-known blood clotting properties (wound, bruises, marks, and scar healing) [247–249].

2.6. Minerals

Seaweeds have a high mineral content, about 8–40% [250–252], and this wide range is dependent on seaweed phylum and species, seaweed oceanic residence time, geographical locations, wave exposure, and seasonal and annual environmental factors [234]. Seaweeds possess most of the mineral elements from the sea, and their content depends on the pH, temperature, and the concentration of the minerals in seawater. Seaweeds have been described as an ideal safe natural source of minerals. Inorganic ions play important roles in different functions of the skin, whereas others can be considered dangerous as a consequence of dermal exposure [253]. Table 5 shows the average mineral content in different type of seaweeds.

Seaweeds contain a variety of mineral elements, macro-elements, and trace elements, which are an excellent mineral source for cosmeceutical benefits for humans. Several minerals (e.g., Ca, Fe, Mg, P, Na, Zn, Cu, and Se) are recognized as necessary for health and well-being. All seaweeds contain high amounts of both macro minerals (Ca, Mg, Na, K, and P) and trace elements (Fe, Zn, I, Cu, Se, and Mn) [234,250,255]. High potassium contents were reported in red macroalgal *Gracilaria* species and the brown macroalgal species *Laminaria digitata*; nevertheless, seaweeds have low Na/K ratios (<1.5) [250]. *Caulerpa veravelensis*, *Ulva lactuca*, and *Sargassum polycystum* contain higher amounts of calcium. Seaweeds have been described as a good source of iodine, which is present in several chemical forms, and brown algae contains greater amounts, up to over 1% wet weight; its accumulation in seaweed tissues could be 30,000 times its concentration in sea water [254,255]. According to Peñalver and coauthors, seaweeds are a primary source of iodine, allowing to achieve daily iodine requirements [234], as it is an essential element in order to maintain thyroid function and health [234,251].

Polefka et al. summarized the scientific evidence available on the benefits and risks of topical application of mineral salts [256]. Seaweeds are, in general, a better source of minerals than sea salts, because the proportion of minerals are closer to those in human skin and body's plasm and the penetration of nutrients is better [39]. Due to this high affinity to human skin, mineral sea salts used in cosmetics are rapidly absorbed, and refresh and replenish or hydrate the skin [39,257]. Several skin care and cosmetic products contain various nutrients and minerals from seaweed, seawater, or sea mud, especially for their therapeutic properties fir psoriasis and other skin-related disorders, and for their beneficial effects on skin (they help to retain water for a longer time, restores skin pH, help in blood circulation, acne repair, and prevention, and have anti-aging effects) [39,257,258]. Alves et al. reported that high concentrated forms of marine minerals and trace elements provide a protective effect against UV radiation [259].

Table 5. Minimum and maximum values (g/100 g or mg/kg dry weight) for macro and micro elements found in edible European macroalgae [234,254].

Element (Concentration)	Brown Algae	Green Algae	Red Algae
Ca (%)	0.89–1.32	0.21–1.87	0.39–45.0
Mg (%)	0.22–1.2	0.12–2.8	0.20–167
P (%)	0.15–0.98	0.21–500	0.10–1.40
K (%)	3.8–11.5	1.1–8.1	0.33–10.2
Na (%)	1.3–7.1	0.52–8.9	1 1–4.3
S (%)	1.33–1.5	0.23–8.5	1 5–4.0
Cu (ppm)	1.1–11.0	1.6–12.1	<0 4–35.0
I (ppm)	0.20–500	20–1000	0.24–1200
Fe (ppm)	15.8–270	17.7–2890	16–1820
Mn (ppm)	<1–52.7	<2–347	<1–748
Zn (ppm)	2.5–52.3	1.98–84	7.2–714.4

2.7. Pigments

Regarding the concentration of pigments, seaweeds are classified into three groups: green (chlorophylls a, b and c), brown (carotenoids), and red (phycobilins as phycoerythrin). In addition, free radical scavenging, inhibiting melanogenesis, and photoprotection are some of the properties of these compounds that make them suitable for skin care [260]. Carotenoids are isoprenoid molecules produced by photosynthetic plants, fungi, and algae. These lipophilic compounds can be chemically classified as carotenes, such as α-carotene, β-carotene, and lycopene, and xanthophylls. Carotenoids are used as colors in foods and as natural color enhancers, in the food, pharmaceutical, and cosmetic industries. Some act as provitamin A, and recently they have attracted considerable interest due to their antioxidant and anti-inflammatory properties [261]. β-Carotene helps to counteract free radicals involved in various diseases and premature aging [28]. In this context, the extracts obtained from three brown seaweeds were assessed to study antioxidant capacities, where fucoxanthin, violaxanthin, â-carotene, cyanidin-3-O-glucoside, and other carotenoid and chlorophyll derivatives were also characterized. The results suggest that these compounds are responsible for antioxidant properties [262].

Fucoxanthin is the main carotenoid in brown algae, this xanthophyll can counteract oxidative stress caused by UV radiation [171] and suppresses tyrosinase activity in UVB-irradiated guinea pig and melanogenesis in UVB-irradiated mice [27]; anti-melanogenic, anti-aging and antioxidant activities were also associated with this compound [40]. Fucoxanthin enhanced the fat burning rate of fat cells in adipose tissue and might be used to treat obesity and reduce the risk of certain disorders, such as type 2 diabetes [26,28,261,263,264]. Some reported actions are summarized in Table 6.

Table 6. Biological activities of algal pigments of interest in cosmeceuticals.

Extract/Compound	Activity	Seaweed	Reference
97% fucoxanthin extract	Antioxidant (DPPH scavenging capacity, reducing power)	*Himanthalia elongata*	[265]
Fucoxanthin	Antioxidant, anti-melanogenesis	Brown seaweeds	[266,267]
	Antiobesity	*Undaria pinnatifida*	[263]
	Skin protective (antiphotodamage, anti-pigmentary, antiphotoaging, anti-wrinkling	*Sargassum siliquastrum*	[268]
	Anti-inflammatory	*Myagropsis myagroides*	[269]
	Tyrosinase activity	*Laminaria japonica*	[266]
	Photoprotective	*Undaria pinnatifida*	[270]
	Antioxidant	*Sargassum fusiforme,*	[271]
Lutein	Whitening; visual disorders and cognition diseases	*Rhodophyta* spp.	[28,272]

3. Technological Functions

According to their functions, cosmetic ingredients are classified as (i) additives; (ii) stabilizing or excipient agents; and (iii) bioactive compounds, with real cosmetic functions [28,35]. Algal components can be used as technical ingredients to improve texture, color or stability of cosmetics, but also as bioactive agents, since they can confer a variety of biological desirable actions, which are applicable in the manufacturing of cosmeceuticals and skin care products [38,273]. Macroalgal components can be included in cosmetics as thickening or gelling agents, antioxidant, and colorants, or as active ingredients in hydrating, antiaging, skin-whitening, and pigmentation reduction products. These dual potentialities are summarized in Figure 1.

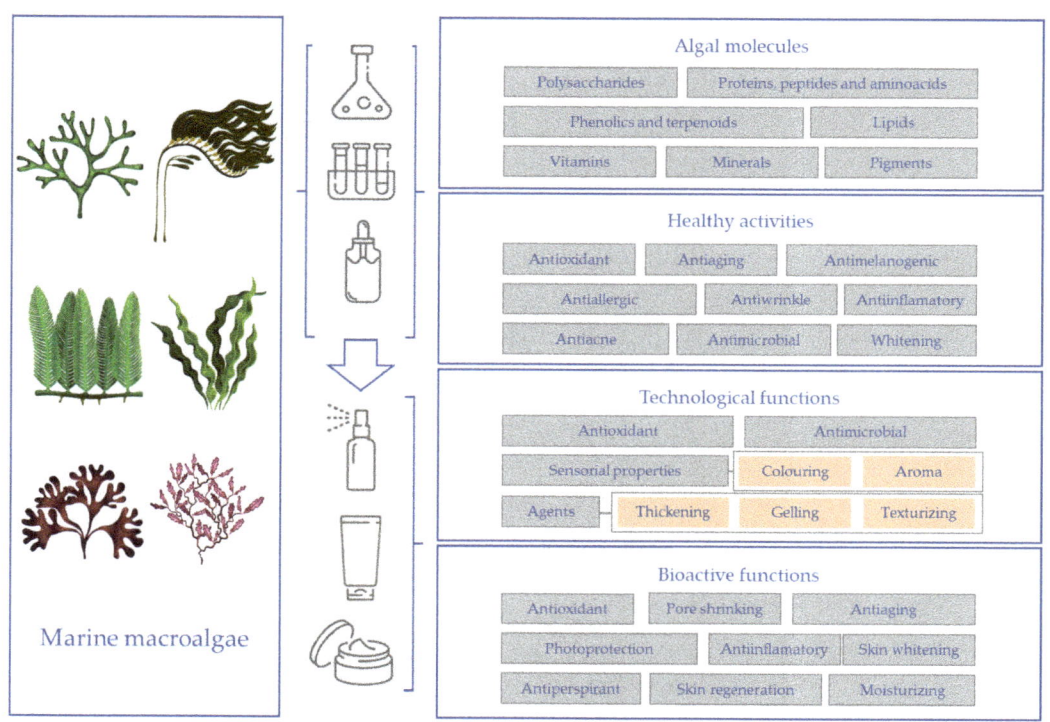

Figure 1. Cosmeceutical potential of algae components.

The incorporation of seaweed components was successful in different physical forms, and are commercially available in soaps, shampoos, sprays, hydrogels, or creams [274,275].

Their efficiency and stability can be enhanced with suitable carrier systems or vesicles, such as liposomes, nano/microparticles, emulsions, hydrogels, etc., designed to carry active agents in commercial products to achieve promoted effects [276–278].

3.1. Antimicrobial Agents

The antimicrobial properties of seaweed components are well known, in particular for food and pharmaceutical industries [279–281]. Extracts from macroalga have shown antibacterial and antifungal activities, the most active components being terpenoids and phlorotannins [27,281], which can avoid the side effects and allergic reactions associated with synthetic drugs [282]. Extracts from brown and green seaweeds proved effective against acne vulgaris [201,283], brown algal extracts against common skin pathogenic bacteria, such as methicillin-resistant *Staphylococcus aureus*, *Staphylococcus aureus* and *Staphylococcus epidermidis* [284–286], green algal extracts showed activity against oral bacteria [78,206], and red algae are active against *Staphylococcus* and *Candida* sp. [28,287–290]. In order to have products with a wider spectrum of protection, mixtures could be a valid approach. Widowati et al. formulated a moisturizer cream with adequate color and odor, using an antibacterial extract obtained from mixtures of *Sargassum duplicatum*, *Sargassum echinocarpum*, and *S. polycystum* extracts, which inhibited the development of bacteria for a longer period of time [291]. All seaweeds contained steroids, quinones, flavonoids, and alkaloids, and saponins were only found in *S. duplicatum*.

3.2. Antioxidants

Since many cosmetic and cosmeceutical formulations contain a lipidic component, they are highly susceptible to lipid peroxidation. The addition of antioxidants is needed to protect from oxidative deterioration, which also maintains the sensorial properties of the cosmetic products, in the context of appearance and odor. The contradictory data on the safety of synthetic chemical antioxidants have incentivized the search and use of natural compounds with antioxidant properties. Seaweeds represent an abundant and widespread source of compounds with confirmed antiradical and reducing properties [173,284–286,292]. Furthermore, they showed the potential to protect and/or retard oxidation of cosmetic products [20] and have a wide range of biological properties. The most efficient algal compounds are phlorotannin-derived fractions, but peptides and polysaccharide fractions also display reducing properties and antiradical capacity [97,293]; the phenolic compounds found in red seaweed can also scavenge free radicals and also show other properties, such as the inhibition of tyrosinase [294].

3.3. Sensorial Properties

The incorporation of different seaweed ingredients has to be evaluated in relation to organoleptic, spreadability, and hedonic tests [295,296]. Seaweed can provide different compounds with coloring compounds as an alternative to synthetic, mineral, and plant dyes, and show lower allergenic properties. Among the major compounds with this property are phycobilins and carotenoids, which cover a wide range of blue, yellow, orange, and red colors [29], as well as other biologically interesting properties [264].

Aroma is a key feature in cosmetics and cosmeceuticals, and the potential of seaweeds to produce terpenoids, carotenoids, fatty acid derivatives, and sulfur compounds is well known [29,297].

3.4. Texturizing

Thickening, gelling, and texturizing agents are used to control viscoelasticity and to form a cohesive internal structure in cosmetic products. Alginate, has been traditionally used in the cosmetic industry as a stabilizer for emulsions and suspensions due to its high stability, and for its thickening and gelling properties [56,57,171,298]. Later, authors indicated that it could be used as a hydrogel for the encapsulation of bioactives, drug delivery systems, and tissue engineering. The use of extreme pH values is not recommended and the concentration of polyvalent metal ions must be controlled in cosmetic formulations using alginates by means of adding sequestrants to avoid altering the viscosity and alginic acid precipitation [28,299]. Agar, a polysaccharide from red algae, can be applied to control both the viscosity and emollience of cosmetic products. Dita et al. confirmed that agar from *Gracilaria* sp. has a gelling agent capable of having a thickening effect on certain products, such as liquid bath soap, as a cocamide DEA (diethanolamine) substitute [300]. Carrageenans are commonly used in cosmetics as stabilizing, thickening, and gelling agents due to their excellent properties, such as gel-forming ability and chemical stability [27,30,58,301]. The rheological behavior of carrageenan and hybrid carrageenans is temperature sensitive and also depends on the structure, sulfate content, or molecular weight [28,302,303]. Carrageenans can be degraded by carrageenases to produce a number of even-numbered carrageenan oligosaccharides, which exhibit different attractive functions, such as anti-inflammation, anti-tumor, anticoagulation, or antithrombosis effects [304].

Bagal-Kestwal et al. summarized the use of carrageenans (κ, λ, and ι with sodium) as binder and emulsion stabilizers, preventing constituent separation in toothpastes in a recent comprehensive review [274]. In a previous work, these carrageenans were proposed as bodying, emulsion stabilizer, thickeners, dispersion media for shampoos, body lotion, and other cosmetic creams, and as an ingredient binder for personal lubricants [305]. Some comprehensive works [278,306] discussed the most recent breakthroughs in the field of skin care and rejuvenation using cosmeceutical facial masks developed using biopolymer-based hydrogels, which are commonly used for sensitive skins with cooling and soothing effects. Tiwari and co-workers explained the potential of biopolymers in the development of topical matrices (cream, ointment, and gel) employed as dosage forms for burn treatments [298]. Later, authors detailed the potential of carrageenans for drugs delivery or alginates for wound dressings due to their hemostatic potential. Wasupalli et al. pointed out the ability of carrageenans to form unique thermoreversible gels that are very useful to encapsulate active compounds in the cosmetic field [302]. Graham et al. corroborated the potential of thermoresponsive polymers, including agarose or carrageenan, to be used in cosmetics [307]. Hu et al. proposed a simple method to prepare hydrophilic−hydrophobic core−shell microparticles using seaweed polymers (alginates, κ-carrageenan, or agarose) with great prospective applications in the protection of unstable compounds and delivery and controlled release of drugs or bioactives in cosmetics [301].

4. Bioactive Functions

4.1. Moisturization

Moisturizer agents help to maintain skin appearance and elasticity, improving its barrier role against harmful environmental factors [28]. Polysaccharides in cosmetics are efficient at maintaining hydration, and algal extracts that are rich in polysaccharides would be an alternative to hydroxy acids [38] and are also promising for their various properties that are beneficial to skin, including antioxidant, anti-melanogenic, and skin anti-aging properties [23,24,41]. Water:propylene glycol (1:1) extracts of *Laminaria japonica* showed skin moisturizing properties in in vivo tests with human skin [28,308]. Wang et al. reported that polysaccharides from this seaweed absorbed and retained more moisture than polysaccharides from both the red algae *Chondrus cripus*, which provides hydrating, moisturizing, and therapeutic effects, and from the green algae *Codium tomentosum*, which can regulate water distribution in skin [28]. Agar is used as a moisturizer for skin and hair [46]. Mineral-rich seaweed extracts may be found in skin moisturizing agents, facial cleansing products, masks, make-up removers, bath additives, and in products to prevent cellulites. Fatty acids, either in the diet or topically applied, are efficient at preventing trans-epidermal water loss [37].

4.2. Skin Whitening

Skin whitening, particularly demanded in Asia, is also desired to achieve fair and flawless skin. Tyrosinase catalyzes two distinct significant reactions in melanin synthesis: the hydroxylation of l-tyrosine to 3,4-dihydroxy-L-phenylalanine, which is oxidized to dopaquinone, and further converted to melanin. Sun exposure increases the synthesis of both tyrosinase and melanosomes. Different seaweed components can be active tyrosinase inhibitors and are commonly proposed for skin whitening [27,192,193,309]; and brown algal extracts are as effective as kojic acid [284–286,310,311]. Similarly, Park et al. reported that *P. yezoensis* extracts could be proposed as a safe and effective agent to enhance skin whitening and prevention or alleviation of skin wrinkle formation. The extracts exhibited a significant decrease in tyrosinase activity, but was less marked than arbutin. However, arbutin could have secondary undesirable effects, whereas these aqueous seaweed extracts promoted collagen production and, in a study with 23 volunteers, they also enhanced skin brightness [312].

Due to the variety of activities, different fractions of seaweeds have been combined to achieve complementary actions, i.e., between phenolics and polysaccharides [313]. In addition, seaweed mixtures can be explored for their dermo-cosmetic potential [195,291,314,315], i.e., a cream mask from a mixture of seaweeds showing antibacterial, cell proliferation, moisture retention, and tyrosinase inhibitory activities, and also high spread and adhesive abilities, being a nonirritant and safe [314]. In addition, combination with other marine ingredients, such as nanomelanin from *Halomonas venusta*, isolated from a marine sponge *Callyspongia* sp., incorporated in a cream fortified with concentrates of seaweed *Gelidium spinosum* showed antioxidant, antimicrobial, and wound healing activity in addition to improved texture [316].

4.3. UV Protection, Antioxidant and Antiaging

Skin aging, causing thinning, dryness, laxity, fragility, enlarged pores, fine lines, and wrinkles, is a complex process of intrinsic and extrinsic aging. Intrinsic aging refers to the natural degradation of the skin, whereas extrinsic aging results from reactive oxygen species (ROS) generated during exposure to UV radiation [28]. Although the human body possesses an endogenous antioxidant system able to block reactive oxygen species, under conditions of oxidative stress, these defenses can be insufficient and may lead to free radical cell damage to proteins, lipids, and DNA. ROS accumulation may be responsible for photoaging complications, such as cutaneous inflammation, erythema, premature aging, melanoma, and skin cancer [317]. UVB-induced decreased cell viability could be restored by eckstolonol treatment through the enzymatic activities of catalase and superoxide dismutase [200]. Ultraviolet B irradiation induces the production of matrix metalloproteinases, and is structurally and functionally related to zinc endopeptidases, capable of digesting extracellular matrix components, such as collagens, proteoglycans, fibronectin, and laminin [64,90]. Sun-damaged skin shows significantly elevated levels of active gelatinases than intrinsically aged skin, since prolonged exposure to UV radiation causes the enzymatic breakage of collagen and elastin fibers, which are responsible for maintaining the elasticity and integrity of skin [6]. Bioactive compounds derived from marine sources [29] and from algae, especially phlorotannins, have potential anti-photoaging agents, preventing UV-induced oxidative stress, and also inhibit the expressions of MMPs in human dermal fibroblasts [27,176,318]. Riani et al. reported antioxidant and anti-collagenase activity of a *Sargassum plagyophyllum* extract as active pharmaceutical ingredient for anti-wrinkle cosmetics [319]. The potential of fucoxanthin was also confirmed, and its incorporation was compatible with other components in homogeneous water creams [295].

Since these compounds are preferentially extracted in organic solvents, different examples of macerated extracts with potential photoprotective action can be found [4,204,320,321]. Since other compounds, such as mycosporine-like amino acids, sulfated polysaccharides, carotenoids, and polyphenols, exhibit photoprotective action though a wide range of biological activities, including ultraviolet absorbing, antioxidant, matrix-metalloproteinase inhibitors and anti-aging activities, crude extracts with complex composition can be promising [322]. Gager et al. reported that the phlorotannin-enriched fractions, extracted by maceration and further purified by a liquid–liquid extraction showed antioxidant and photoprotective activities comparable to those of commercial molecules and the anti-aging activity of the obtained fraction was higher than that of epigallocatechin gallate [204]. The efficiency of mixtures of components has been described. Hameury et al. [323] confirmed that an association of ingredients from marine origin revealed activity on the epidermis and the dermis, by regulation of proteins involved in gene expression, cell survival and metabolism, inflammatory processes, dermal extracellular matrix synthesis, melanogenesis and keratinocyte proliferation, migration, and differentiation, thus helping to prevent the visible signs of skin aging.

5. Patents

Seaweeds and their components have been claimed as functional, sensorial, and biological agents in the formulation of cosmetics, cosmeceuticals, and nutricosmetics. Some representative examples on their utilization in the formulation of products with different claimed actions are summarized in Table 7.

Table 7. Examples of patents claiming the use of seaweed and seaweed components in cosmetic, cosmeceutical, and nutricosmetics formulations to confer different properties.

Activity	Applicant Company	References
\multicolumn{3}{Functional and sensorial}
Emulsifying, water retention, gelling	Asahi Denka Kogyo Kk; Health Care Ltd.; Ichimaru Pharcos Inc; Iwasekenjiro Shoten Kk; Lg Household & Amp Lvxinyan Guangdong Bio Tech Co. Ltd.	[324–327]
Film forming	Kowa Techno Search Kk	[328]
Improved water solubility and imparting excellent feeling of use	Artnature Co. Ltd.; Kanebo Ltd.; Koosee Kk; Kyoei Kagaku Kogyo Kk; Natura Cosmeticos Sa; Toyo Shinyaku Co. Ltd.;	[329–333]
Stabilization system	Yantai New Era Health Industry Daily Chemical Co. Ltd.	[334]
Biological		
Anti-aging and antistress	Givenchy Parfums; Hanbul Cosmetics Co. Ltd.; Hainan Hairun Biolog Technology Co. Ltd. Shengfeng Yantai Agricultural Tech Co. Ltd.	[335–339]
Anti-inflammatory	Explzn Inc; Yantai Yucheng Enterprise Man Consulting Co. Ltd.	[340,341]
Antimicrobial	Nippon Enu Yuu Esu Kk	[342]
Antioxidant	Gelyma; Jeollanamdo	[343,344]
Antiperspirant, desodorant	Japan Natural Lab Co. Ltd.	[345]
Anti-wrinkle	Mamachi Co. Ltd.	[346]
Bood circulation	Kowa Techno Search Kk	[328]
Hair and scalp care and treatment, hair growth	Clean Sea Co. Ltd.; Henkel Ag & Co Kgaa; Kose Corp; Nantong Snakebite Therapy Res Inst; Pinebio Co. Ltd.; Sako Kk; Shirako Co. Ltd.; Lion Corp	[347–354]
Moisturizing	Amazonebio Co. Ltd.; Clarins; Jingmen Nuoweiying New Material Tech Co Ltd.; Kracie Home Products Ltd.; Qingdao Better Biolog Science & Technology Co Ltd.	[308,355–358]
Oil control, acne prevention and removal of acne marks	Yantai New Era Health Ind Daily Chemical Co. Ltd.; Guangzhou Yuanmeisheng Cosmetic Co. Ltd.; Shanghai Bonaquan Cosmetics Co. Ltd.; Suzhou Cosmetic Materials Co. Ltd.; Tubio; Yantai New Era Health Ind Daily Chemical Co. Ltd.	[359–363]
Pore shrinking, cleaning and minimizing	Foshan Aai Cosmetic Health Care Product Co. Ltd.; South China Sea Inst Oceanology; Rongding Guangdong Biotechnology Co. Ltd.; Kose Corp	[364–366]
Prevention and amelioration of aged and rough skin	Anhui Shuanglu Flour Co. Ltd.; Dzintars As; Explzn Inc; Guangzhou Saliai Stemcell Science & Technology Co. Ltd.; Kyoei Chemical Ind; Nox Bellcow Zs Nonwoven Chemical Ltd.; Shanghai Bonaquan Cosmetics Co. Ltd.; Wuhu Chuanshi Information Tech Co. Ltd.	[360,367–373]

Table 7. Cont.

Activity	Applicant Company	References
Protecting from pollution	Codif International Sa	[374]
Safe melanin production and whitening	Ichimaru Pharcos Inc; Shenzhen Sanda Cosmetics Co. Ltd.	[375,376]
Skin regeneration and epidermal cell repair	Beihai Yuanlong Pearl Company Ltd.; Jeonnam Bioindustry Found; Hexie Tech Co. Ltd.; Mokpo Marin Food Industry Res Center; Yantai New Era Health Industry Daily Chemical Co. Ltd.	[334,377–379]
Sunscreen and anti-sun tan	Lg Household & Health Care Ltd.; Mikimoto Seiyaku Kk; Miin	[380–382]
Weight-reduction and slimming	Kanebo Ltd.; Sekisui Plastics	[383,384]
Whitening	Ichimaru Pharcos Inc; Lion Corp; Mikimoto Seiyaku Kk; World Costec Co. Ltd.	[385–389]
Mixed Effects, More Than One Of The Following Actions		
Antiaging, anti-allergic, anti-inflammatory, antioxidant, anti-wrinkle; cleaning, moisturizing, repairing, sunscreen, whitening	Amorepacific Corp; Baiyun Lianjia Fine Chemical Factory; Ecomine Co. Ltd.; Foshan Chancheng Relakongjian Biotechnology Co. Ltd.; Guangdong Darz Group Co. Ltd.; Guangzhou Baiyun Lianjia Fine Chemical Factory; Guangzhou Keneng Cosmetic Res Co. Ltd.; Guangzhou Xibao Daily Chemical Co. Ltd.; Hainan Shiboli Biotechnology Co. Ltd.; I2b Co. Ltd.; Jeollanamdo; Kaiso Shigen Kenkyusho Kk; Pola Chem Ind Inc.	[344,390–398]

Seaweeds can be used either fresh or fermented [349,363,399], and are usually incorporated as extracts, but also a pure single compounds, such as P-334 and DP-334 from *Porphyra dentata* [378], can be found. Both single species and seaweed mixtures have been found [359,386,387,400]. In addition, seaweed extracts can be combined with extracts from terrestrial plants, medicinal herbs, mushroom, microalgae, and fish [401–406], as well as with conventional ingredients [332,350,351,407–410] or even gold [372]. These mixtures of species and combination with other raw materials during manufacturing of cosmetics can be adopted to generate synergistic effects [335,359,375,411].

A variety of formulations has been found, including liposomes [355] and nano-liposome emulsions for improving the stability of extracts and its compatibility in the cosmetic system, reaching a deep layer of skin and minimizing sensitization responses by direct contact with epidemic cells [334]. Not only have creams been the object of patents, but other specific products, such as masks [412], disposable glove-shaped hand films [357], or mist compositions with fine particles that are widely dispersed when sprayed [413].

Seaweed fractions can confer functional properties or technical properties, such as thickening [346] and emulsifying properties of the polysaccharides, alginate, agar, and carrageenan [324], which also can impart water retention ability, conferring a smooth or moist humectant feeling without imparting stickiness [325,329]. Particularly, in hair cosmetics, they can provide a glossy and elastic feeling for hair and a moist feeling for the scalp [333,350]. Sensorial properties, such as suppressing the stickiness or stiffness of hair, facilitating hairdressing, the extensibility and spread on hair and producing a good feeling in its use, which are desirable for these types of products [330]. Seaweed components can also replace different additives, such as antimicrobials [342] or conventional ultraviolet ray blockers [382].

Seaweed components are interesting in the formulation of different hygienic products, including deodorants, shampoos [330,349,414,415], and cleaning supplies [328,416], especially water washing-free cleaning agents without surfactants. Other proposed formulations of cosmetics were aimed at skin condition [417] and moisturizing [403,410] improvements. Cosmeceuticals containing seaweeds are non-irritants [376], and can perform different functions, such as improving psoriasis and preventing skin problems, especially atopic dermatitis [393], hyperpigmentation [375,401,402,408], acne [410], wrinkles [406], and hair loss [351,401,402]. Many products formulated claims of a plurality of skin care effects, i.e., moisturizing, repair, and anti-aging [338,339,418] or melanin-formation inhibitory action, alleviation of skin stains and freckles, amelioration of roughened and dry skins, and conferring skins gloss and tension [387].

A number of nutricosmetics have been designed to be used in common foods and beverages to improve skin appearance and firmness [386,387], but also claim to improve immunity, strengthening the body's constitution and improving skin antioxidant capacity [368], losing weight, and beautifying skin [419].

Other patents have claimed pollution-free, safe, sanitary, ecological, environmentally friendly and energy-saving preparation processes [338,339,374,377,419] and also purification and deodorization stages [380,419–423].

6. Conclusions and Future Trends

Cosmetics, cosmeceuticals, and nutricosmetics are daily-use products that are gaining increasing commercial importance for improving the appearance of skin and for treating various dermatologic conditions. Seaweeds are a source of valuable components for the formulation of products due to the variety of functional, sensorial and biological properties they can confer. A diverse group of biologically active compounds, including vitamins, minerals, amino acids, carbohydrates, and lipids, can be extracted from seaweeds to develop conventional and novel cosmeceutical products. The possibility of offering a vast array of activities makes seaweeds a highly attractive renewable and versatile resource, and the importance of extraction and purification processes should also be considered. Other important aspects requiring study are in relation to greener extraction of bioactives, their chemical and biological characterization, as well as stabilization and delivery into novel products. As with other ingredients and applications, quality control and standardization are required for the commercial use of seaweed bioactives.

Author Contributions: Conceptualization, E.F. and H.D.; resources, M.D.T., E.F. and H.D.; writing—original draft preparation, M.P.C., E.M.B., L.L.-H., T.F.-A., N.F.-F., M.D.T., E.F. and H.D.; writing—review and editing, N.F.-F., M.D.T., E.F. and H.D.; project administration, H.D.; funding acquisition, M.D.T. and H.D. All authors have read and agreed to the published version of the manuscript.

Funding: This work has received financial support from the Ministry of Science, Innovation, and Universities of Spain (RTI2018-096376-B-I00) and the Xunta de Galicia (Centro singular de investigación de Galicia accreditation 2019–2022) and the European Union (European Regional Development Fund-ERDF)—Ref. ED431G2019/06.

Institutional Review Board Statement: Not applicable.

Informed Consent Statement: Not applicable.

Data Availability Statement: Data are available in the original papers cited.

Conflicts of Interest: The authors declare no conflict of interest.

References

1. Soulioti, I.; Diomidous, M.; Theodosopoulou, H.; Violaki, N.; Plessa, H.; Charalambidou, M.; Pistolis, J.; Plessas, S.T. Cosmetics: History, products, industry, legislation, regulations and implications in public health. *Rev. Clin. Pharmacol. Pharmacokinet.* **2013**, *27*, 5–15.
2. Pangestuti, R.; Shin, K.-H.; Kim, S.-K. Anti-photoaging and potential skin health benefits of seaweeds. *Mar. Drugs* **2021**, *19*, 172. [CrossRef] [PubMed]
3. Pimentel, F.B.; Alves, R.C.; Rodrigues, F.; Oliveira, M.B.P.P. Macroalgae-Derived Ingredients for Cosmetic Industry—An Update. *Cosmetics* **2018**, *5*, 2. [CrossRef]
4. Resende, D.I.S.P.; Ferreira, M.; Magalhães, C. Trends in the use of marine ingredients in anti-aging cosmetics. *Algal Res.* **2021**, *55*, 102273. [CrossRef]
5. Aslam, A.; Bahadar, A.; Liaquat, R.; Saleem, M.; Waqas, A.; Zwawi, M. Algae as an attractive source for cosmetics to counter environmental stress. *Sci. Total Environ.* **2021**, *772*, 144905. [CrossRef]
6. Preetha, J.P.; Karthika, K. Cosmeceuticals—An evolution. *Int. J. Chemtech Res.* **2009**, *1*, 1217–1223.
7. Chaudhari, P.M.; Kawade, P.V.; Funne, S.M. Cosmeceuticals-a review. *Int. J. Pharm. Technol.* **2011**, *3*, 774–798.
8. Draelos, Z.D. Cosmeceuticals: Efficacy and influence on skin tone. *Dermatol. Clin.* **2014**, *32*, 137–143. [CrossRef]

9. Querellou, J.; Børresen, T.; Boyen, C.; Dobson, A.; Höfle, M.G.; Ianora, A.; Jaspars, M.; Kijjoa, A.; Olafsen, J.; Rigos, G.; et al. Marine Biotechnology: Realising the Full Potential of Europe. In *EurOCEAN—Challenges for Marine Research in the Next Decade*; McDonough, N., Ed.; VLIZ Special Publication: Oostende, Belgium, 2010; Volume 47, p. 21.
10. Brandt, F.S.; Cazzaniga, A.; Hann, M. Cosmeceuticals: Current trends and market analysis. *Semin. Cutan. Med. Surg.* **2011**, *30*, 141–143. [CrossRef]
11. Pham, A.K.; Dinulos, J.G. Cosmeceuticals for children: Should you care? *Curr. Opin. Pediatr.* **2014**, *26*, 446–451. [CrossRef]
12. De Lacerda, D.; Thioly-Bensoussan, D.; Burke, K. Cosmeceuticals for Men. Available online: https://pubmed.ncbi.nlm.nih.gov/24308151/ (accessed on 28 September 2021).
13. Draelos, Z.D. Cosmeceuticals for Male Skin. *Dermatol. Clin.* **2018**, *36*, 17–20. [CrossRef]
14. Lin, T.J. Evolution of cosmetics: Increased need for experimental clinical medicine. *J. Exp. Clin. Med.* **2010**, *2*, 49–52. [CrossRef]
15. Faria-Silva, C.; Ascenso, A.; Costa, A.M.; Marto, J.; Carvalheiro, M.; Ribeiro, H.M.; Simões, S. Feeding the skin: A new trend in food and cosmetics convergence. *Trends Food Sci. Technol.* **2020**, *95*, 21–32. [CrossRef]
16. Pereira, L. Seaweeds as Source of Bioactive Substances and Skin Care Therapy—Cosmeceuticals, Algotheraphy, and Thalassotherapy. *Cosmetics* **2018**, *5*, 68. [CrossRef]
17. Sotelo, C.G.; Blanco, M.; Ramos, P.; Vazquez, J.A.; Perez-Martin, R.I. Sustainable sources from aquatic organisms for cosmeceuticals ingredients. *Cosmetics* **2021**, *8*, 48. [CrossRef]
18. Zárate, R.; Portillo, E.; Teixidó, S.; de Carvalho, M.A.A.P.; Nunes, N.; Ferraz, S.; Seca, A.M.L.; Rosa, G.P.; Barreto, M.C. Pharmacological and cosmeceutical potential of Seaweed Beach-casts of Macaronesia. *Appl. Sci.* **2020**, *10*, 5831 [CrossRef]
19. Félix, R.; Carmona, A.M.; Félix, C.; Novais, S.C.; Lemos, M.F.L. Industry-friendly hydroethanolic extraction protocols for *Grateloupia turuturu* UV-shielding and antioxidant compounds. *Appl. Sci.* **2020**, *10*, 5304. [CrossRef]
20. Balboa, E.M.; Soto, M.L.; Nogueira, D.R.; González-López, N.; Conde, E.; Moure, A.; Vinardell, M.P.; Mitjans, M.; Domínguez, H. Potential of antioxidant extracts produced by aqueous processing of renewable resources for the formulation of cosmetics. *Ind. Crop. Prod.* **2014**, *58*, 104–110. [CrossRef]
21. Dolorosa, M.T.; Nurjanah; Purwaningsih, S.; Anwar, E. Utilization of *Kappaphycus alvarezii* and *Sargassum plagyophyllum* from Banten as cosmetic creams. *IOP Conf. Ser. Earth Environ. Sci.* **2019**, *404*, 012008. [CrossRef]
22. Wahyuni, T. The Potential and Application of *Eucheuma* sp. For Solid Soap: A Review. *IOP Conf. Ser. Earth Environ. Sci.* **2021**, *750*, 012048. [CrossRef]
23. Jesumani, V.; Du, H.; Aslam, M.; Fei, P.; Huang, N. Potential use of seaweed bioactive compounds in skincare—A review. *Mar. Drugs* **2019**, *17*, 688. [CrossRef] [PubMed]
24. Jesumani, V.; Du, H.; Fei, P.; Zheng, C.; Cheong, K.-L.; Huang, N. Unravelling property of polysaccharides from *Sargassum* sp. as an anti-wrinkle and skin whitening property. *Int. J. Biol. Macromol.* **2019**, *140*, 216–224. [CrossRef] [PubMed]
25. Lordan, S.; Ross, R.P.; Stanton, C. Marine bioactives as functional food ingredients: Potential to reduce the incidence of chronic diseases. *Mar. Drugs* **2011**, *9*, 1056–1100. [CrossRef]
26. Gellenbeck, K.W. Utilization of algal materials for nutraceutical and cosmeceutical applications—What do manufacturers need to know? *J. Appl. Phycol.* **2012**, *24*, 309–313. [CrossRef]
27. Thomas, N.V.; Kim, S. Beneficial effects of marine algal compounds in cosmeceuticals. *Mar. Drugs* **2013**, *11*, 146–164. [CrossRef] [PubMed]
28. Wang, H.M.D.; Chen, C.C.; Huynh, P.; Chang, J.S. Exploring the potential of using algae in cosmetics. *Biores. Technol.* **2015**, *184*, 355–362. [CrossRef]
29. Couteau, C.; Coiffard, L. Phycocosmetics and other marine cosmetics, specific cosmetics formulated using marine resources. *Mar. Drugs* **2020**, *18*, 322. [CrossRef]
30. Kharkwal, H.; Joshi, D.; Panthari, P.; Pant, M.K.; Kharkwal, A.C. Algae as future drugs. *Asian J. Pharm. Clin. Res.* **2012**, *5*, 1–4.
31. Senevirathne, W.S.M.; Kim, S.K. Cosmeceuticals from Algae. In *Functional Ingredients from Algae for Foods and Nutraceuticals*, 1st ed.; Domínguez, H., Ed.; Woodhead Publishing: Cambridge, UK, 2013; pp. 694–713.
32. Vo, T.; Ngo, D.; Kang, K.; Jung, W. Kim, S. The beneficial properties of marine polysaccharides in alleviation of allergic responses. *Mol. Nutr. Food Res.* **2015**, *59*, 129–138. [CrossRef] [PubMed]
33. Salehi, B.; Sharifi-Rad, J.; Seca, A.M.L.; Pinto, D.C.G.A.; Michalak, I.; Trincone, A.; Mishra, A.P.; Nigam, M.; Zam, W.; Martins, N. Current Trends on Seaweeds: Looking at Chemical Composition, Phytopharmacology, and Cosmetic Applications. *Molecules* **2019**, *24*, 4182. [CrossRef]
34. Morais, T.; Cotas, J.; Pacheco, D.; Pereira, L. Seaweeds compounds: An ecosustainable source of cosmetic ingredients? *Cosmetics* **2021**, *8*, 8. [CrossRef]
35. Bedoux, G.; Hardouin, K.; Burlot, A.S.; Bourgougnon, N. Bioactive components from seaweeds: Cosmetic applications and future development. *Adv. Bot. Res.* **2014**, *71*, 345–378.
36. Agatonovic-Kustrin, S.; Morton, D.W. Cosmeceuticals derived from bioactive substances found in marine algae. *J. Oceanogr. Mar. Res.* **2013**, *1*, 106.
37. Couteau, C.; Coiffard, L. Seaweed Application in Cosmetics in Seaweed. In *Health and Disease Prevention*; Fleurence, J., Levine, I., Eds.; Nikki Levy. Elsevier Inc.: Amsterdam, The Netherlands, 2016; pp. 423–441.
38. Kim, S.K.; Ravichandran, Y.D.; Khan, S.B.; Kim, Y.T. Prospective of the cosmeceuticals derived from marine organisms. *Biotechnol. Bioproc. Engineer.* **2008**, *13*, 511–523 [CrossRef]

39. Kim, S.K. Review: Marine cosmeceuticals. *J. Cosmet. Dermatol.* **2014**, *13*, 56–67. [CrossRef] [PubMed]
40. Thiyagarasaiyar, K.; Goh, B.-H.; Jeon, Y.-J.; Yow, Y.-Y. Algae Metabolites in Cosmeceutical: An Overview of Current Applications and Challenges. *Mar. Drugs* **2020**, *18*, 323. [CrossRef] [PubMed]
41. Ahmed, A.B.A.; Adel, M.; Karimi, P.; Peidayesh, M. Pharmaceutical, cosmeceutical, and traditional applications of marine carbohydrates. *Adv. Food Nutr. Res.* **2014**, *73*, 197–220.
42. Kim, J.H.; Lee, J.-E.; Kim, K.H.; Kang, N.J. Beneficial effects of marine algae-derived carbohydrates for skin health. *Mar. Drugs* **2018**, *16*, 459. [CrossRef]
43. Shanura Fernando, I.P.; Asanka Sanjeewa, K.K.; Samarakoon, K.W.; Kim, H.S.; Gunasekara, U.K.D.S.S.; Park, Y.J.; Abeytungaa, D.T.U.; Lee, W.W.; Jeon, Y.-J. The potential of fucoidans from *Chnoospora minima* and *Sargassum polycystum* in cosmetics: Antioxidant, anti-inflammatory, skin-whitening, and antiwrinkle activities. *J. Appl. Phycol.* **2018**, *30*, 3223–3232. [CrossRef]
44. Morya, V.; Kim, J.; Kim, E. Algal fucoidan: Structural and size-dependent bioactivities and their perspectives. *Appl. Microbiol. Biotechnol.* **2012**, *93*, 71–82. [CrossRef]
45. Casas, M.P.; Rodríguez-Hermida, V.; Pérez-Larrán, P.; Conde, E.; Liveri, M.T.; Ribeiro, D.; Fernandes, E.; Domínguez, H. In vitro bioactive properties of phlorotannins recovered from hydrothermal treatment of *Sargassum muticum*. *Sep. Purif. Technol.* **2016**, *167*, 117–126. [CrossRef]
46. Ruocco, N.; Costantini, S.; Guariniello, S.; Costantini, M. Polysaccharides from the marine environment with pharmacological, cosmeceutical and nutraceutical potential. *Molecules* **2016**, *21*, 551. [CrossRef]
47. Lee, Y.-E.; Kim, H.; Seo, C.; Park, T.; Lee, K.B.; Yoo, S.-Y.; Hong, S.-C.; Kim, J.T.; Lee, J. Marine polysaccharides: Therapeutic efficacy and biomedical applications. *Arch. Pharm. Res.* **2017**, *40*, 1006–1020. [CrossRef]
48. Sanjeewa, K.K.A.; Kang, N.; Ahn, G.; Jee, Y.; Kim, Y.T.; Jeon, Y.J. Bioactive potentials of sulfated polysaccharides isolated from brown seaweed *Sargassum* spp in related to human health applications: A review. *Food Hydrocoll.* **2018**, *81*, 200–208. [CrossRef]
49. Fernando, I.P.S.; Kim, K.N.; Kim, D.; Jeon, Y.J. Algal polysaccharides: Potential bioactive substances for cosmeceutical applications. *Crit. Rev. Biotechnol.* **2019**, *39*, 99–113. [CrossRef] [PubMed]
50. Cikoš, A.M.; Jerković, I.; Molnar, M.; Šubarić, D.; Jokić, S. New trends for macroalgal natural products applications. *Nat. Prod. Res.* **2021**, *35*, 1180–1191. [CrossRef] [PubMed]
51. Fournière, M.; Bedoux, G.; Lebonvallet, N.; Lescchiera, R.; Goff-Pain, C.L.; Bourgougnon, N.; Latire, T. Poly-and oligosaccharide *ulva* sp. Fractions from enzyme-assisted extraction modulate the metabolism of extracellular matrix in human skin fibroblasts: Potential in anti-aging dermo-cosmetic applications. *Mar. Drugs* **2021**, *19*, 156. [CrossRef] [PubMed]
52. Wong, T.; Brault, L.; Gasparotto, E.; Vallée, R.; Morvan, P.Y.; Ferrières, V.; Nugier-Chauvin, C. Formation of Amphiphilic Molecules from the Most Common Marine Polysaccharides, toward a Sustainable Alternative? *Molecules* **2021**, *26*, 4445. [CrossRef]
53. Xu, S.-Y.; Kan, J.; Hu, Z.; Liu, Y.; Du, H.; Pang, G.-C.; Cheong, K.-L. Quantification of Neoagaro-Oligosaccharide Production through Enzymatic Hydrolysis and Its Anti-Oxidant Activities. *Molecules* **2018**, *23*, 1354. [CrossRef]
54. Zhang, W.; Jin, W.; Duan, D.; Zhang, Q. Structural analysis and anti-complement activity of polysaccharides extracted from *Grateloupia livida* (Harv.) Yamada. *J. Oceanol. Limnol.* **2019**, *37*, 806–814. [CrossRef]
55. Zhang, Y.H.; Song, X.N.; Lin, Y.; Xiao, Q.; Du, X.P.; Chen, Y.H.; Xiao, A.F. Antioxidant capacity and prebiotic effects of *Gracilaria neoagaro* oligosaccharides prepared by agarase hydrolysis. *Int. J. Biol. Macromol.* **2019**, *137*, 177–186. [CrossRef]
56. Sachan, N.K.; Pushkar, S.; Jha, A.; Bhattcharya, A. Sodium alginate: The wonder polymer for controlled drug delivery. *J. Pharm. Res.* **2009**, *2*, 1191–1199.
57. Priyadarshani, I.; Rath, B. Commercial and industrial applications of micro algae—A review. *J. Algal Biomass Util.* **2012**, *3*, 89–100.
58. Xue, C.; Yu, G.; Hirata, T.; Terao, J.; Lin, H. Antioxidative activities of several marine polysaccharides evaluated in a phosphatidylcholine-liposomal suspension and organic solvents. *Biosci. Biotechnol. Biochem.* **1998**, *62*, 206–209. [CrossRef] [PubMed]
59. Thevanayagam, H.; Mohamed, S.M.; Chu, W.-L. Assessment of UVB-photoprotective and antioxidative activities of carrageenan in keratinocytes. *J. Appl. Phycol.* **2014**, *26*, 1813–1821. [CrossRef]
60. Sun, Z.; Mohamed, M.A.A.; Park, S.Y.; Yi, T.H. Fucosterol protects cobalt chloride induced inflammation by the inhibition of hypoxia-inducible factor through PI3K/Akt pathway. *Int. Immunopharmacol.* **2015**, *29*, 642–647. [CrossRef] [PubMed]
61. Fernando, I.P.S.; Jayawardena, T.U.; Kim, H.S.; Vaas, A.; De Silva, H.I.C.; Nanayakkara, C.M.; Abeytunga, D.T.U.; Lee, W.; Ahn, G.; Lee, D.S.; et al. A keratinocyte and integrated fibroblast culture model for studying particulate matter-induced skin lesions and therapeutic intervention of fucosterol. *Life Sci.* **2019**, *233*, 116714. [CrossRef] [PubMed]
62. Xie, X.-T.; Zhang, X.; Liu, Y.; Chen, X.-Q.; Cheong, K.-L. Quantification of 3,6-anhydro-galactose in red seaweed polysaccharides and their potential skin-whitening activity. *3 Biotech* **2020**, *10*, 189. [CrossRef]
63. Senni, K.; Gueniche, F.; Foucault-Bertaud, A.; Igondjo-Tchen, S.; Fioretti, F.; Colliec-Jouault, S.; Durand, P.; Guezennec, J.; Godeau, G.; Letourneur, D. Fucoidan a sulfated polysaccharide from brown algae is a potent modulator of connective tissue proteolysis. *Arch. Biochem. Biophys.* **2006**, *445*, 56–64. [CrossRef]
64. Moon, H.J.; Lee, S.H.; Ku, M.J.; Yu, B.C.; Jeon, M.J.; Jeong, S.H.; Stonik, V.A.; Zvyagintseca, T.N.; Ermakova, S.P.; Lee, Y.P. Fucoidan inhibits UVB-induced MMP-1 promoter expression and down regulation of type I procollagen synthesis in human skin fibroblasts. *Eur. J. Dermatol.* **2009**, *19*, 129–134. [CrossRef]

65. Wang, L.; Oh, J.-Y.; Lee, W.; Jeon, Y.-J. Fucoidan isolated from *Hizikia fusiforme* suppresses ultraviolet B-induced photodamage by down-regulating the expressions of matrix metalloproteinases and pro-inflammatory cytokines via inhibiting NF-κB, AP-1, and MAPK signaling pathways. *Int. J. Biol. Macromol.* **2021**, *166*, 751–759. [CrossRef]
66. Su, W.; Wang, L.; Fu, X.; Ni, L.; Duan, D.; Xu, J.; Gao, X. Protective effect of a fucose-rich fucoidan isolated from Saccharina japonica against ultraviolet B-induced photodamage in vitro in human keratinocytes and in vivo in Zebrafish. *Mar. Drugs* **2020**, *18*, 316. [CrossRef] [PubMed]
67. Wang, L.; Jayawardena, T.U.; Yang, H.-W.; Lee, H.-G.; Jeon, Y.-J. The potential of sulfated polysaccharides isolated from the brown seaweed *Ecklonia maxima* in cosmetics: Antioxidant, anti-melanogenesis, and photoprotective activities. *Antioxidants* **2020**, *9*, 724. [CrossRef] [PubMed]
68. Ayoub, A.; Pereira, J.M.; Rioux, L.; Turgeon, S.L.; Beaulieu, M.; Moulin, V.J. Role of seaweed *Laminaran* from *Saccharina longicruris* on matrix deposition during dermal tissue-engineered production. *Int. J. Biol. Macromol.* **2015**, *75*, 13–20. [CrossRef]
69. Ozanne, H.; Toumi, H.; Roubinet, B.; Landemarre, L.; Lespessailles, E.; Daniellou, R.; Cesaro, A. Laminarin Effects, a β-(1,3)-Glucan, on Skin Cell Inflammation and Oxidation. *Cosmetics* **2020**, *7*, 66. [CrossRef]
70. Jiang, N.; Li, B.; Wang, X.; Xu, X.; Liu, X.; Li, W.; Chang, X.; Li, H.; Qi, H. The antioxidant and antihyperlipidemic activities of phosphorylated polysaccharide from *Ulva pertusa*. *Int. J. Biol. Macromol.* **2020**, *145*, 1059–1065. [CrossRef]
71. Yu, B.; Bi, D.; Yao, L.; Li, T.; Gu, L.; Xu, H.; Li, X.; Li, H.; Hu, Z.; Xu, X. The inhibitory activity of alginate against allergic reactions in an ovalbumin-induced mouse model. *Food Funct.* **2020**, *11*, 2704–2713. [CrossRef]
72. Szekalska, M.; Sosnowska, K.; Tomczykowa, M.; Winnicka, K.; Kasacka, I.; Tomczyk, M. In vivo anti-inflammatory and anti-allergic activities of cynaroside evaluated by using hydrogel formulations. *Biomed. Pharmacother.* **2020**, *121*, 109681. [CrossRef]
73. Holdt, S.L.; Kraan, S. Bioactive compounds in seaweed: Functional food applications and legislation. *J. Appl. Phycol.* **2011**, *23*, 543–597. [CrossRef]
74. Xing, M.; Cao, Q.; Wang, Y.; Xiao, H.; Zhao, J.; Zhang, Q.; Ji, A.; Song, S. Advances in Research on the Bioactivity of Alginate Oligosaccharides. *Mar. Drugs* **2020**, *18*, 144. [CrossRef]
75. Deville, C.; Gharbi, M.; Dandrifosse, G.; Peulen, O. Study on the effects of laminarin, a polysaccharide from seaweed, on gut characteristics. *J. Sci. Food Agric.* **2007**, *87*, 1717–1725. [CrossRef]
76. Shannon, E.; Conlon, M.; Hayes, M. Seaweed Components as Potential Modulators of the Gut Microbiota. *Mar. Drugs* **2021**, *19*, 358. [CrossRef]
77. Choi, J.; Ha, Y.; Joo, C.; Cho, K.K.; Kim, S.; Choi, I.S. Inhibition of oral pathogens and collagenase activity by seaweed extracts. *J. Environ. Biol.* **2012**, *33*, 115–121
78. Gómez-Mascaraque, L.G.; Martínez-Sanz, M.; Martínez-López, R.; Martínez-Abad, A.; Panikuttira, B.; López-Rubio, A.; Tuohy, M.G.; Hogan, S.A.; Brodkorb, A. Characterization and gelling properties of a bioactive extract from *Ascophyllum nodosum* obtained using a chemical-free approach. *Curr. Res. Food Sci.* **2021**, *4*, 354–364. [CrossRef] [PubMed]
79. Huang, Y.; Jiang, H.; Mao, X.; Ci, F. Laminarin and Laminarin Oligosaccharides Originating from Brown Algae: Preparation, Biological Activities, and Potential Applications. *J. Ocean Univ. China* **2021**, *20*, 641–653. [CrossRef]
80. Kadam, S.U.; Tiwari, B.K.; O'Donnell, C.P. Extraction, structure and biofunctional activities of laminarin from brown algae. *Int. J. Food Sci. Technol.* **2015**, *50*, 24–31. [CrossRef]
81. Costa, A.M.S.; Rodrigues, J.M.M.; Pérez-Madrigal, M.M.; Dove, A.P.; Mano, J.F. Modular Functionalization of Laminarin to Create Value-Added Naturally Derived Macromolecules. *J. Am. Chem. Soc.* **2020**, *142*, 19689–19697. [CrossRef] [PubMed]
82. Li, J.; Cai, C.; Yang, C.; Li, J.; Sun, T.; Yu, G. Recent advances in pharmaceutical potential of brown algal polysaccharides and their derivatives. *Curr. Pharm. Des.* **2019**, *25*, 1290–1311. [CrossRef]
83. Tümen Erden, S.; Ekentok Atici, C.; Cömez, B.; Sezer, A.D. Preparation and in vitro characterization of laminarin based hydrogels. *J. Res. Pharm.* **2021**, *25*, 164–172.
84. Zargarzadeh, M.; Amaral, A.J.R.; Custódio, C.A.; Mano, J.F. Biomedical applications of laminarin. *Carbohydr. Polym.* **2020**, *232*, 115774. [CrossRef]
85. Narayanaswamy, R.; Jo, B.W.; Choi, S.K.; Ismail, I.S. Fucoidan: Versatile cosmetic ingredient. An overview. *J. Appl. Cosmetol.* **2013**, *31*, 131–138.
86. Baweja, P.; Kumar, S.; Sahoo, D.; Levine, I. Biology of Seaweeds in Seaweed. In *Health and Disease Prevention*; Fleurence, J., Levine, I., Eds.; Nikki Levy Elsevier Inc.: Amsterdam, The Netherlands, 2016; pp. 41–106.
87. Li, N.; Zhang, Q.; Song, J. Toxicological evaluation of fucoidan extracted from *Laminaria japonica* in Wistar rats. *Food Chem. Toxicol.* **2005**, *43*, 421–426. [CrossRef]
88. Citkowska, A.; Szekalska, M.; Winnicka, K. Possibilities of fucoidan utilization in the development of pharmaceutical dosage forms. *Mar. Drugs* **2019**, *17*, 458. [CrossRef]
89. Jiao, G.L.; Yu, G.L.; Zhang, J.Z.; Ewart, H.S. Chemical structures and bioactivities of sulfated polysaccharides from marine algae. *Mar. Drugs* **2011**, *9*, 196–223. [CrossRef]
90. Wijesinghe, W.; Jeon, Y. Biological activities and potential industrial applications of fucose rich sulfated polysaccharides and fucoidans isolated from brown seaweeds: A review. *Carbohydr. Polym.* **2012**, *88*, 13–20. [CrossRef]
91. Kartik, A.; Akhil, D. Lakshmi, D.; Panchamoorthy Gopinath, K.; Arun, J.; Sivaramakrishnan, R.; Pugazhendhi, A. A critical review on production of biopolymers from algae biomass and their applications. *Bioresour. Technol.* **2021**, *329*, 124868. [CrossRef] [PubMed]

92. Xue, C.-H.; Fang, Y.; Lin, H.; Chen, L.; Li, Z.-J.; Deng, D.; Lu, C.-X. Chemical characters and antioxidative properties of sulfated polysaccharides from *Laminaria japonica*. *J. Appl. Phycol.* **2001**, *13*, 67–70. [CrossRef]
93. Kim, S.M.; Kang, K.; Jeon, J.S.; Jho, E.H.; Kim, C.Y.; Nho, C.W.; Um, B.H. Isolation of phlorotannins from *Eisenia bicyclis* and their hepatoprotective effect against oxidative stress induced by tert-butyl hyperoxide. *Appl. Biochem. Biotechnol.* **2011**, *165*, 1296–1307. [CrossRef] [PubMed]
94. Li, Y.; Wang, X.; Jiang, Y.; Wang, J.; Hwang, H.; Yang, X.; Wang, P. Structure characterization of low molecular weight sulfate *Ulva* polysaccharide and the effect of its derivative on iron deficiency anemia. *Int. J. Biol. Macromol.* **2019**, *126*, 747–754. [CrossRef]
95. Senni, K.; Pereira, J.; Gueniche, F.; Delbarre-Ladrat, C.; Sinquin, C.; Ratiskol, J.; Godeau, G.; Fischer, A.-M.; Helley, D.; Colliec-Jouault, S. Marine polysaccharides: A source of bioactive molecules for cell therapy and tissue engineering. *Mar. Drugs* **2011**, *9*, 1664–1681. [CrossRef] [PubMed]
96. Ali Karami, M.; Sharif Makhmalzadeh, B.; Pooranian, M.; Rezai, A. Preparation and optimization of silibinin-loaded chitosan–fucoidan hydrogel: An in vivo evaluation of skin protection against UVB. *Pharm. Dev. Technol.* **2021**, *26*, 209–219. [CrossRef]
97. Costa, L.S.; Fidelis, G.P.; Telles, C.B.S.; Dantas-Santos, N.; Camara, R.B.G.; Cordeiro, S.L.; Costa, M.S.; Almetida-Lima, J.; Oliveira, R.M.; Alburquerque, I.R.; et al. Antioxidant and antiproliferative activities of heterofucans from the seaweed *Sargassum filipendula*. *Mar. Drugs* **2011**, *9*, 952–966. [CrossRef] [PubMed]
98. Qiao, L.; Li, Y.; Chi, Y.; Ji, Y.; Gao, Y.; Hwang, H.; Aker, W.G.; Wang, P. Rheological properties, gelling behavior and texture characteristics of polysaccharide from *Enteromorpha prolifera*. *Carbohydr. Polym.* **2016**, *136*, 1307–1314. [CrossRef] [PubMed]
99. Lin, G.-P.; Wu, D.-S.; Xiao, X.-W.; Huang, Q.-Y.; Chen, H.-B.; Liu, D.; Fu, H.; Chen, X.-H.; Zhao, C. Structural characterization and antioxidant effect of green alga *Enteromorpha prolifera* polysaccharide in Caenorhabditis elegans via modulation of microRNAs. *Int. J. Biol. Macromol.* **2020**, *150*, 1084–1092. [CrossRef]
100. Adrien, A.; Bonnet, A.; Dufour, D.; Badouin, S.; Maugard, T.; Bridiau, N. Pilot production of ulvans from *Ulva* sp. and their effects on hyaluronan and collagen production in cultured dermal fibroblasts. *Carbohydr. Polym.* **2017**, *157*, 1306–1314. [CrossRef]
101. Lahaye, M.; Robic, A. Structure and function properties of Ulvan, a polysaccharide from green seaweeds. *Biomacromol* **2007**, *8*, 1765–1774. [CrossRef]
102. Mo'o, F.R.C.; Wilar, G.; Devkota, H.P.; Wathoni, N. Ulvan, a polysaccharide from Macroalga *Ulva* sp.: A review of chemistry, biological activities and potential for food and biomedical applications. *Appl. Sci.* **2020**, *10*, 5488. [CrossRef]
103. Kidgell, J.T.; Carnachan, S.M.; Magnusson, M.; Lawton, R.J.; Sims, I.M.; Hinkley, S.F.R.; de Nys, R.; Glasson, C.R.K. Are all ulvans equal? A comparative assessment of the chemical and gelling properties of ulvan from blade and filamentous Ulva. *Carbohyd. Polym.* **2021**, *264*, 118010. [CrossRef] [PubMed]
104. Li, B.; Xu, H.; Wang, X.; Wang, Y.; Jiang, N.; Qi, H.; Liu, X. Antioxidant and antihyperlipidemic activities of high sulfate content purified polysaccharide from *Ulva pertusa*. *Int. J. Biol. Macromol.* **2020**, *146*, 756–762. [CrossRef]
105. Chen, X.; Fu, X.; Huang, L.; Xu, J.; Gao, X. Agar oligosaccharides: A review of preparation, structures, bioactivities and application. *Carbohydr. Polym.* **2021**, *265*, 118076.
106. Aziz, E.; Batool, R.; Khan, M.U.; Rauf, A.; Akhtar, W.; Heydary, M.; Rehman, S.; Shahzad, T.; Malik, A.; Mosavat, S.-H.; et al. An overview on red algae bioactive compounds and their pharmaceutical applications. *J. Altern. Complement. Med.* **2021**, *17*, 20190203.
107. Laurienzo, P. Marine polysaccharides in pharmaceutical applications: An overview. *Mar. Drugs* **2010**, *8*, 2435–2465. [CrossRef] [PubMed]
108. Ghanbarzadeh, M.; Golmoradizadeh, A.; Homaei, A. Carrageenans and carrageenases: Versatile polysaccharides and promising marine enzymes. *Phytochem. Rev.* **2018**, *17*, 535–571. [CrossRef]
109. Isaka, S.; Cho, K.; Nakazono, S.; Abu, R.; Ueno, M.; Kim, D.; Oda, T. Antioxidant and anti-inflammatory activities of porphyrin isolated from discolored nori (*Porphyra yezoensis*). *Int. J. Biol. Macromol.* **2015**, *74*, 68–75. [CrossRef]
110. Beaumont, M.; Tran, R.; Vera, G.; Niedrist, D.; Rousset, A.; Pierre, R.; Shastri, V.P.; Forget, A. Hydrogel-Forming Algae Polysaccharides: From Seaweed to Biomedical Applications. *Biomacromolecules* **2021**, *22*, 1027–1052. [CrossRef]
111. Kwon, M.; Nam, T. Porphyran induces apoptosis related signal pathway in AGS gastric cancer cell lines. *Life Sci.* **2006**, *79*, 1956–1962. [CrossRef]
112. Pacheco-Quito, E.-M.; Ruiz-Caro, R.; Veiga, M.-D. Carrageenan: Drug Delivery Systems and Other Biomedical Applications. *Mar. Drugs* **2020**, *18*, 583. [CrossRef] [PubMed]
113. Qiu, Y.; Jiang, H.; Fu, L.; Ci, F.; Mao, X. Porphyran and oligo-porphyran originating from red algae *Porphyra*: Preparation, biological activities, and potential applications. *Food Chem.* **2021**, *349*, 129209. [CrossRef]
114. Araujo, I.W.F.; Vanderlei, E.S.O.; Rodrigues, J.A.G.; Coura, C.O.; Quindere, A.L.G.; Fontes, B.P.; Queiroz, I.N.L.; Jorge, R.J.B.; Bezerra, M.M.; Silva, A.A.R.; et al. Effects of a sulfated polysaccharide isolated from the red seaweed *Solieria filiformis* on models of nociception and inflammation. *Carbohydr. Polym.* **2011**, *86*, 1207–1215. [CrossRef]
115. Zhang, Y.; Tian, R.; Wu, H.; Li, X.; Li, S.; Bian, L. Evaluation of acute and sub-chronic toxicity of *Lithothamnion* sp. in mice and rats. *Toxicol. Rep.* **2020**, *7*, 852–858. [CrossRef]
116. Cheong, K.-L.; Qiu, H.-M.; Du, H.; Liu, Y.; Khan, B.M. Oligosaccharides derived from red seaweed: Production, properties, and potential health and cosmetic application. *Molecules* **2018**, *23*, 245. [CrossRef]
117. Bleakley, S.; Hayes, M. Algal proteins: Extraction, application, and challenges concerning production. *Foods* **2017**, *6*, 33. [CrossRef] [PubMed]

118. Fleurence, J. Seaweed Proteins. In *Proteins in Food Processing*; Yada, R.Y., Ed.; Woodhead Publishing Limited: Cambridge, UK, 2004; pp. 197–213.
119. Gressler, V.; Fujii, M.T.; Martins, A.P.; Colepicolo, P.; Mancini-Filho, J.; Pinto, E. Biochemical composition of two red seaweed species grown on the Brazilian coast. *J. Sci. Food Agric.* 2011, 91, 1687–1692. [CrossRef]
120. Cheung, R.C.F.; Ng, T.B.; Wong, J.H. Marine peptides: Bioactivities and applications. *Mar. Drugs* 2015, 13, 4006–4043. [CrossRef] [PubMed]
121. Qasim, R. Amino acids composition of some common seaweeds. *Pak. J. Pharmac. Sci.* 1991, 4, 49–54.
122. Wong, K.H.; Cheung, P.C.K. Nutritional evaluation of some subtropical red and green seaweeds. Part II. In vitro protein digestibility and amino acid profiles of protein concentrates. *Food Chem.* 2001, 72, 11–17. [CrossRef]
123. Matanjun, P.; Mohamed, S.; Mustapha, N.M.; Muhammad, K. Nutrient content of tropical edible seaweeds, *Eucheuma cottoni*, *Caulerpa lentillifera* and *Sargassum polycysum*. *J. Appl. Phycol.* 2009, 21, 75–80. [CrossRef]
124. Admassu, H.; Abdalbasit, M.; Gasmalla, A.; Yang, R.; Zhao, W. Bioactive peptides derived from seaweed protein and their health benefits: Antihypertensive, antioxidant, and antidiabetic properties. *J. Food Sci.* 2018, 83, 6–16. [CrossRef]
125. Meisel, H. Multifunctional peptides encrypted in milk proteins. *Biofactors* 2004, 21, 55–61. [CrossRef]
126. Murray, B.A.; FitzGerald, R.J. Angiotensin converting enzyme inhibitory peptides derived from food proteins: Biochemistry, bioactivity and production. *Curr. Pharmac. Des.* 2007, 13, 773–791. [CrossRef]
127. Harnedy, P.A.; FitzGerald, R.J. Bioactive proteins, peptides, and amino acids from macroalgae. *J. Phycol.* 2011, 47, 218–232. [CrossRef]
128. Indumathi, P.; Mehta, A. A novel anticoagulant peptide from the nori hydrolysate. *J. Funct. Foods* 2016, 20, 606–617. [CrossRef]
129. Jo, C.; Khan, F.F.; Khan, M.I.; Iqbal, J. Marine bioactive peptides: Types, structures, and physiological functions. *Food Rev. Int.* 2016, 33, 44–61. [CrossRef]
130. Lafarga, T.; Acién-Fernández, F.G.; Garcia-Vaquero, M. Bioactive peptides and carbohydrates from seaweed for food applications: Natural occurrence, isolation, purification, and identification. *Algal Res.* 2020, 48, 101909. [CrossRef]
131. Sridhar, K.; Inbaraj, B.S.; Chen, B.-H. Recent developments on production, purification and biological activity of marine peptides. *Food Res. Int.* 2021, 47, 110468. [CrossRef]
132. Pangestuti, R.; Kim, S.K. Seaweed Proteins, Peptides, and Amino Acids. In *Seaweed Sustainability: Food and Non-Food Applications*; Tiwari, B.K., Toy, D.J., Eds.; Academic Press: San Diego, CA, USA, 2015; pp. 125–140.
133. Yanshin, N.; Kushnareva, A.; Lemesheva, V.; Birkemeyer, C.; Tarakhovskaya, E. Chemical composition and potential practical application of 15 red algal species from the White Sea Coast (the Arctic Ocean). *Molecules* 2021, 26, 2489. [CrossRef]
134. Lee, H.-A.; Kim, I.-H.; Nam, T.-J. Bioactive peptide from *Pyropia yezoensis* and its anti-inflammatory activities. *Int. J. Molec. Med.* 2015, 36, 1701–1706. [CrossRef]
135. Ryu, J.; Park, S.J.; Kim, I.H.; Choi, Y.H.; Nam, T.J. Protective effect of porphyra-334 on UVA-induced photoaging in human skin fibroblasts. *Int. J. Mol. Medic.* 2014, 34, 796–803. [CrossRef] [PubMed]
136. Romarís-Hortas, V.; Bermejo-Barrera, P.; Moreda-Piñeiro, A. Ultrasound-assisted enzymatic hydrolysis for iodinated amino acid extraction from edible seaweed before reversed-phase high performance liquid chromatography-inductively coupled plasma-mass spectrometry. *J. Chromatogr. A* 2013, 1309, 33–40. [CrossRef]
137. Shick, J.M.; Dunlap, W.C.; Buettner, G.R. Ultraviolet (UV) Protection in Marine Organisms II, Biosynthesis, Accumulation, and Sunscreening Function of Mycosporine-Like Amino Acids. In *Free Radicals in Chemistry, Biology and Medicine*; Yoshikawa, S., Toyokuni, S., Yamamoto, Y., Naito, Y., Eds.; OICA International: London, UK, 2000; pp. 215–228.
138. Bedoux, G.; Hardouin, K.; Marty, C.; Taupin, L.; Vandanjon, L.; Bourgougnon, N. Chemical characterization and photoprotective activity measurement of extracts from the red macroalga *Solieria chordalis*. *Bot. Mar.* 2014, 57, 291–301. [CrossRef]
139. Dunlap, W.C.; Yamamoto, Y. Small-molecule antioxidants in marine organisms: Antioxidant activity of mycosporine-glycine. *Compar. Biochem. Physiol.* 1995, 112, 105–114. [CrossRef]
140. Bandaranayake, W.M. Mycosporines: Are they nature's sunscreens? *Nat. Prod. Rep.* 1998, 15, 159–172. [CrossRef]
141. Conde, F.R.; Churio, M.S.; Previtali, C.M. The photoprotector mechanism of mycosporine-like amino acids. Excited-state properties and photostability of porphyra-334 in aqueous solution. *J. Photochem. Photobiol. B Biol.* 2000, 56, 139–144. [CrossRef]
142. Gröniger, A.; Sinha, R.P.; Klisch, M.; Häder, D.P. Photoprotective compounds in cyanobacteria, phytoplankton and macroalgae—A database. *J. Photochem. Photobiol. B Biol.* 2000, 58, 115–122. [CrossRef]
143. Adams, N.L.; Shick, J.M. Mycosporine-like amino acids prevent UVB-induced abnormalities during early development of the green sea urchin *Strongylocentrotus droebachiensis*. *Mar. Biol.* 2001, 138, 267–280. [CrossRef]
144. Singh, S.P.; Kumari, S.; Rastogi, R.P.; Singh, K.L.; Sinha, R.P. Mycosporine-like amino acids (MAAs): Chemical structure, biosynthesis and significance as UV-absorbing/screening compounds. *Indian J. Experim. Biol.* 2008, 46, 7–17.
145. Karsten, U.; Sawall, T.; Wiencke, C. A survey of the distribution of UV-absorbing substances in tropical macroalgae. *Phycol. Res.* 2006, 46, 271–279.
146. Rastogi, R.P.; Sonani, R.R.; Madamwar, D. UV Photoprotectants from Algae—Synthesis and Bio-Functionalities. In *Algal Green Chemistry*; Rastogi, R.P., Madamwar, D., Pandey, A., Eds.; Elsevier: Amsterdam, The Netherlands, 2017; pp. 17–38.
147. Orfanoudaki, M.; Hartmann, A. Chemical profiling of mycosporine-like amino acids in twenty-three red algal species. *J. Phycol.* 2019, 55, 393–403. [CrossRef]

148. Gianeti, M.D.; Maia Campos, P.M.B.G. Efficacy evaluation of a multifunctional cosmetic formulation: The benefits of a combination of active antioxidant substances. *Molecules* **2014**, *19*, 18268–18282. [CrossRef]
149. Leandro, A.; Pereira, L.; Gonçalves, A.M.M. Diverse applications of marine macroalgae. *Mar. Drugs* **2020**, *18*, 17. [CrossRef] [PubMed]
150. Chrapusta, E.; Kaminski, A.; Duchnik, K.; Bober, B.; Adamski, M.; Bialczyk, J. Mycosporine-like amino acids: Potential health and beauty ingredients. *Mar. Drugs* **2017**, *15*, 326. [CrossRef] [PubMed]
151. Schmid, D.; Schürch, C.; Zülli, F. UV-A sunscreen from red algae for protection against premature skin aging. *Cosmetics* **2004**, *2004*, 139–143.
152. Rangel, K.C.; Villela, L.Z.; Pereira, K.D.C.; Debonsi, H.M.; Gaspar, L.R. Assessment of the photoprotective potential and toxicity of Antarctic red macroalgae extracts from *Curdiea racovitzae* and *Iridaea cordata* for cosmetic use. *Algal Res.* **2020**, *50*, 101984. [CrossRef]
153. Barceló-Villalobos, M.; Figueroa, F.L.; Korbee, N.; Álvarez-Gómez, F.; Abreu, M.H. Production of Mycosporine-Like amino acids from *Gracilaria vermiculophylla* (Rhodophyta) cultured through one year in an integrated multi-trophic aquaculture (IMTA) system. *Mar. Biotechnol.* **2017**, *19*, 246–254. [CrossRef] [PubMed]
154. Athukorala, Y.; Trang, S.; Kwok, C.; Yuan, Y.V. Antiproliferative and antioxidant activities and mycosporine-Like amino acid profiles of wild-Harvested and cultivated edible Canadian marine red macroalgae. *Molecules* **2016**, *21*, 119. [CrossRef] [PubMed]
155. Pliego-Cortés, H.; Bedoux, G.; Boulho, R.; Taupin, L.; Freile-Pelegrín, Y.; Bourgougnon, N.; Robledo, D. Stress tolerance and photoadaptation to solar radiation in *Rhodymenia pseudopalmata* (Rhodophyta) through mycosporine-like amino acids, phenolic compounds, and pigments in an Integrated Multi-Trophic Aquaculture System. *Algal Res.* **2019**, *41*, 101542. [CrossRef]
156. Leelapornpisid, P.; Mungmai, L.; Sirithunyalug, B.; Jiranusornkul, S.; Peerapornpisal, Y. A novel moisturizer extracted from freshwater macroalga [*Rhizoclonium hieroglyphicum* (C. Agardh) Kützing] for skin care cosmetic. *Chiang Mai J. Sci.* **2014**, *41*, 1195–1207.
157. Francavilla, M.; Franchi, M.; Monteleone, M.; Caroppo, C. The red seaweed *Gracilaria gracilis* as a multi products source. *Mar. Drugs* **2013**, *11*, 3754–3776. [CrossRef] [PubMed]
158. Fan, X.; Bai, L.; Mao, X.; Zhang, X. Novel peptides with anti-proliferation activity from the *Porphyra haitanesis* hydrolysate. *Process Biochem.* **2017**, *60*, 98–107. [CrossRef]
159. Verdy, C.; Branka, J.E.; Mekideche, N. Quantitative assessment of lactate and progerin production in normal human cutaneous cells during normal ageing: Effect of an *Alaria esculenta* extract. *Int. J. Cosmet. Sci.* **2011**, *33*, 462–466. [CrossRef]
160. Arad, S.; Yaron, A. Natural pigments from red microalgae for use in foods and cosmetics. *Trends Food Sci. Technol.* **1992**, *3*, 92–97. [CrossRef]
161. Bermejo, R.; Talavera, E.M.; del Valle, C.; Alvarez-Pez, J.M. C-phycocyanin incorporated into reverse micelles: A fluorescence study. *Colloids Surf. B Biointerfaces* **2000**, *18*, 51–59. [CrossRef]
162. Chronakis, I.S. Biosolar proteins from aquatic algae. *Dev. Food Sci.* **2000**, *41*, 39–75. [CrossRef]
163. Rossano, R.; Ungaro, N.; D'Ambrosio, A.; Liuzzi, G.M.; Riccio, P. Extracting and purifying R-phycoeythrin from Mediterranean red algae *Corallina elongata* Ellis and Solander. *J. Biotecnol.* **2003**, *101*, 289–296. [CrossRef]
164. Sekar, S.; Chandramohan, M. Phycobiliproteins as a commodity: Trends in applied research, patents and commercialization. *J. Appl. Phycol.* **2008**, *20*, 113–136. [CrossRef]
165. Viskari, P.J.; Colyer, C.L. Rapid extraction of phycobiliproteins from cultures cyanobacteria samples. *Anal. Biochem.* **2003**, *319*, 263–271. [CrossRef]
166. Martins, M.; Vieira, F.A.; Correia, I.; Ferreira, R.A.S.; Abreu, H.; Coutinho, J.A.P.; Ventura, S.P.M. Recovery of phycobiliproteins from the red macroalga *Gracilaria* sp. using ionic liquid aqueous solutions. *Green Chem.* **2016**, *18*, 4287–4296. [CrossRef]
167. Saluri, M.; Kaldmäe, M.; Rospu, M.; Sirkel, H.; Paalme, T.; Landreh, M.; Tuvikene, R. Spatial variation and structural characteristics of phycobiliproteins from the red algae *Furcellaria lumbricalis* and *Coccotylus truncatus*. *Algal Res.* **2020**, *52*, 102058. [CrossRef]
168. Osório, C.; Machado, S.; Peixoto, J.; Bessada, S.; Pimentel, F.B.; Alves, R.C.; Oliveira, M.B.P.P. Pigments content (chlorophylls, fucoxanthin and phycobiliproteins) of different commercial dried algae. *Separations* **2020**, *7*, 33. [CrossRef]
169. Fernando, I.P.S.; Lee, W.; Ahn, G. Marine algal flavonoids and phlorotannins; an intriguing frontier of biofunctional secondary metabolites. *Crit. Rev. Biotechnol.* **2021**, 1–23. [CrossRef] [PubMed]
170. Shrestha, A.; Pradhan, R.; Ghotekar, S.; Dahikar, S.; Marasini, B.P. Phytochemical Analysis and Anti-Microbial Activity of Desmostachya Bipinnata: A review. *J. Med. Chem. Sci.* **2021**, *4*, 36–41.
171. Wijesinghe, W.; Jeon, Y. Biological activities and potential cosmeceutical applications of bioactive components from brown seaweeds: A review. *Phytochem. Rev.* **2011**, *10*, 431–443. [CrossRef]
172. Ferreres, F.; Lopes, G.; Gil-Izquierdo, A.; Andrade, P.B.; Sousa, C.; Mouga, T.; Valentão, P. Phlorotannin extracts from fucales characterized by HPLC-DAD-ESI-MSn: Approaches to hyaluronidase inhibitory capacity and antioxidant properties. *Mar. Drugs* **2012**, *10*, 2766–2781. [CrossRef]
173. Balboa, E.M.; Conde, E.; Moure, A.; Falqué, E.; Domínguez, H. In vitro antioxidant properties of crude extracts and compounds from brown algae. *Food Chem.* **2013**, *138*, 1764–1785. [CrossRef] [PubMed]
174. Phasanasophon, K.; Kim, S. Antioxidant and Cosmeceutical Activities of *Agarum cribrosum* Phlorotannin Extracted by Ultrasound Treatment. *Nat. Prod. Commun.* **2018**, *13*, 565–570. [CrossRef]

175. Gheda, S.; Naby, M.A.; Mohamed, T.; Pereira, L.; Khamis, A. Antidiabetic and antioxidant activity of phlorotannins extracted from the brown seaweed *Cystoseira compressa* in streptozotocin-induced diabetic rats. *Environ. Sci. Pollut. Res.* **2021**, *28*, 22886–22901. [CrossRef] [PubMed]
176. Joe, M.; Kim, S.; Choi, H.; Shin, W.; Park, G.; Kang, D.; Kim, Y.K. The inhibitory effects of eckol and dieckol from *Ecklonia stolonifera* on the expression of matrix metalloproteinase-1 in human dermal fibroblasts. *Biol. Pharm. Bull.* **2006**, *29*, 1735–1739. [CrossRef] [PubMed]
177. Le, Q.; Li, Y.; Qian, Z.; Kim, M.; Kim, S. Inhibitory effects of polyphenols isolated from marine alga *Ecklonia cava* on histamine release. *Process Biochem.* **2009**, *44*, 168–176. [CrossRef]
178. Barbosa, M.; Lopes, G. Valentão, P.; Ferreres, F.; Gil-Izquierdo, A.; Pereira, D.M.; Andrade, P.B. Edible seaweeds' phlorotannins in allergy: A natural multi-target approach. *Food Chem.* **2018**, *265*, 233–241. [CrossRef]
179. Sugiura, Y.; Kinoshita, Y.; Misumi, S.; Yamatani, H.; Katsuzaki, H.; Hayashi, Y.; Murase, N. Correlation between the seasonal variations in phlorotannin content and the antiallergic effects of the brown alga *Ecklonia cava* subsp. *stolonifera*. *Algal Res.* **2021**, *58*, 102398. [CrossRef]
180. Barbosa, M.; Lopes, G.; Andrade, P.-B.; Valentão, P. Bioprospecting of brown seaweeds for biotechnological applications: Phlorotannin actions in inflammation and allergy network. *Trends Food Sci. Technol.* **2019**, *86*, 153–171. [CrossRef]
181. Catarino, M.D.; Amarante, S.J.; Mateus, N.; Silva, A.M.S.; Cardoso, S.M. Brown algae phlorotannins: A marine alternative to break the oxidative stress, inflammation and cancer network. *Foods* **2021**, *10*, 1478. [CrossRef] [PubMed]
182. Kang, H.S.; Kim, H.R.; Byun, D.S.; Son, B.W.; Nam, T.J.; Choi, J.S. Tyrosinase inhibitors isolated from the edible brown alga *Ecklonia stolonifera*. *Arch. Pharm. Res.* **2004**, *27*, 1226–1232. [CrossRef] [PubMed]
183. Heo, S.J.; Ko, S.; Cha, S.H.; Kang, D.H.; Park, H.S.; Choi, Y.U.; Kim, D.; Jung, W.K.; Yeon, Y.J. Effect of phlorotannins isolated from *Ecklonia cava* on melanogenesis and their protective effect against photo-oxidative stress induced by UV-B radiation. *Toxicol. Vitr.* **2009**, *23*, 1123–1130. [CrossRef] [PubMed]
184. Kang, S.M.; Heo, S.J.; Kim, K.N.; Lee, S.H.; Yang, H.M.; Kim, A.D.; Jeon, Y.J. Molecular docking studies of a phlorotannin, dieckol isolated from *Ecklonia cava* with tyrosinase inhibitory activity. *Bioorg. Med. Chem.* **2012**, *20*, 311–316. [CrossRef] [PubMed]
185. Kim, J.H.; Lee, S.; Park, S.; Park, J.S.; Kim, Y.H.; Yang, S.Y. Slow-Binding Inhibition of Tyrosinase by *Ecklonia cava* Phlorotannins. *Mar. Drugs* **2019**, *17*, 359. [CrossRef] [PubMed]
186. Susano, P.; Silva, J.; Alves, C.; Martins, A.; Gaspar, H.; Pinteus, S. Mouga, T.; Goettert, M.I.; Petrovski, Ž.; Branco, L.B.; et al. Unravelling the Dermatological Potential of the Brown Seaweed *Carpomitra costata*. *Mar. Drugs* **2021**, *19*, 135. [CrossRef]
187. Hwang, H.; Chen, T.; Nines, R.G. Shin, H.; Stoner, G.D. Photochemoprevention of UVB-induced skin carcinogenesis in SKH-1 mice by brown algae polyphenols. *Int. J. Cancer* **2006**, *119*, 2742–2749. [CrossRef]
188. Hwang, E.; Park, S.-Y.; Sun, Z.-W.; Shin, H.-S.; Lee, D.-G.; Yi, T.H. The protective effects of fucosterol against skin damage in UVB-Irradiated human dermal fibroblasts. *Mar. Biotechnol.* **2014**, *16*, 361–370. [CrossRef]
189. Handajani, F.; Prabowo, S. *Sargassum duplicatum* extract reduced artritis severity score and periarticular tissue matrix metalloproteinase-1 (MMP-1) expression in ajuvan artritis exposed to cold stressor. *Sys. Rev. Pharm.* **2020**, *11*, 302–307.
190. Ryu, B.; Ahn, B.-N.; Kang, K.-H.; Kim, Y.-S.; Li, Y.-X.; Kong, C.-S.; Kim, S.-K.; Kim, D.G. Dioxinodehydroeckol protects human keratinocyte cells from UVB-induced apoptosis modulated by related genes Bax/Bcl-2 and caspase pathway. *J. Photochem. Photobiol. B* **2015**, *153*, 352–357. [CrossRef]
191. Vo, T.S.; Kim, S.-K.; Ryu, B.; Ngo, D.H.; Yoon, N.-Y.; Bach, L.G.; Hang, N.T.N.; Ngo, D.N. The suppressive activity of fucofuroeckol-a derived from brown algal *Ecklonia stolonifera okamura* on UVB-induced mast cell degranulation. *Mar. Drugs* **2018**, *16*, 1. [CrossRef]
192. Manandhar, B.; Paudel, P.; Seong, S.H.; Jung, H.A.; Choi, J.S. Characterizing eckol as a therapeutic aid: A systematic review. *Mar. Drugs* **2019**, *17*, 361. [CrossRef] [PubMed]
193. Manandhar, B.; Wagle, A.; Seong, S.H.; Paudel, P.; Kim, H.-R.; Jung, H.A.; Choi, J.S. Phlorotannins with potential anti-tyrosinase and antioxidant activity isolated from the marine seaweed *Ecklonia stolonifera*. *Antioxidants* **2019**, *8*, 240. [CrossRef]
194. Sanjeewa, K.K.A.; Kim, E.-A.; Son, K.-T.; Jeon, Y.-J. Bioactive properties and potentials cosmeceutical applications of phlorotannins isolated from brown seaweeds: A review. *J. Photochem. Photobiol. B* **2016**, *162*, 100–105. [CrossRef] [PubMed]
195. Freitas, R.; Martins, A.; Silva, J.; Alves, C.; Pinteus, S.; Alves, J.; Teodoro, F.; Ribeiro, H.M.; Gonçalves, L.; Petrovski, Ž.; et al. Highlighting the Biological Potential of the Brown Seaweed *Fucus spiralis* for Skin Applications. *Antioxidants* **2020**, *9*, 611.
196. Arunkumar, K.; Raj, R.; Raja, R.; Carvalho, I.S. Brown seaweeds as a source of anti-hyaluronidase compounds. *S. Afr. J. Bot.* **2021**, *139*, 470–477. [CrossRef]
197. Ko, S.; Lee, M.; Lee, J.; Lee, S.; Lim, Y.; Jeon, Y. Dieckol, a phlorotannin isolated from a brown seaweed, *Ecklonia cava*, inhibits adipogenesis through AMP-activated protein kinase (AMPK) activation in 3T3-L1 preadipocytes. *Environ. Toxicol. Pharmacol.* **2013**, *36*, 1253–1260. [CrossRef]
198. Eom, S.H.; Lee, E.H.; Park, K.; Kwon, J.Y.; Kim, P.H.; Jung, W.K. Kim, Y.M. Ecklol from *Eisenia bicyclis* inhibits inflammation through the Akt/NF-κB signaling in *Propionibacterium acnes*-induced human keratinocyte Hacat cells. *J. Food Biochem.* **2017**, *41*, 12312. [CrossRef]
199. Hermund, D.B.; Plaza, M.; Turner, C.; Jónsdóttir, R.; Kristinsson, H.G.; Jacobsen, C.; Nielsen, K.F. Structure dependent antioxidant capacity of phlorotannins from Icelandic *Fucus vesiculosus* by UHPLC-DAD-ECD-QTOFMS. *Food Chem.* **2018**, *240*, 904–909.

200. Jang, J.; Ye, B.-R.; Heo, S.-J.; Oh, C.; Kang, D.-H.; Kim, J.H.; Affan, A.; Yoon, K.-T.; Choi, Y.-U.; Park, S.C.; et al. Photo-oxidative stress by ultraviolet-B radiation and antioxidative defense of eckstolonol in human keratinocytes. *Environ. Toxicol. Pharmacol.* **2012**, *34*, 926–934. [CrossRef]
201. Lee, J.-H.; Eom, S.-H.; Lee, E.-H.; Jung, Y.-J.; Kim, H.-J.; Jo, M.-R.; Son, K.-T.; Lee, H.-J.; Kim, J.H.; Lee, M.-S.; et al. In vitro antibacterial and synergistic effect of phlorotannins isolated from edible brown seaweed *Eisenia bicyclis* against acne-related bacteria. *Algae* **2014**, *29*, 47–55. [CrossRef]
202. Sugiura, Y.; Matsuda, K.; Yamada, Y.; Nishikawa, M.; Shioya, K.; Katsuzaki, H.; Imai, K.; Amano, H. Isolation of a new anti-allergic phlorotannin, phlorofucofuroeckol-B, from an edible brown alga, *Eisenia arborea*. *Biosci. Biotechnol. Biochem.* **2006**, *70*, 2807–2811. [CrossRef]
203. Le Lann, K.; Surget, G.; Couteau, C.; Coiffard, L.; Cerantola, S.; Gaillard, F.; Larnicol, M.; Zubia, M.; Gerard, F.; Poupart, N.; et al. Sunscreen, antioxidant, and bactericide capacities of phlorotannins from the brown macroalga *Halidrys siliquosa*. *J. Appl. Phycol.* **2016**, *28*, 3547–3559. [CrossRef]
204. Gager, L.; Connan, S.; Molla, M.; Couteau, C.; Arbona, J.F.; Coiffard, L.; Cérantola, S.; Stiger-Pouvreau, V. Active phlorotannins from seven brown seaweeds commercially harvested in Brittany (France) detected by ^{1}H NMR and in vitro assays: Temporal variation and potential valorization in cosmetic applications. *J. Appl. Phycol.* **2020**, *32*, 2375–2386. [CrossRef]
205. Lee, J.H.; Ko, J.-Y.; Samarakoon, K.; Oh, J.-Y.; Heo, S.-J.; Kim, C.-Y.; Nah, J.-W.; Jang, M.-K.; Lee, J.-S.; Jeon, Y.-J. Preparative isolation of sargachromanol E from *Sargassum siliquastrum* by centrifugal partition chromatography and its anti-inflammatory activity. *Food Chem. Toxicol.* **2013**, *62*, 54–60. [CrossRef] [PubMed]
206. Kim, J.; Ahn, B.; Kong, C.; Kim, S. The chromenesargachromanol E inhibits ultraviolet A-induced ageing of skin in human dermal fibroblasts. *Br. J. Dermatol.* **2013**, *168*, 968–976. [CrossRef] [PubMed]
207. Balboa, E.M.; Li, Y.; Ahn, B.; Eom, S.; Domínguez, H.; Jiménez, C.; Rodríguez, J. Photodamage attenuation effect by a tetraprenyl-toluquinol chromane meroterpenoid isolated from *Sargassum muticum*. *J. Photochem. Photobiol. B* **2015**, *148*, 51–58. [CrossRef]
208. Azam, M.S.; Choi, J.; Lee, M.-S.; Kim, H.-R. Hypopigmenting Effects of Brown Algae-Derived Phytochemicals: A Review on Molecular Mechanisms. *Mar. Drugs* **2017**, *15*, 297. [CrossRef]
209. Hamid, N.; Ma, Q.; Boulom, S.; Liu, T.; Zheng, Z.; Balbas, J.; Robertson, J. Seaweed Minor Constituents. In *Seaweed Sustainability: Food and Non-Food Applications*; Tiwari, B.K., Troy, D., Eds.; Academic Press: London, UK, 2015; pp. 193–242.
210. Stiger-Pouvreau, V.; Zubia, M. Macroalgal diversity for sustainable biotechnological development in French tropical overseas territories. *Bot. Mar.* **2020**, *63*, 17–41. [CrossRef]
211. Neto, R.T.; Marçal, C.; Queirós, A.S.; Abreu, H.; Silva, A.M.S.; Cardoso, S.M. Screening of *Ulva rigida*, *Gracilaria* sp., *Fucus vesiculosus* and *Saccharina latissima* as Functional Ingredients. *Int. J. Mol. Sci.* **2018**, *19*, 2987. [CrossRef]
212. Biris-Dorhoi, E.-S.; Michiu, D.; Pop, C.R.; Rotar, A.M.; Tofana, M.; Pop, O.L.; Socaci, S.A.; Farcas, A.C. Macroalgae—A Sustainable Source of Chemical Compounds with Biological Activities. *Nutrients* **2020**, *12*, 3085. [CrossRef] [PubMed]
213. Kumari, P.; Kumar, M.; Reddy, C.R.K.; Jha, B. Algal Lipids, Fatty Acids and Sterols. In *Functional Ingredients from Algae for Foods and Nutraceuticals*; Domínguez, H., Ed.; Woodhead Publishing: Cambridge, UK, 2013; pp. 87–134.
214. Lever, J.; Brkljača, R.; Kraft, G.; Urban, S. Natural Products of Marine Macroalgae from South Eastern Australia, with Emphasis on the Port Phillip Bay and Heads Regions of Victoria. *Mar. Drugs* **2020**, *18*, 142. [CrossRef]
215. Saadaoui, I.; Rasheed, R.; Abdulrahman, N.; Bounnit, T.; Cherif, M.; Al Jabri, H.; Mraiche, F. Algae-Derived Bioactive Compounds with Anti-Lung Cancer Potential. *Mar. Drugs* **2020**, *18*, 197. [CrossRef] [PubMed]
216. Plaza, M.; Cifuentes, A.; Ibáñez, E. In the search of new functional food ingredients from algae. *Trends Food Sci. Technol.* **2008**, *19*, 31–39. [CrossRef]
217. Gómez-Zorita, S.; González-Arceo, M.; Trepiana, J.; Eseberri, I.; Fernández-Quintela, A.; Milton-Laskibar, I.; Aguirre, L.; González, M.; Portillo, M.P. Anti-Obesity Effects of Macroalgae. *Nutrients* **2020**, *12*, 2378. [CrossRef] [PubMed]
218. Lange, K.W.; Hauser, J.; Nakamura, Y.; Kanaya, S. Dietary seaweeds and obesity. *Food Sci. Hum. Wellness* **2015**, *4*, 87–96. [CrossRef]
219. Lee, S.; Lee, Y.S.; Jung, S.H.; Kang, S.S.; Shin, K.H. Anti-oxidant activities of fucosterol from the marine algae *Pelvetia siliquosa*. *Arch. Pharm. Res.* **2003**, *26*, 719–722. [CrossRef] [PubMed]
220. Abdul, Q.A.; Choi, R.J.; Jung, H.A.; Choi, J.S. Health benefit of fucosterol from marine algae: A review. *J. Sci. Food Agric.* **2016**, *96*, 1856–1866. [CrossRef]
221. Hannan, M.A.; Sohag, A.A.M.; Dash, R.; Haque, M.N.; Mohibbullah, M.; Oktaviani, D.F.; Hossain, M.T.; Choi, H.J.; Moon, I.S. Phytosterols of marine algae: Insights into the potential health benefits and molecular pharmacology. *Phytomedicine* **2020**, *69*, 153201. [CrossRef]
222. Perumal, P.; Sowmiya, R.; Prasanna Kumar, S.; Ravikumar, S.; Deepak, P.; Balasubramani, G. Isolation, structural elucidation and antiplasmodial activity of fucosterol compound from brown seaweed, *Sargassum linearifolium* against malarial parasite *Plasmodium falciparum*. *Nat. Prod. Res.* **2017**, *32*, 1316–1319. [CrossRef]
223. Sugawara, T.; Kushiro, M.; Zhang, H.; Nara, E.; Ono, H.; Nagao, A. Lysophosphatidylcholine enhances carotenoid uptake from mixed micelles by Caco-2 human intestinal cells. *J. Nutr.* **2001**, *131*, 2921–2927. [CrossRef]
224. Okada, T.; Mizuno, Y.; Sibayama, S.; Hosokawa, M.; Miyashita, H. Antiobesity effects of *Undaria* lipid capsules prepared with scallop phospholipids. *J. Food Sci.* **2011**, *76*, 2–6. [CrossRef]
225. Rexliene, J.; Sridhar, J. Extraction and characterization of essential oil from Portieria hornemannii with applications in antibacterial edible films. *Res. J. Biotechnol.* **2021**, *16*, 81–89.

226. Lee, H.J.; Dang, H.T.; Kang, G.J.; Yang, E.J.; Park, S.S.; Yoon, W.J.; Jung, J.H.; Kang, H.K.; Yoo, E.S. Two enone fatty acids isolated from *Gracilaria verrucosa* suppress the production of inflammatory mediators by down-regulating NF-êB and STAT1 activity in lipopolysaccharide-stimulated raw 264.7 cells. *Arch. Pharm. Res.* **2009**, *32*, 453–462. [CrossRef] [PubMed]
227. Patra, J.K.; Das, G.; Baek, K. Chemical composition and antioxidant and antibacterial activities of an essential oil extracted from an edible seaweed, *Laminaria japonica* L. *Molecules* **2015**, *20*, 12093–12113. [CrossRef] [PubMed]
228. Lee, Y.; Shin, K.; Jung, S.; Lee, S. Effects of the extracts from the marine algae *Pelvetia siliquosa* on hyperlipidemia in rats. *Korean J. Pharmacogn.* **2004**, *35*, 143–146.
229. Zhangfan, M.; Xiaoling, S.; Ping, D.; Gaoli, L.; Shize, P.; Xiangran, S.; Haifeng, H.; Li, P.; Jie, H. Fucosterol exerts antiproliferative effects on human lung cancer cells by inducing apoptosis, cel cycle arrest and targeting of Raf/MEK/ERK signaling pathway. *Phytomedicine* **2019**, *61*, 152809.
230. Richard, D.; Kefi, K.; Barbe, U.; Bausero, P.; Visioli, F. Polyunsaturated fatty acids as antioxidants. *Pharmacol. Res.* **2008**, *57*, 451–455. [CrossRef]
231. Mohy El-Din, S.M. Fatty acid profiling as bioindicator of chemical stress in marine *Pterocladia capillacea*, *Sargassum hornschuchii* and *Ulva lactuca*. *Int. J Environ. Sci. Technol.* **2018**, *15*, 791–800. [CrossRef]
232. Calandra, I.P.; Simonetti, S. Nutritional supplements in dermocosmetology. *Ann. Ital. Dermatol. Clin. Sper.* **1995**, *49*, 49–56.
233. Jacob, L.; Baker, C.; Farris, P. Vitamin-based cosmeceuticals. *Cosmet. Dermatol.* **2012**, *25*, 405.
234. Peñalver, R.; Lorenzo, J.M.; Ros, G.; Amarowicz, R.; Pateiro, M.; Nieto, G. Seaweeds as a Functional Ingredient for a Healthy Diet. *Mar. Drugs* **2020**, *18*, 301. [CrossRef]
235. Kafi, R.; Kwak, H.S.R.; Schumacher, W.E.; Cho, S.; Hanft, V.N.; Hamilton, T.A.; King, A.L.; Neal, J.D.; Varani, J.; Fisher, G.J.; et al. Improvement of naturally aged skin with vitamin a (retinol). *Arch. Dermatol.* **2007**, *143*, 606–612. [CrossRef] [PubMed]
236. Searle, T.; Al-Niaimi, F.; Ali, F.R. The top 10 cosmeceuticals for facial hyperpigmentation. *Dermatol. Ther.* **2020**, *33*, 14095. [CrossRef] [PubMed]
237. Bissett, D.L.; Oblong, J.E.; Goodman, L.J. Topical Vitamins. In *Cosmetic Dermatology: Products and Procedures*; Draelos, Z.D., Ed.; Wiley & Sons, Ltd.: Hoboken, NJ, USA, 2015; pp. 336–345.
238. Kilinç, B.; Semra, C.; Gamze, T.; Hatice, T.; Koru, E. Seaweeds for Food and Industrial Applications. In *Food Industry*; Muzzalupo, I., Ed.; InTech: Rijeka, Croatia, 2013; pp. 735–748.
239. Campiche, R.; Curpen, S.J.; Lutchmanen-Kolanthan, V.; Gougeon, S.; Cherel, M.; Laurent, G.; Gempeler, M.; Schuetz, R. Pigmentation effects of blue light irradiation on skin and how to protect against them. *Int. J. Cosmet. Sci.* **2020**, *42*, 399–406. [CrossRef] [PubMed]
240. Kim, S.K.; Bhatnagar, I. Physical, chemical, and biological properties of wonder kelp-*Laminaria*. *Adv. Food Nutr. Res.* **2011**, *64*, 85–96. [PubMed]
241. Watanabe, F.; Yabuta, Y.; Bito, T.; Teng, F. Vitamin B12-containing plant food sources for vegetarians. *Nutrients* **2014**, *6*, 1861–1873. [CrossRef]
242. Bito, T.; Tanioka, Y.; Watanabe, F. Characterization of vitamin B12 compounds from marine foods. *Fish. Sci.* **2018**, *84*, 747–755. [CrossRef]
243. Manela-Azulay, M.; Bagatin, E. Cosmeceuticals vitamins. *Clin. Dermatol.* **2009**, *27*, 469–474. [CrossRef]
244. Lorencini, M.; Brohem, C.A.; Dieamant, G.C.; Zanchin, N.I.; Maibach, H.I. Active ingredients against human epidermal aging. *Ageing Res. Rev.* **2014**, *15*, 100–115. [CrossRef]
245. Paiva, L.; Lima, E.; Neto, A.I.; Marcone, M.; Baptista, J. Health-promoting ingredients from four selected Azorean macroalgae. *Food Res. Int.* **2016**, *89*, 432–438. [CrossRef] [PubMed]
246. Mercurio, D.G.; Wagemaker, T.A.L.; Alves, V.M.; Benevenuto, C.G.; Gaspar, L.R.; Maia Campos, P.M.B.G. In vivo photoprotective effects of cosmetic formulations containing UV filters, vitamins, *Ginkgo biloba* and red algae extracts. *J. Photochem. Photobiol. B* **2015**, *153*, 121–126. [CrossRef]
247. Sumi, H.; Osada, K.; Yatagai, C.; Naito, S.; Yanagisawa, Y. High concentration of vitamin K1 proved in the seaweeds and sweet potato leaves. *J.-Jpn. Soc. Food Sci. Technol.* **2003**, *50*, 63–66. [CrossRef]
248. Kamao, M.; Suhara, Y.; Tsugawa, N.; Uwano, M.; Yamaguchi, N.; Uenishi, K.; Ishida, H.; Sasaki, S.; Okano, T. Vitamin K content of foods and dietary vitamin K intake in Japanese young women. *J. Nutr. Sci. Vitaminol.* **2007**, *53*, 464–470. [CrossRef]
249. Del Mondo, A.; Smerilli, A.; Sané, E.; Sansone, C.; Brunet, C. Challenging microalgal vitamins for human health. *Microb. Cell Factories* **2020**, *19*, 201. [CrossRef] [PubMed]
250. Rupérez, P. Mineral content of edible marine seaweeds. *Food Chem.* **2002**, *79*, 23–26. [CrossRef]
251. Circuncisão, A.R.; Catarino, M.D.; Cardoso, S.M.; Silva, A.M.S. Minerals from Macroalgae Origin: Health Benefits and Risks for Consumers. *Mar. Drugs* **2018**, *16*, 400. [CrossRef]
252. Lozano Muñoz, I.; Díaz, N.F. Minerals in edible seaweed: Health benefits and food safety issues. *Crit. Rev. Food Sci. Nutr.* **2020**, *18*, 1–16. [CrossRef] [PubMed]
253. Tarnowska, M.; Briancon, S.; Resende de Azevedo, J.; Chevalier, Y.; Bolzinger, M.-A. Inorganic ions in the skin: Allies or enemies? *Int. J. Pharm.* **2020**, *591*, 119991. [CrossRef]
254. Kraan, S. Pigments and Minor Compounds in Algae. In *Functional Ingredients from Algae for Foods and Nutraceuticals*; Domínguez, H., Ed.; Woodhead Publishing: Cambridge, UK, 2013; pp. 205–251.

255. Mohamed, S.; Hashim, S.N.; Rahman, H.A. Seaweeds: A sustainable functional food for complementary and alternative therapy. *Trends Food Sci. Technol.* **2012**, *23*, 83–96. [CrossRef]
256. Polefka, T.G.; Bianchini, R.J.; Shapiro, S. Interaction of mineral salts with the skin: A literature survey. *Int. J. Cosmet. Sci.* **2012**, *34*, 416–423. [CrossRef]
257. Martins, A.; Vieira, H.; Gaspar, H.; Santos, S. Review: Marketed marine natural products in the pharmaceutical and cosmeceutical industries: Tips for success. *Mar. Drugs* **2014**, *12*, 1066–1101. [CrossRef]
258. Guillerme, J.-B.; Couteau, C.; Coiffard, L. Applications for Marine Resources in Cosmetics. *Cosmetics* **2017**, *4*, 35. [CrossRef]
259. Alves, A.; Sousa, E.; Sousa, E.; Kijjoa, A.; Pinto, M. Marine-derived compounds with potential use as cosmeceuticals and nutricosmetics. *Molecules* **2020**, *25*, 2536. [CrossRef] [PubMed]
260. Chakdar, H.; Pabbi, S. Algal Pigments for Human Health and Cosmeceuticals. In *Algal Green Chemistry*; Rastogi, R.P., Madamwar, D., Pandey, A., Eds.; Elsevier: Amsterdam, The Netherlands, 2017; pp. 171–188.
261. Christaki, E.; Bonos, E.; Giannenasa, I.; Florou-Paneria, P. Functional properties of carotenoids originating from algae. *J. Sci. Food Agric.* **2013**, *93*, 5–11. [CrossRef]
262. Rajauria, G. In-Vitro Antioxidant Properties of Lipophilic Antioxidant Compounds from 3 Brown Seaweed. *Antioxidants* **2019**, *8*, 596. [CrossRef] [PubMed]
263. Maeda, H.; Hosokawa, M.; Sashima, T.; Funayama, K.; Miyashita, K. Fucoxanthin from edible seaweed, *Undaria pinnatifida*, shows antiobesity effect through UCP1 expression in white adipose tissues. *Biochem. Biophys. Res. Commun.* **2005**, *332*, 392–397. [CrossRef] [PubMed]
264. Gammone, M.A.; D'Orazio, N. Anti-obesity activity of the marine carotenoid fucoxanthin. *Mar. Drugs* **2015**, *13*, 2196–2214. [CrossRef] [PubMed]
265. Rajauria, G.; Foley, B.; Abu-Ghannam, N. Characterization of dietary fucoxanthin from *Himanthalia elongata* brown seaweed. *Food Res. Int.* **2017**, *99*, 995–1001. [CrossRef]
266. Shimoda, H.; Tanaka, J.; Shan, S.; Maoka, T. Anti-pigmentary activity of fucoxanthin and its influence on skin mRNA expression of melanogenic molecules. *J. Pharm. Pharmacol.* **2010**, *62*, 1137–1145. [CrossRef]
267. Peng, J.; Yuan, J.P.; Wu, C.F.; Wang, J.H. Fucoxanthin, a marine carotenoid present in brown seaweeds and diatoms: Metabolism and bioactivities relevant to human health. *Mar. Drugs* **2011**, *9*, 1806–1828. [CrossRef] [PubMed]
268. Heo, S.; Jeon, Y. Protective effect of fucoxanthin isolated from *Sargassum siliquastrum* on UV-B induced cell damage. *J. Photochem. Photobiol. B* **2009**, *95*, 101–107. [CrossRef] [PubMed]
269. Heo, S.-J.; Yoon, W.-J.; Kim, K.-N.; Ahn, G.-N.; Kang, S.-M.; Kang, D.-H.; Affan, A.; Oh, C.; Jung, W.-K.; Jeon, Y.-J. Evaluation of anti-inflammatory effect of fucoxanthin isolated from brown algae in lipopolysaccharide-stimulated RAW 264.7 macrophages. *Food Chem. Toxicol.* **2010**, *48*, 2045–2051. [CrossRef]
270. Matsui, M.; Tanaka, K.; Higashiguchi, N.; Okawa, H.; Yamada, Y.; Tanaka, K.; Taira, S.; Aoyama, T.; Takanishi, M.; Natsume, C.; et al. Protective and therapeutic effects of fucoxanthin against sunburn caused by UV irradiation. *J. Pharmacol. Sci.* **2016**, *132*, 55–64. [CrossRef] [PubMed]
271. Nie, J.; Chen, D.; Lu, Y.; Dai, Z. Effects of various blanching methods on fucoxanthin degradation kinetics, antioxidant activity, pigment composition, and sensory quality of *Sargassum fusiforme*. *LWT-Food Sci. Tecnol.* **2021**, *143*, 111179. [CrossRef]
272. Jia, Y.P.; Sun, L.; Yu, H.S.; Liang, L.P.; Li, W.; Ding, H.; Song, X.B.; Zhang, L.J. The Pharmacological Effects of Lutein and Zeaxanthin on Visual Disorders and Cognition Diseases. *Molecules* **2017**, *22*, 610. [CrossRef] [PubMed]
273. Naser, W. The cosmetic effects of various natural biofunctional ingredients against skin aging: A review. *Int. J. Appl. Pharm.* **2021**, *13*, 10–18. [CrossRef]
274. Bagal-Kestwal, D.R.; Pan, M.-H.; Chiang, B.-H. Properties and Applications of Gelatin, Pectin, and Carrageenan Gels. In *Bio Monomers for Green Polymeric Composite Materials*; Visakh, P.M., Bayraktar, O., Menon, G., Eds.; John Wiley & Sons Ltd.: Hoboken, NJ, USA, 2019; pp. 117–140.
275. Tarman, K.; Ain, N.H.; Sulistiawati, S.; Hardjito, L.; Sadi, U. Biological process to valorise marine algae. *IOP Conf. Ser. Earth Environ. Sci.* **2020**, *414*, 012026. [CrossRef]
276. Li, D.; Wu, Z.; Martini, N.; Wen, J. Advanced carrier systems in cosmetics and cosmeceuticals: A review. *J. Cosmet. Sci.* **2011**, *62*, 549–563.
277. Peng, J.; Xu, W.; Ni, D.; Zhang, W.; Zhang, T.; Guang, C.; Mu, W. Preparation of a novel water-soluble gel from *Erwinia amylovora* levan. *Int. J. Biol. Macromol.* **2019**, *122*, 469–478. [CrossRef]
278. Prima, N.R.; Andriyono, S. Techniques of additional *Kappaphycus alvarezii* on seaweed face mask production. *IOP Conf. Ser. Earth Environ. Sci.* **2021**, *679*, 012021. [CrossRef]
279. Eom, S.; Kim, Y.; Kim, S. Antimicrobial effect of phlorotannins from marine brown algae. *Food Chem. Toxicol.* **2012**, *50*, 3251–3255. [CrossRef]
280. Abu-Ghannam, N.; Rajauria, G. Antimicrobial Activity of Compounds Isolated from Algae. In *Functional Ingredients from Algae for Foods and Nutraceuticals*; Domínguez, H., Ed.; Woodhead Publishing: Cambridge, UK, 2013; pp. 287–306.
281. Pérez, M.J.; Falqué, E.; Domínguez, H. Antimicrobial action of compounds from marine seaweed. *Mar. Drugs* **2016**, *14*, 52. [CrossRef] [PubMed]

282. Lopes, G.; Sousa, C.; Silva, L.R.; Pinto, E.; Andrade, P.B.; Bernardo, J.; Mouga, T.; Valentão, P. Can phlorotannins purified extracts constitute a novel pharmacological alternative for microbial infections with associated inflammatory conditions? *PLoS ONE* 2012, 7, 31145. [CrossRef]
283. Amiguet, V.T.; Jewell, L.E.; Mao, H.; Sharma, M.; Hudson, J.B.; Durst, T.; Allard, M.; Rochefort, G.; Arnason, J.T. Antibacterial properties of a glycolipid-rich extract and active principle from Nunavik collections of the macroalgae *Fucus evanescens* C. Agardh (Fucaceae). *Can. J. Microbiol.* 2011, 57, 745–749. [CrossRef] [PubMed]
284. Arguelles, E.D.L.R.; Sapin, A.B. Bioprospecting of *Turbinaria ornata* (Fucales, phaeophyceae) for cosmetic application. Antioxidant, tyrosinase inhibition and antibacterial activities. *J. Int. Soc. Southeas. Asian Agric. Sci.* 2020, 26, 30–41.
285. Arguelles, E.R.; Sapin, A.B. Bioactive properties of Sargassum siliquosum J. Agardh (Fucales, Ochrophyta) and its potential as source of skin-lightening active ingredient for cosmetic application. *J. Appl. Pharm. Sci.* 2020, 10, 51–58.
286. Arguelles, E.L.R. Evaluation of antioxidant capacity, tyrosinase inhibition, and antibacterial activities of brown seaweed, *Sargassum ilicifolium* (Turner) c. agardh 1820 for cosmeceutical application. *J. Fish. Environ.* 2021, 45, 64–77.
287. Kim, I.H.; Lee, D.G.; Lee, S.H.; Ha, J.M.; Ha, B.J.; Kim, S.K.; Le, J.H. Antibacterial activity of *Ulva lactuca* against methicillin-resistant *Staphylococcus aureus* (MRSA). *Biotechnol. Bioprocess Eng.* 2007, 12, 579–582. [CrossRef]
288. Pierre, G.; Sopena, V.; Juin, C.; Mastouri, A.; Graber, M.; Maugard, T. Antibacterial activity of a sulfated galactan extracted from the marine alga *Chaetomorpha aerea* against *Staphylococcus aureus*. *Biotechnol. Bioprocess Eng.* 2011, 16, 937–945. [CrossRef]
289. Ha, Y.; Choi, J.; Lee, E.; Moon, H.E.; Cho, K.K.; Choi, I.S. Inhibitory effects of seaweed extracts on the growth of the vaginal bacterium *Gardnerella vaginalis*. *J. Environ. Biol.* 2014, 35, 537–542. [PubMed]
290. Wei, Y.; Liu, Q.; Yu, J.; Feng, Q.; Zhao, L.; Song, H.; Wang, W. Antibacterial mode of action of 1, 8-dihydroxy-anthraquinone from porphyrahaitanensis against *Staphylococcus aureus*. *Nat. Prod. Res.* 2015, 29, 976–979. [CrossRef]
291. Widowati, I.; Suprijanto, J.; Trianto A.; Puspita, M.; Bedoux, G.; Bourgougnon, N. Antibacterial activity and proximate analysis of Sargassum extracts as cosmetic additives in a moisturizer cream. *AACL Bioflux* 2019, 12, 1961–1969.
292. Poyato, C.; Thomsen, B.R.; Hermund, D.B.; Ansorena, D.; Astiasarán I.; Jónsdóttir, R.; Kristinsson, H.G.; Jacobsen, C. Antioxidant effect of water and acetone extracts of *Fucus vesiculosus* on oxidative stability of skin care emulsions. *Eur. J. Lipid Sci. Technol.* 2017, 119, 1600072. [CrossRef]
293. Paiva, A.A.D.O.; Castro, A.J.G.; Nascimento, M.S.; Will, L.S.E.P.; Santos, N.D.; Araújo, R.M.; Xavier, C.A.C.; Rocha, F.A.; Leite, E.L. Antioxidant and anti-inflammatory effect of polysaccharides from *Lobophora variegata* on zymosan-induced arthritis in rats. *Int. Immunopharmacol.* 2011, 11, 1241–1250. [CrossRef]
294. Nursid, M.; Khatulistiani, T.S.; Noviendri, D.; Hapsari, F.; Hardiyati, T. Total phenolic content, antioxidant activity and tyrosinase inhibitor from marine red algae extract collected from Kupang, East Nusa Tenggara. *IOP Conf. Ser. Earth Environ. Sci.* 2020, 493, 012013. [CrossRef]
295. Sari, D.S.P.; Saputra, E.; Alamsjah, M.A. Potential of fucoxanthin content in *Sargassum* sp. On sunscreen cream preparation. *Int. J. Recent Technol. Eng.* 2019, 7, 448–451.
296. Fransiska, D.; Darmawan, M.; Sinurat, E.; Sedayu, B.B.; WArdana, Y.W.; Herdiana, Y.; Setiana, G.P. Characteristics of Oil in Water (o/w) Type Lotions Incorporated with Kappa/Iota Carrageenan. *IOP Conf. Ser. Earth Environ. Sci.* 2021, 715, 012030. [CrossRef]
297. Cunha, S.C.; Fernandes, J.O.; Vallecillos, L.; Cano-Sancho, G.; Domingo, J.L.; Pocurull, E.; Borrull, F.; Mauvault, A.L.; Ferrari, E.; Fernández-Tejedor, M.; et al. Co-occurrence of musk fragrances and UV-filters in seafood and macroalgae collected in European hotspots. *Environ. Res.* 2015, 143, 65–71. [CrossRef]
298. Tiwari, R.; Tiwari, G.; Lahiri, A.; Vadivelan, R.; Rai, A.K. Localized delivery of drugs through medical textiles for treatment of burns: A perspective approach. *Adv. Pharm. Bull.* 2021, 11, 248–260
299. Mohan, R.; Singh, S.; Kumar, G.; Srivastava, M. Evaluation of gelling behavior of natural gums and their formulation prospects. *Indian J. Pharm. Educ. Res.* 2020, 54, 1016–1023. [CrossRef]
300. Dita, L.R.; Sudarno, S.; Triastuti, J. Utilization of agar *Gracilaria* sp. as a natural thickener on liquid bath soap formulation. *IOP Conf. Ser. Earth Environ. Sci.* 2020, 441, 012021. [CrossRef]
301. Hu, B.; Han, L.; Ma, R.; Phillips, G.O.; Nishinari, K.; Fang, Y. All-natural food-grade hydrophilic–hydrophobic core–shell microparticles: Facile fabrication based on gel-network-restricted antisolvent method. *ACS Appl. Mater. Interfaces* 2019, 11, 11936–11946. [CrossRef] [PubMed]
302. Wasupalli, G.K.; Verma, D. Polysaccharides as Biomaterials. In *Fundamental Biomaterials: Polymers*; Thomas, S.; Balakrishnan, P.; Sreekala, M.R., Eds.; Woodhead Publishing: Cambridge, UK, 2018; pp. 37–70.
303. Tafuro, G.; Costantini, A.; Baratto, G.; Francescato, S.; Busata, L.; Semenzato, A. Characterization of polysaccharidic associations for cosmetic use: Rheology and texture analysis. *Cosmetics* 2021, 8, 32. [CrossRef]
304. Zhu, B.; Ni, F.; Sun, Y.; Zhu, X.; Yin, H.; Yao, Z.; Du, Y. Insight into carrageenases: Major review of sources, category, property, purification method, structure, and applications. *Crit. Rev. Biotechnol.* 2018, 38, 1261–1276. [CrossRef]
305. Vilela, A.; Cosme, F.; Pinto, T. Emulsions, Foams, and Suspensions: The Microscience of the Beverage Industry. *Beverages* 2018, 4, 25. [CrossRef]
306. Nilforoushzadeh, M.A.; Amirkhani, M.A.; Zarrintaj, P.; Salehi Moghaddam, A.; Mehrabi, T.; Alavi, S.; Mollapour Sisakht, M. Skin care and rejuvenation by cosmeceutical facial mask. *J. Cosmet. Dermatol.* 2018, 17, 693–702. [CrossRef]
307. Graham, S.; Marina, F.F.; Blencowe, A. Thermoresponsive polysaccharides and their thermoreversible physical hydrogel networks. *Carbohydr. Polym.* 2019, 207, 143–159. [CrossRef] [PubMed]

308. Choi, J.; Moon, W.S.; Choi, J.N.; Do, K.H.; Moon, S.H.; Cho, K.K.; Han, C.J.; Choi, I.S. Effects of seaweed *Laminaria japonica* extracts on skin moisturizing activity in vivo. *Int. J. Cosmet. Sci.* **2013**, *64*, 193–205.
309. Dolorosa, M.T.; Nurjanah; Purwaningsih, S.; Anwar, E.; Hidayat, T. Tyrosinase inhibitory activity of *Sargassum plagyophyllum* and *Eucheuma cottonii* methanol extracts. *IOP Conf. Ser. Earth Environ. Sci.* **2019**, *278*, 012020. [CrossRef]
310. Cha, S.H.; Ko, S.C.; Kim, D.; Jeon, Y.J. Screening of marine algae for potential tyrosinase inhibitor: Those inhibitors reduced tyrosinase activity and melanin synthesis in zebrafish. *J. Dermatol.* **2011**, *38*, 354–363. [CrossRef] [PubMed]
311. Chan, Y.Y.; Kim, K.H.; Cheah, S.H. Inhibitory effects of *Sargassum polycystum* on tyrosinase activity and melanin formation in B16F10 murine melanoma cells. *J. Ethnopharmacol.* **2011**, *137*, 1183–1188. [CrossRef]
312. Park, J.; Lee, H.; Choi, S.; Pandey, L.K.; Depuydt, S.; De Saeger, J.; Park, J.-T.; Han, T. Extracts of red seaweed, *Pyropia yezoensis*, inhibit melanogenesis but stimulate collagen synthesis. *J. Appl. Phycol.* **2021**, *33*, 653–662. [CrossRef]
313. Jesumani, V.; Du, H.; Pei, P.; Aslam, M.; Huang, N. Comparative study on skin protection activity of polyphenol-rich extract and polysaccharide-rich extract from *Sargassum vachellianum*. *PLoS ONE* **2020**, *15*, e0227308.
314. Thu, N.T.H.; Anh, H.T.L.; Hien, H.T.M.; Ha, N.C.; Tam, L.T.; Khoi, T.X.; Duc, T.M.; Hong, D.D. Preparation and evaluation of cream mask from Vietnamese seaweeds. *J. Cosmet. Sci.* **2018**, *69*, 447–462. [PubMed]
315. Pratama, G.; Yanuarti, R.; Ilhamdy, A.F.; Suhana, M.P. Formulation of sunscreen cream from *Eucheuma cottonii* and *Kaempferia galanga* (zingiberaceae). *IOP Conf. Ser. Earth Environ. Sci.* **2019**, *278*, 012062. [CrossRef]
316. Poulose, N.; Sajayan, A.; Ravindran, A.; Sreechithra, T.V.; Vardhan, V.; Selvin, J.; Kiran, G.S. Photoprotective effect of nanomelanin-seaweed concentrate in formulated cosmetic cream: With improved antioxidant and wound healing properties. *J. Photochem. Photobiol. B* **2020**, *205*, 111816. [CrossRef] [PubMed]
317. Pallela, R. Antioxidants from Marine Organisms and Skin Care. In *Systems Biology of Free Radicals and Antioxidants*; Laher, I., Ed.; Springer: Berlin/Heidelberg, Germany, 2014; pp. 3771–3783.
318. Raikou, V.; Protopapa, E.; Kefala, V. Photo-protection from marine organisms. *Rev. Clin. Pharmacol. Pharmacokinet.* **2011**, *25*, 131–136.
319. Riani Mansauda, K.L.; Anwar, E.; Nurhayati, T. Antioxidant and anti-collagenase activity of sargassum plagyophyllum extract as an anti-wrinkle cosmetic ingredient. *Pharmacogn. Mag.* **2018**, *10*, 932–936.
320. Kasitowati, R.D.; Wahyudi, A.; Asmara, R.; Aliviyanti, D.; Iranawati, F.; Panjaitan, M.A.P.; Pratiwi, D.C.; Arsad, S. Identification photoprotective activity of marine seaweed: *Eucheuma* sp. *IOP Conf. Ser. Earth Environ. Sci.* **2021**, *679*, 012014. [CrossRef]
321. Sami, F.J.; Soekamto, N.H.; Firdaus; Latip, J. Bioactivity profile of three types of seaweed as an antioxidant, uv-protection as sunscreen and their correlation activity. *Food Res.* **2021**, *5*, 441–447. [CrossRef]
322. Pangestuti, R.; Siahaan, E.A.; Kim, S.-K. Photoprotective substances derived from marine algae. *Mar. Drugs* **2018**, *16*, 399. [CrossRef] [PubMed]
323. Hameury, S.; Borderie, L.; Monneuse, J.-M.; Skorski, G.; Pradines, D. Prediction of skin anti-aging clinical benefits of an association of ingredients from marine and maritime origins: Ex vivo evaluation using a label-free quantitative proteomic and customized data processing approach. *J. Cosmet. Dermatol.* **2019**, *18*, 355–370. [CrossRef]
324. Uji, Y.; Shibayama, J.; Shirakawa, Y. Oil-In-Water Type Emulsified Composition for External Skin Use. JPH0366281B2, 16 October 1991.
325. Ando, H.; Ando, Y. Cosmetic Containing Agar Oligosaccharide and/or Its Esterified Substance. JP3223038B2, 29 October 2001.
326. Kang, N.G.; Park, B.G. Solid-Type Cosmetic Composition for Moisturizing. KR20120019409A, 6 March 2012.
327. Luo, Q.; Peng, Y. Powder-Containing Oil-in-Water Type Solid-State Cosmetic Composition and Preparation Method and Application Thereof. CN110664628A, 10 January 2020.
328. Kawagishi, F.; Yamada, K.; Yokota, S. Pack Cosmetic. JPH11302124A, 2 November 1999.
329. Hasunuma, K.; Saito, M. Powdery Pack Cosmetic. JPH08217631A, 27 August 1996.
330. Nakagaki, E.; Suzuki, T. Hair Cosmetic. JP2779926B2, 23 July 1998.
331. Sawaki, S.; Yamada, K. Water-Soluble Powdery Cosmetic. JP2889922B2, 10 May 1999.
332. Pedroso De Oliveira, A.P. A Base Composition for Preparing Multi-Functional Formulations for Skin Care and Process for the Preparation Thereof. MXPA04009861A, 18 April 2005.
333. Igarashi, Y.; Kobayashi, M.; Oka, S.; Takagaki, K. Scalp and Hair Cosmetic. JP2015030670A, 16 February 2015.
334. Bi, L.; Pan, S.; Shao, X.; Sui, H.; Zhao, L.; Zou, P. Nano-Liposome Emulsion and Preparation Method Thereof. CN103876982A, 25 June 2014.
335. Billiotte, J.-C.; Dampeirou, C. Cosmetic Skin Firming Compsn. For Combating Effects of Stress and Ageing. CH686997A5, 30 August 1996.
336. Kim, K.B.; Ko, H.J.; Lee, D.H.; Lee, G.S.; Pyo, H.B. Ulva Spp Seaweed Hydrolysates That Have High Glucuronic Acid Cotent, Preparation Method Thereof and Antiaging Cosmetic Composition Containing the Same. KR101356535B1, 29 January 2014.
337. Kong, Q.; Zhou, L. Anti-Aging Cosmetic Containing Seaweed Extract and Preparation Method Thereof. CN105030587A, 11 November 2015.
338. Yao, Z. Marine Bioactive Cosmetic. CN112426381A, 2 March 2021.
339. Yao, Z. Marine Bioactive Cosmetic. CN112451429A, 9 March 2021.
340. Yang, H. Seaweed-Containing Cosmetic Additive and Preparation Method and Application Thereof. CN107669588A, 9 February 2018.
341. Min, G.H. Functional Cosmetic Composition for Anti-Dust and Anti-Inflammatory Containing Natural Extract as an Effective Ingredient and Functional Cosmetic Including the Same. KR101988489B1, 12 June 2019.

342. Kawashima, Y.; Uchibori, T. Antimicrobial Agent. JP2879590B2, 5 April 1999.
343. Andre, G.; Pellegrini, L.; Pellegrini. M. Use of Undaria Pinnatifida Seaweed Extract in Cosmetic or Dermatological Compositions for Protecting the Skin and Visible Organs from the Harmful Effects of Oxygen Radicals and Atmospheric Pollution. FR2837383A1, 26 September 2003.
344. Gwon, S.B.; Jo, J.H.; Joo, W.H.; Kim, E.H.; Lee, J.H.; Lee, J.H.; Park, S.H.; Ryu, G.Y. Antioxidant and Whitening Functional Cosmetics. KR101351387B1, 14 January 2014.
345. Imada, K.; Mitsui, Y. Anti-Perspiration and Deodorization Cosmetic, and Method for Producing the Same. JP2008184395A, 14 August 2008.
346. Park, D.I. Cosmetic Composition that Is Effective against Wrinkles. KR20120119797A, 31 October 2012.
347. Hagino, H.; Saito, M. Cosmetics. US2004131580A1, 8 July 2004.
348. Subuchi, H. Hair Shampoo, Hair Treatment, Hair-Growing Agent and Cosmetic Cream. JP2006008599A, 12 January 2006.
349. Holtkoetter, O.; Scheunemann, V.; Schulze Zur Wiesche, E. Hair Treatment Agent. EP2457556A2, 23 November 2011.
350. Aono, M.; Yamaoka, Y. Scalp and Hair Cosmetic. JP2012184220A, 27 September 2012.
351. Cha, Y.J.; Hong, Y.C.; Hong, Y.K.; Kim, Y.J. Cosmetic Manufacturing Method Using Natural Originated Material and Cosmetic Thereof. KR20150063336A, 9 June 2015.
352. Cheng, G.; Cheng, J. Nano-Element Shampoo. CN104739747A, 1 July 2015.
353. Kim, K.E. Kelp, Deep Cleansing, Shampoo, Cosmetics. KR20110013349A, 10 February 2011.
354. Egawa, M.; Nakamura, R. Skin Care Method. JP2015043973A, 12 March 2015.
355. Courtin, O. Cosmetic Composition for Combating the Adverse Effects of Agents in the Atmosphere. FR2688137A1, 10 September 1993.
356. Ishii, K. Combined Cosmetic. JP2011032200A, 17 February 2011.
357. Wu, X. Cosmetic Hand Film. CN202682386U, 23 January 2013.
358. Han, J.; Zhao, Y. Moisturizing and Oil-Controlling Cosmetic Composition and Preparation Method of Composition. CN111407684A, 14 July 2020.
359. Bi, L.; Mou, W.; Sui, H.; Yang, J.; Yu, J.; Zhao, L.; Zou, P. Seaweed Composition with Oil-Control Function and Cosmetic Thereof. CN108904340A, 30 November 2013.
360. Li, Y. Liquid Cosmetic Formula and Preparation Method Thereof. CN112022768A, 4 December 2020.
361. Qian, F. Oil-Control Acne-Preventive Cosmetic with Pure Herbal Essence and Preparation Method Thereof. CN111888287A, 6 November 2020.
362. Chen, J.; Jin, Z.; Ouyang, Z.; Quar, C.; Yu, G.; Zhang, F. Preparing Method of Traditional Chinese Medicine Anti-Acne Cosmetic. CN108434039A, 24 August 2018.
363. Kim, D.S. Cosmetic Composition Comprising the Ozonized Oil and Fermented Extract of Seaweed. KR20180013659A, 7 February 2018.
364. Hua, C.; Huili, S.; Xin, C.; Zhigang, C. Marine Biological Function Cosmetic for Minimizing Pores. CN102178636A, 14 September 2011.
365. Chen, Y.; Yang, S.; Zhou, Z. Production Process of Moisturizing Lotion with Pore Cleaning Function. CN111991324A, 28 August 2020.
366. Nakamura, R. Pore-Shrinking Agent. JP2015030675A, 16 February 2015.
367. Chun, J.U. Composition Having Anti-Wrinkle Effects Using the Natural Plant Extract and Cosmetic Composition Comprising the Same. KR101952695B1, 27 February 2019.
368. Wang, J. Making Method of Anti-Wrinkle Beautifying Seaweed-Containing Flour. CN105685784A, 22 June 2016.
369. Yu, K. Anti-Aging Composition and Cosmetic Product Containing Same. CN109431888A, 8 March 2019.
370. Chen, H.; Chen, L.; Ge, X.; Wang, Y.; Yue, K. Composition Capable of Resisting Aging and Fading Spots and Cosmetic Containing Composition. CN108670927A, 19 October 2018.
371. Osawa, Y.; Sawaki, S.; Tamaoki, S. Elastin-Like Agent and Cosmetic Containing the Same. JP2003342150A, 3 December 2003.
372. Deng, Y. Vitamin B (VB) Face Cream Cosmetic Containing 24K Gold. CN102824285A, 19 December 2012.
373. Gerčikovs, I.; Lando, O. Cosmetic Preparation for Taking Care of the Feet Skin. LV14321A, 20 April 2011.
374. Gedouin, A.; Vallee, R. Production of Cosmetic Composition for Protecting Skin from Effects of Atmospheric Pollution. FR2779953A1, 24 December 1999.
375. Hori, M.; Nishibe, Y.; Tanaka, K. Cosmetic Composition. JP2003104835A, 9 April 2003.
376. Yang, Z. Seaweed Extraction Liquid, Preparation Method of Seaweed Extraction Liquid, Whitening Composition and Preparation Method of Whitening Composition. CN108324601A, 27 July 2018.
377. Li, Y.; Pei, Q.; Shi, C.; Shi, H.; Shi, Z. Pearl Cosmetic Cellular Liquor and Preparation Method Thereof. CN106265463A, 4 January 2017.
378. Choi, C.Y.; Choi, S.J.; Im, S.J.; Jeong, C.S.; Jeong, J.C.; Jo, A.; Kang, H.W.; Kim, H.G.; Kim, J.Y.; Kim, J.Y.; et al. Pharmaceutical Composition and Cosmetic Composition for Skin Regeneration Comprising Active Ingredient Extracted and Isolated from Porphyra Dentata. WO2020175754A1, 3 September 2020.
379. Yang, G.; Zhao, J.; Zhao, Y. Facial Beautifying Composition and Preparation Method Thereof. CN111544369A, 18 August 2020.
380. Takabayashi, M. Anti-Suntan Cosmetic and its Production. JP3568979B2, 22 September 2004.
381. Paik, H.K. Cosmetic Compositions Containing Natural Ultraviolet Intercepting Agent Based Seaweed from Jeju Island. KR20140089997A, 16 July 2014.
382. Han, J.S.; Lee, E.J.; Lee, J.W.; Oh, J.Y.; Park, S.G. Sunscreen Cosmetic Composition. KR20170004842A, 11 January 2017.
383. Murakami, M.; Ota, K.; Saito, M.; Sumida, Y. Weight-Reducing Composition and Method for Reducing Weight. JPH08104618A, 23 April 1996.

384. Azuma, T.; Hayashi, Y.; Ishihata, S.; Kuroda, A.; Sakai, K.; Sato, S. Sheetlike Pack Cosmetic for Body. JP2001019615A, 23 January 2001.
385. Takabayashi, M. Beautifying and Whitening Cosmetic. JP2970767B2, 2 November 1999.
386. Kawai, N.; Tanaka, K.; Wakamatsu, K. Cosmetic Composition. JP2001139419A, 22 May 2001.
387. Kawai, N.; Tanaka, K.; Wakamatsu, K. Cosmetic Composition. JP2001302491A, 31 October 2001.
388. Adachi, K.; Kotake, Y.; Suzuki, Y. Preparation for External Use for Skin. JP3460904B2, 27 October 2003.
389. Kang, S.W.; Kim, E.J.; Kim, S.J. Skin Moisturizing and Funtional Composition Containing Fermented Seeweed. KR20190029897A, 21 March 2019.
390. Han, S.H.; Hong, Y.J.; Kim, H.C.; Kim, Y.J. Cosmetic Composition Containing Gulfweed Extract, Sea Staghorn Extract, and Brown Seaweed Extract. WO2012070835A2, 31 May 2012.
391. Ahn, D.H.; Kim, J.Y.; Moon, J.N.; Moon, W.S. Cosmetic Composition Containing Seaweed Extract. WO2015099280A1, 2 July 2015.
392. Zhou, Y. Cosmetic Preparation with Anti-Allergic and Repairing Effects and Preparation Method Thereof. CN108578353A, 28 September 2018.
393. Kang, D.H.; Kim, M.G.; Lee, B.H. Beauty Expenses Composite Containing Seaweed Extract. KR20150022365A, 4 March 2015.
394. Cong, L.; Gao, H.; Li, C.; Lin, S.; Liu, D.; Liu, P.; Mao, Y.; Zhang, C.; Zhang, W. Sunscreen Cosmetic Composition and Method for Preparing Seaweed Sunscreen Components of Composition. CN104644511A, 27 May 2015.
395. Cai, C.; Li, Y.; Wang, H. Facial Mask for Removing Freckles, Whitening and Relieving Sunburn and Preparation Method of Facial Mask. CN106619272A, 10 May 2017.
396. Kawakubo, A.; Kouno, S.; Matsuka, S.; Motoyoshi, K.; Ninomiya, M.; Ota, Y. Photo-Aging Resister and Skin Cosmetic Containing the Resister. JP3432033B2, 28 July 2003.
397. Gan, X.; Zhang, K. Eye-Beautifying Firming Eye Cream Cosmetic and Preparation Method Thereof. CN109875933A, 14 June 2019.
398. Choi, J.B.; Jo, J.H.; Joo, W.H.; Kim, E.H.; Lee, J.H.; Lee, J.H.; Ryu, G.Y. Antioxidant And Whitening Functional Cosmetics. KR101413328B1, 1 July 2014.
399. Li, K.; Liang, Y.; Wang, T.; Yue, Q.; Zhao, L. Method for Preparing Seaweed Fermentation Solution by Virtue of Probiotics Fermentation and Application of Seaweed Fermentation Solution in Cosmetics. CN108653059A, 16 October 2018.
400. Choi, B.S.; Choi, J.H.; Chun, H.S.; Kim, S.; Kim, S.J.; Lee, H.J.; Park, E.T.; Park, S.E. Food Composition Comprising Algae Extracts and the Use Thereof. KR20130054518A, 27 May 2013.
401. Hirose, K.; Hirose, Y. Composition Having Bleaching Activity and Cosmetic Containing the Same. JP2006036680A, 9 February 2006.
402. Hirose, K.; Hirose, Y. Composition Having Hair Loss Preventing Action and Hair Loss Preventing Cosmetic Containing the Same. JP2006052151A, 23 February 2006.
403. Zhang, R. Pure Natural Moisturizing Cosmetic. CN103690407A, 2 April 2014.
404. Park, J.W. Cosmetic Composition for Spa Comprising Natural Mixture as Effective Component. KR20180024141A, 8 March 2018.
405. Ku, W.L.; Lee, H.J. Cosmetic Composition Using Pine Tree and Seaweeds and Manufacturing Method of it. KR20200122677A, 28 October 2020.
406. Park, S.L. Cosmetic Composition for Anti-Wrinkle Activity Comprising Fermented Soybean Paste and Seaweed Extracts as Active Ingredient. KR20200080500A, 7 July 2020.
407. Oouma, T.; Takekoshi, Y.; Takahashi, T. Cosmetics. US2002009472A1, 24 January 2002.
408. Choi, K.J. Cosmetics Composition. KR20090126670A, 9 December 2009.
409. Guo, Z. Cosmetic Containing Active Peptide. CN105982831A, 5 October 2016.
410. Qiu, H.Y.; BI, H.Y.; Chen, X.; Chen, W.Y.; Du, L.N.; Jin, Y.G. Curcumin Hydrogel Combined with Photodynamics to Treat Acne. *J. Int. Pharm. Res.* **2017**, *44*, 1125–1130.
411. Cho, J.H. Cosmetic Composition Contained Seaweeds Extract with Silver Nano-Particles Colloid. KR20080035090A, 23 April 2008.
412. Chen, J.; Chen, J. Anti-Inflammatory Sedation Patch Mask. CN112402339A, 26 February 2021.
413. Kim, J.E.; Yang, Y.J. Mist Containing Seaweed Extract. KR20180080058A, 11 July 2018.
414. Fukuhara, K.; Kamiyama, K. Hair Cosmetic. JP2005272396A, 6 October 2005.
415. Kim, K.E. Kelp Shampco, Pock, Cosmetics. KR20110006337A, 20 January 2011.
416. Chen, F.; Li, Y.; Wang, X. Washing Cosmetic Containing Seaweed Extract-Carrageen. CN104434696A, 25 March 2015.
417. Sato, Y.; Sigihara, Y. Cosmetic Composition, Screening Method, and Cosmetic Method. WO2019098352A1, 23 May 2019.
418. Huang, J.; Li, C.; Lin, S.; Liu, D.; Ma, J.; Qian, J.; Xiang, Q. Water-Free Washing-Free Gold Seaweed Cleaning Oil. CN109431878A, 8 March 2019.
419. Chen, H.C. Diet Cosmetic Food and Its Production. CN101028075A, 5 September 2007.
420. Takahashi, N. Production of Cosmetic or Bathing Agent. JPS62286907A, 12 December 1987.
421. Hashimoto, H.; Hiraki, Y.; Ichioka, M.; Inami, M.; Kamiyama, S.; Kono, H.; Nagaoka, M.; Yoshikawa, S. Highly Pure Fucoidan and Preparation Thereof. JP2000351801A, 10 October 2000.
422. Kusuoku, H.; Nishizawa, Y.; Shibuya, Y. Purification of Seaweed Extract. JP2000109407A, 18 April 2000.
423. Kusuoku, H.; Nishizawa, Y.; Shibuya, Y. Method for Purifying Seaweed Extract. JP2005145983A, 9 June 2005.

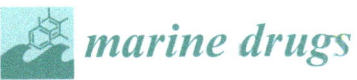

Review

Seaweed Protein Hydrolysates and Bioactive Peptides: Extraction, Purification, and Applications

Javier Echave [1,†], Maria Fraga-Corral [1,2,†], Pascual Garcia-Perez [1], Jelena Popović-Djordjević [3], Edina H. Avdović [4], Milanka Radulović [5], Jianbo Xiao [1,6], Miguel A. Prieto [1,2,*] and Jesus Simal-Gandara [1,*]

1. Nutrition and Bromatology Group, Analytical and Food Chemistry Department, Faculty of Food Science and Technology, Ourense Campus, University of Vigo, E-32004 Ourense, Spain; javier.echave@uvigo.es (J.E.); mfraga@uvigo.es (M.F.-C.); pasgarcia@uvigo.es (P.G.-P.); jianboxiao@uvigo.es (J.X.)
2. Centro de Investigação de Montanha (CIMO), Instituto Politécnico de Bragança, Campus de Santa Apolonia, 5300-253 Bragança, Portugal
3. Department of Chemistry and Biochemistry, Faculty of Agriculture, University of Belgrade, 11080 Belgrade, Serbia; jelenadj@agrif.bg.ac.rs
4. Department of Science, Institute for Information Technologies Kragujevac, University of Kragujevac, 34000 Kragujevac, Serbia; edina.avdovic@pmf.ac.rs
5. Department of Bio-Medical Sciences, State University of Novi Pazar, Vuka Karadžića bb, 36300 Novi Pazar, Serbia; mradulovic@np.ac.rs
6. International Research Center for Food Nutrition and Safety, Jiangsu University, Zhenjiang 212013, China
* Correspondence: mprieto@uvigo.es (M.A.P.); jsimal@uvigo.es (J.S.-G.)
† These authors contributed equally to the publication.

Citation: Echave, J.; Fraga-Corral, M.; Garcia-Perez, P.; Popović-Djordjević, J.; H. Avdović, E.; Radulović, M.; Xiao, J.; A. Prieto, M.; Simal-Gandara, J. Seaweed Protein Hydrolysates and Bioactive Peptides: Extraction, Purification, and Applications. *Mar. Drugs* **2021**, *19*, 500. https://doi.org/10.3390/md19090500

Academic Editor: Marc Diederich

Received: 13 August 2021
Accepted: 28 August 2021
Published: 31 August 2021

Publisher's Note: MDPI stays neutral with regard to jurisdictional claims in published maps and institutional affiliations.

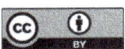

Copyright: © 2021 by the authors. Licensee MDPI, Basel, Switzerland. This article is an open access article distributed under the terms and conditions of the Creative Commons Attribution (CC BY) license (https://creativecommons.org/licenses/by/4.0/).

Abstract: Seaweeds are industrially exploited for obtaining pigments, polysaccharides, or phenolic compounds with application in diverse fields. Nevertheless, their rich composition in fiber, minerals, and proteins, has pointed them as a useful source of these components. Seaweed proteins are nutritionally valuable and include several specific enzymes, glycoproteins, cell wall-attached proteins, phycobiliproteins, lectins, or peptides. Extraction of seaweed proteins requires the application of disruptive methods due to the heterogeneous cell wall composition of each macroalgae group. Hence, non-protein molecules like phenolics or polysaccharides may also be co-extracted, affecting the extraction yield. Therefore, depending on the macroalgae and target protein characteristics, the sample pretreatment, extraction and purification techniques must be carefully chosen. Traditional methods like solid–liquid or enzyme-assisted extraction (SLE or EAE) have proven successful. However, alternative techniques as ultrasound- or microwave-assisted extraction (UAE or MAE) can be more efficient. To obtain protein hydrolysates, these proteins are subjected to hydrolyzation reactions, whether with proteases or physical or chemical treatments that disrupt the proteins native folding. These hydrolysates and derived peptides are accounted for bioactive properties, like antioxidant, anti-inflammatory, antimicrobial, or antihypertensive activities, which can be applied to different sectors. In this work, current methods and challenges for protein extraction and purification from seaweeds are addressed, focusing on their potential industrial applications in the food, cosmetic, and pharmaceutical industries.

Keywords: seaweed; protein; extraction; bioactive peptides; industrial application

1. Introduction

Seaweeds are considered an important source of macronutrients, especially proteins and lipids, and micronutrients, represented by vitamins and minerals, together with dietary fiber and other minoritarian constituents, as it is the case of polyphenols. This rich variety of biomolecules turns macroalgae into a well appreciated resource for the extraction of natural ingredients aimed to the development of nutraceuticals, functional food, cosmetics, pharmaceutical products, or animal feeding, among others [1]. Furthermore, the estimated rise of the global population for 2050 is an international concern since it is expected a parallel increase of protein demand. In this sense, seaweed may stand for a potential source of proteins [2]. Indeed, macroalgae have been reported to annually produce higher protein yield per surface area (2.5–7.5 annual tons per hectare) than terrestrial plants (around 1 to 2 tons per hectare for soybean, legumes, or wheat) [3]. The protein content in seaweeds is variable among red (Rhodophyta), brown (Ochrophyta), and green (Chlorophyta) seaweeds. For instance, red seaweeds are considered the most prominent source of proteins, with protein content representing between 19 and 44% of dry weight (dw), while the green and brown ones exhibit lower protein amounts, around 20% or 10% of dry weight, respectively [4]. These values are comparable and even slightly higher than those of legumes (20–30%), cereals (10–15%), or nuts (20–30%) [5].

As previously reported, the protein concentration in algal sources depends on several factors, including interspecific variations, geographical location, environmental conditions, and seasonal variations [6]. The maximal protein contents have been described between winter and the beginning of spring, while minimal levels were reported by summer and early fall [7]. Besides, macroalgae, as it occurs with terrestrial plants, are highly susceptible to the presence of different biotic and abiotic stress signals, which contribute to the regulation of protein expression and the biosynthesis of specialized metabolites.

Regarding the variability of the protein profile of macroalgae, they show a rich source of several types of seaweed protein (SP) and derivatives—such as peptides, enzymes, glycoproteins, lectins, and mycosporine-like amino acids (MAAs), as well as phycobiliproteins, characteristic of red seaweeds [4]. Understanding the quality of proteins, in terms of amino acid composition and digestibility, is a fundamental step facing their use for human consumption. Thus, concerning amino acid composition, proteins of high quality are those holding high proportions of essential amino acids (EAAs), due to the impossibility of being synthesized by the human body. In the case of SP, the most abundant amino acids are glycine, alanine, arginine, proline, glutamic, and aspartic acids, while tryptophan, cysteine and lysine are present in a lower extent. The sum of aspartic and glutamic acids content in macroalgae may stand for about 30% of the total amino acids (Table 1). Consequently, the combination of macroalgae ingest with other protein-enriched foods is regarded as an optimal approach for a high-quality intake of proteins [8]. On the other hand, protein quality depends on their digestibility. Indeed, the higher proportion of poorly digestible amino acids the lower nutritional value of SP. Besides, digestibility can be altered by distinct factors, such as the presence of anti-nutritional molecules like some polysaccharides or tannin derivates, among others [3,8]. In recent years, scientific works have analyzed both the amino acids profile and the digestibility of macroalgal proteins to accurately predict their nutritional quality (Table 1). In general terms, algal proteins display a rich free amino acid profile and remarkable digestibility rates, mostly higher than 70% and thus, comparable to those of grains (69–84%), legumes (72–92%), fruits (72–92%), and vegetables (68–80%) [3].

Therefore, macroalgae stand for a sustainable source of proteins that can be applied as ingredients for human and animal consumption. In fact, seaweed have been consumed since ancient times, mostly in Asian countries, and nowadays, they may be used for fortifying food or feed matrixes either with low protein content or poor amino acidic profile. They can be also used as natural food preservatives or additives to improve the organoleptic properties of food products while minimizing the side effects associated to their synthetic analogues [9]. Indeed, food grade phycobiliproteins are generally recognized as safe (GRAS), which point them as target compounds for their direct application in food industry.

Table 1. Average protein content, essential amino acidic composition, and digestibility of few representative seaweed sources.

Species	Protein (% dw)	EAA Composition (% TAA)	EAA (% prot.)	Digestibility	Reference
Rhodophyta					
Gracilaria gracilis	31–45%	R 1.3, H 0.2, K 1.6, T 1.7, I 2.3, L 1.9, V 3.1, M 0.2, F 1.7, C 0.4, P 1.0, A 1.9, Y 1.3, D 2.6, E 2.4, G 1.1, S 1.6	14%	68% (in vivo)	[8,10]
Palmaria palmata	55%	T 4.1, V 5.4, M 2.0, I 4.3, L 7.2, K 5.7, F 4.7, W 0.9, H 1.7, S 6.2, Q + E 14.9, P 7.9, G 5.8, A 8.8, C 2.5, D + N 9.7, Y 2.7, R 5.6	36%	56% (pancreatin)	[8,11]
Porphyra sp.	31%	D 8.5, T 5.3, S 4.9, E 10.2, G 5.1, A 6.2, V 5.2, I 3.3, L 5.9, Y 3.4, F 3.5, H 2.6, K 5.2, R 5.9, P 3.6, C 1.3, M 1.8, W 0.7	51%	57% (pepsin), 56% (pancreatin), 78% (pronase)	[8,12]
Clorophyta					
Cladophora rupestris	12%	A 5.5, R 6.5, N 15.3, E 15.3, G 6.7, H 1.4, I 3.6, L 7.2, K 7.4, M 1.8, F 4.5, P 5.7, S 4.3, T 5.1, Y 4.3, V 5.8	13.9%	N.A.	[13]
Codium fragile	11%	D 0.3, E 1.1, S 0.5, H 0.1, G 0.5, T 0.6, R 0.4, A 0.6, Y 0.4, V 1.4, M 0.9, C 0.1, I 0.4, L 0.7, F 0.5, L 0.5	5.4%	N.A.	[14]
Ulva sp.	27%	D 1.3, E 1.5, S 0.8, H 0.1, G 0.8, T 0.8, R 0.5, A 1.1, Y 0.4, V 0.3, M 0.7, I 0.5, L 1.0, F 1.2, K 0.7	12%	17% (pepsin), 67% (pancreatin), 95% (pronase)	[8,15]
Ochrophyta					
Fucus serratus	4%	A 5.8, R 4.4, N 14.0, E 1596, G 5.8, H 1.7, I 4.0, L 6.3, K 5.5, M 1.9, F 5.0, P 4.0, S 5.6, T 5.5, Y 3.7, V 5.6	4.6%	N.A.	[13]
Sargassum fusiformis	12%	D 9.1, T 4.1, S 5.6, E 18.7, G 4.8, A 4.3, V 4.9, I 4.0, L 6.7, Y 2.8, F 4.6, H 2.6, K 3.1, R 4.5, P 3.8, C 0.9, M 1.6, W 0.4	10.9%	N.A.	[12]
Undaria pinnatifida	19.8%	D 8.7, T 4.4, S 4.0, E 14.5, G 5.1, A 4.7, V 5.2, I 4.1, L 7.4, Y 2.9, F 4.7, H 2.5, K 5.6, R 5.2, P 3.6, C 0.9, M 1.7, W 0.5	35.5%	24% (pepsin), 48% (pancreatin), 87% (pronase)	[8,12]

Abbreviations: dw: Dry weight, N.A: Not analyzed, prot: Protein, EAA: Essential amino acids, TAA: Total amino acids.

For instance, phycobiliproteins from *Neoporphyra haitanensis* (formerly *Porphyra haitanensis*) were investigated for their further inclusion in liposome–meat systems. They have a high EAA content (43%) and significant antioxidant capacity, able to reduce lipid peroxidation [16]. In the same way, SP have been involved in the development of functional products, as reported for the protein hydrolysates from *Palmaria palmata*, which were incorporated into bread to keep its renin inhibitory activity after baking, thus preserving its cardiovascular protective properties. Hence, the fortification of commonly consumed products makes SP excellent carriers of bioactive compounds, showing a wide range of health benefits [17].

In this sense, several biological activities have been associated to SP, hydrolysates, or peptides that are of great interest for other industrial sectors, such as pharmacology or cosmetics. SP can be found inside cell cytoplasm and/or attached to macroalgae cell wall polysaccharides (e.g., ulvan, alginate, carrageenan ...) forming diverse complexes. These polymers are mostly composed of glucans of different nature depending on the species, and preeminently xylan-based polysaccharides, which are highly resistant to hydrolysis [18]. Hence, disrupting these cell wall polysaccharides is an essential process that must be conducted to obtain and further process SP. To obtain SP hydrolysates, these proteins must be degraded either by physical (energy) or chemical methods (e.g., endoproteases, pH-induced degradation). For example, *P. palmata*, was used to obtain a protein hydrolysate with the ability of improving glycemia and insulin production when assessed in vivo, as the specific Alcalase/Flavourzyme protein hydrolysate enhanced the glucose tolerance and satiety. Thus, these *P. palmata* protein hydrolysates were suggested as potential molecules for managing two chronic diseases with a worldwide increasing prevalence: obesity and type-2 diabetes mellitus [19]. Another work based on proteins extracted from the same species proved their antiproliferative capacity against five human cancer cell lines derived from breast (MCF-7), liver (HepG-2), gastric (SGC-7901), lung (A549), and colon cancers (HT-29), with half inhibitory concentrations (IC_{50}) ranging between 192 and 317 µg/mL [20]. In the field of cosmetics, MAAs are of great interest for the formulation of sunscreens, thanks to their low molecular weight, hydrosolubility, and chemical stability towards light and heat. Arginine, which can be found at higher concentrations in *Palmaria* and *Porphyra* species, is also a highly appreciated amino acid in cosmetics for being a precursor of urea, a widely used cosmetic ingredient [21].

Therefore, macroalgae represent a sustainable and natural source of high-quality proteins and protein-derived molecules. Their multiple applications as food, nutraceutical or drug ingredients revealed them as cost-effective and profitable molecules for their use in various industries. Moreover, SP hydrolysates have displayed increased bioactive properties in comparison to whole proteins. Herein, available methods of SP extraction, purification, and hydrolysate production will be discussed in the following sections.

2. Extraction Technologies

Prior to hydrolysate or peptide production, SP must be released and isolated from the rest of biomass components, which requires disruption of the seaweed cell wall polysaccharides. This implies that macroalgae biomass must be subjected to a pretreatment stage prior extraction, involving different disruptive techniques, that would aid to improve the extraction yield. A combinatorial approach including a coordinate pretreatment and extraction technique increases protein recovery [22]. Pretreatment methods aim at breaking cell walls to release the intracellular fraction of biological samples, including free and cell wall-attached proteins, depending on the system of choice. Extensively used pretreatment methods thus include mechanical grinding, osmotic shock (OS), alkaline treatment, freeze-thaw, or ultrasonic sonication [4]. Since seaweeds are marine organisms, they are susceptible to strong osmotic pressures, and their cell walls may be broken by allowing the seaweed biomass to be transferred into hypotonic solutions. This may be achieved using ultrapure or de-ionized water to induce OS [23]. In the same manner, a combination of sonication and OS has been proven to increase SP yield and extractability [24]. Nonetheless, one of the most valuable pretreatment methods involves the application of glucanases to the extraction mix to maximize SP yield [25]. Using fresh, dried or freeze-dried seaweed samples may also influence the resulting SP yield, although yield variations are not significant. Drying tests on several *Sargassum* species revealed that freeze-dried seaweeds subjected to classical SLE yielded slightly more extractable protein in comparison to oven-dried [26]. However, Angell et al. found out that using fresh pulped *Ulva ohnoi* blades yielded as much as by two-fold the extractable proteins, applying the same SLE method, but following a sample management closer to that of terrestrial plants [27]. In the same manner, heat treatment exerts a differential effect on SP extractability depending on the algal biomass. For example, in the study carried out by O'Connor et al., autoclave treatment (>121 °C) resulted in higher SP yields for *P. palmata* but not for *F. vesiculosus* or *Alaria esculenta* [24]. In summary, diverse pretreatment and extraction options must be specifically studied and assessed for each seaweed species, reaching meaningful rates of SP yield, stability, or digestibility.

Extraction methods currently available for protein extraction include solid–liquid extraction (SLE), enzyme-assisted extraction (EAE), pulse-electric field (PEF), high hydrostatic pressure extraction (HHPE), ultrasound-assisted extraction (UAE), and microwave-assisted extraction (MAE). In general terms, solubilization is a paramount factor that modulates protein extraction, which depends on different physicochemical conditions. In fact, proteins can be extracted by their solubilization at different pH values, involving the sequential use of differently buffered solutions. Nevertheless, proteins are generally co-extracted with other interferents, such as sugar or phenolic compounds [25,28], forcing the application of protein precipitation to achieve the isolation and purification of the extracted SP. Moreover, except for EAE, extraction methods promote an unspecific protein hydrolysis, which is also accompanied by the liberation of intracellular proteases from cell walls that may further degrade protein structures. Protein integrity is also affected by the precipitation method of choice, aimed at reaching the protein isoelectric point (IP) by acidifying the medium pH and causing the 'salting-out' effect, improving protein solubility using salts like ammonium sulphate, $(NH_4)_2SO_4$ [29]. Yet, protein stability is not a top priority feature for hydrolysate production. Thereafter, more disruptive methods may be used to that aim, such as MAE, PFE, or UAE.

2.1. Solid–Liquid Extraction

SLE is the most traditional method used for SP extraction, involving the use of different solvents, such as distilled water, buffered solutions, and lysis surfactant-containing solutions [30]. Nonetheless, about food applications, the use of either non-toxic or easy-to-remove reagents must be employed for SP extraction. Thus, demineralized and de-ionized water are the most extensively used solvents for the application of SLE methods, as they lead to performance of OS, helping protein extraction in a cost-effective and easy manner [31]. However, this method should be optimized to improve its efficiency, modulating different factors, such as the algal biomass/solvent ratio (w:v), temperature, or time.

Temperature is a key parameter in SP extraction, as it influences protein integrity, enzymatic activity, and solubility of other cellular constituents, such as cell wall polysaccharides [24]. Indeed, hot water has been classically selected to extract algal polysaccharides by SLE, also promoting the co-extraction of proteins. Therefore, SP aqueous extraction requires low temperatures (around 4 °C) to ensure protein integrity, whereas higher temperatures can be applied for protein hydrolysate production, thus involving heat-assisted extraction (HAE) or a combination with enzymatic pretreatments [32]. Due to the heterogeneous protein composition of algal extracts, SLE procedures are generally based on two sequential extraction procedures to meet the solubility requirements of different acidic and alkaline proteins, which includes an initial OS stage followed by the application of an alkaline NaOH solution [16,27]. The process is considered food-grade, as NaOH is used for protein extraction from various food matrices [28]. A reducing agent, normally 2-mercaptoethanol, is usually added to the alkaline solution to minimize potential protein degradation, although it has been reported as a toxic compound and has been increasingly replaced by N-acetyl-L-cysteine (NAC) for food purposes [22]. That shift on pH extraction has shown beneficial results on protein extraction, obtaining enhanced extraction yields, as it was seen on the combination of acidic SLE followed by alkaline SP extraction from *Ascophyllum nodosum* [33]. Moreover, the application of pH-shift combined with IP precipitation, reaching pH values between 2 and 4 ensures a maximum yield with this extraction method [29]. Combining these methods, a 14% protein yield (w/w) was obtained from *Porphyra dioica* [34]. Besides the combination of OS and an SLE extraction of alkaline-soluble proteins with NaOH, the use of a lysis solution holding urea, detergent and other reactants, allowed for extracting 11.8% (w/v) of protein from *Ulva* sp. [31]. While SP extraction yields by SLE may be near the total protein content of seaweed species, it is also a very time-consuming method [32].

2.2. Enzyme-Assisted Extraction

EAE is one of the most studied techniques used to disrupt macroalgal cell walls. The application of targeted polysaccharide-digesting enzymes, such as cellulases, hemicellulases, β-glucanases, and xylanases has been described as a food-grade approach to breakdown the macroalgae cell wall. Thus, commercial enzyme cocktails have been proven to be successful for this purpose [25]. However, seaweed cell wall composition can vary among phyla and species and, therefore, a right choice of carbohydrase(s), together with the optimization of operating conditions (enzyme:substrate ratio (E:S), temperature, pH) of individual enzymes or cocktails must be proved prior to large-scale extraction to maximize protein recovery. In general, EAE has been mostly studied on red and green seaweeds, because of their simpler composition with respect to brown seaweeds. A greater protein yield has been reported on *Solieria chordalis*, *Ulva* sp. and *Sargassum muticum* seaweeds when using EAE and traditional SLE [35]. In accordance with a study comparing EAE using cellulase, hemicellulose, and a mixture of both to *P. palmata* and *S. chordalis* while testing HHPE, showed that cellulase alone was generally more effective and further enhanced SP yield in combination with HHPE [36]. In other study, the use of cellulase-assisted extraction (using commercially available CellicCTec3®) on brown and red seaweeds, *Macrocystis pyrifera* and *Chondracanthus chamissoi*, led to significantly higher protein yields compared to SLE, 36.10% and 74.60% respectively (Table 2), as a result of the optimization of the extraction process through a central composite experimental design [37]. Other authors reported that a higher yield of alkaline soluble protein was recovered from *P. palmata* following treatment with a combination of commercial glucanase cocktails (Shearzyme and Celluclast) [22]. This resulted in a total protein recovery of 8.39% when compared to that obtained following OS and mechanical shear (6.77% and 6.92%, respectively). Therefore, EAE employing glucanases may achieve high protein yield, although the co-extraction of other components (i.e., phenolics) may also occur [25].

Table 2. Source, protein yield, pre-treatment, extraction, and purification methods described. Protein yields are indicated as % of algal biomass dw.

Source	Pretreatment	Extraction Method	Precipitation and Purification	Yield (% dw)	Reference
		Rhodophyta			
Palmaria palmata	Freeze-dried OS, (1: 20), 16 h, 4 °C // EPr, Celluclast + Shearzyme (E:S 4.8 × 10^3 U/100 g), pH 5, 24 h, 40 °C	SLE ak, 0.12 M NaOH + 0.1 mg/L NAC, 1 h, 25 °C	Pr: IP, pH 4, 1N HCl	11.57%	[22]
	Freeze dried	EAE (E:S 0.5) Celluclast 0.2% + Alcalase 0.2%, pH 4.5, 14 h, 50 °C // SLE ak, 0.1 M NaOH + 1 g/L NAC, 1.5 h, 25 °C	Pr: IP, pH 3, 5M HCl	13.7%	[28]
	Dried, milled Hydrated (6%) Tris-HCl, pH 5, 16 h, 4 °C	EAE-HHPE, Hemicellulase (E:S 0.05), pH 4.5, 400 MPa, 20 min 40 °C	-	6.3%	[36]
Soliera chordalis	Dried, milled Hydrated (6%) Tris-HCl, pH 5, 16 h, 4 °C	EAE-HHPE, Hemicellulase (E:S 0.05), pH 4.5, 400 MPa, 20 min, 40 °C	-	3.4%	[36]
Porphyra dioica	Freeze dried OS, (1: 20), 16 h, 4 °C	SLE ak, NaOH 0.12 M, 1 h, 25 °C	Pr: IP, pH 4.5 1M HCl	14.28%	[34]
Neoporphyra haitanensis	Freeze dried	UAE ak, 400 W, 40 kHz, 0.01% NaOH, 20 min, 35 °C	Pr: (NH$_4$)$_2$SO$_4$, 40%, 4 h, 4 °C	3.8%	[38]
Chondrus crispus	Freeze dried	UAE, $_d$W (1:20), 42 Hz, 1 h, 4 °C	Pr: (NH$_4$)$_2$SO$_4$, 80%, 1 h, 4 °C Pu: DI, 3.5 kDa	~6.7%	[24]
	Freeze dried	HHPE, $_d$W (1:20) 600 MPa, 4 min, 4 °C	Pu: Filtered, 100 µm nylon bag	~3.1%	

Table 2. Cont.

Source	Pretreatment	Extraction Method	Precipitation and Purification	Yield (% dw)	Reference
Condracanthus chamissoi	Oven dried (60 °C) 0.1 M NaOAc buffer, pH 4.5, 10 min, 50 °C	EAE Cellic CTec3 (E:S 0.1, 1.64 U/mg), pH 4.5, 15 h, 50 °C	Pr: Cold acetone (1: 4), 2 h	6.35%	[37]
Clorophyta					
Ulva sp.	Oven dried (60 °C), freeze dried, milled	UAE ak (2×), (1:10), 1M NaOH, sonication (Hz non specified), 2 h, 25 °C	Pu: Filtered (0.45 μm) // DI, 2 kDa // IEC, Tris buffer, pH 9.5 // DI 2 kDa	5.4%	[39]
	Freeze dried, milled	SLE (1:20), lysis solution (8 M urea, 2% Tween, 1% PVP, 30 mM DTT), 16 h, 4 °C	Pu: DI, 6–8 kDa, 4 °C, 16 h	11.88%	[31]
	Untreated	PFE aq, $_d$W, 50 kV, 50 pulses, 0.5 Hz, 34 kJ // Mechanical press	Pr: DI, 100–500 kDa	4.7%	[23]
Ulva ohnoi	Oven dried (55 °C), milled	SLE aq, $_d$W (1: 20), 16 h, 30 °C // SLE 1M NaOH, pH 12, 30 °C, 2 h	Pr: IP, pH 2.25, 10% v/v HCl	12.28%	[27]
	Fresh, pulped	SLE aq, $_d$W (1:20), 16 h, 30 °C // Filtration (100 μm) // SLE 1M NaOH, pH 12, 30 °C, 2 h // Filtration (100 μm)	Pr: IP, pH 2.25, 10% v/v HCl	17.13%	
	OS (1:10), 30 min, 40 °C // 0.05M HCl, 1 h, 85 °C	MAE aq, $_d$W (1:34), 5 min., 123 °C	Pr: IP, pH 2.25, 10% v/v HCl	11.3%	[40]
Ulva compressa	Oven dried (60 °C), milled OS (1: 20), 16 h, 35 °C	SLE ak, 1M NaOH, pH 12 + 0.5% 2-mercaptoethanol, 2 h, 25 °C	Pr: $(NH_4)_2SO_4$ 80% Pu: DI (kDa n.s.)	6.48%	[41]
Ochrophyta					
Ascophyllum nodosum	Oven dried (40 °C) UPr, $_d$W (1: 20), 750 W, 20kHz, 10 min, 4 °C	SLE ak (1:15) 0.4M NaOH 1 h, 4°C // SLE ac (1:15) 0.4M HCl 1 h, 4 °C	Pu: HPSEC, 150–300 Å, 15 min, 40 °C	4.23%	[33]
Alaria esculenta	Freeze dried, milled	HAE aq Autoclave, $_d$W (1:20), 0.101 MPa, 2 × 15 min, 124 °C	Pu: Filtered, 100 μm muslin bag	~2.4%	[24]
Sargassum patens	Freeze dried OS, (1:20), 16 h, 35 °C	SLE ak, 1M NaOH, pH 12 + 0.5% 2-mercaptoethanol, 2 h, 25 °C	Pr: $(NH_4)_2SO_4$ 85% Pu: DI (kDa n.s.)	8.2%	[26]
Macrocystis pyrifera	Oven dried (60 °C) 0.1 M NaOAc buffer, pH 4.5, 10 min, 50 °C	EAE Cellic CTec3 (E:S 0.1, 1.64 U/mg), pH 4.5, 16 h, 50 °C	Pr: Cold acetone (1:4), 2 h	7.39%	[37]
Undaria pinnatifida	Dried, powdered	SLE aq, $_d$W (1:3), 20 min, 93 °C	Pu: HPLC, Develosil ODS-5 column, 25% CH_3CN + 0.05% CF_3COOH	12%	[42]
Fucus vesiculosus	Freeze dried, milled	UAE aq, $_d$W (1:20), 42 Hz, 1 h, 4 °C	Pr: $(NH_4)_2SO_4$, 80%, 1 h, 4 °C Pu: DI 3.5 kDa	~1.8%	[24]

Abbreviations: OS: Osmotic shock, EPr: Enzymatic pretreatment, Upr: Ultrasonic treatment, //: sequential procedures, SLE: Solid-liquid extraction, aq: Aquose, ak: Alkaline, ac: Acid, Pr: Precipitation, Pu: Purification, $_d$W: Deionized water, DI: Dialysis, NAC: N-acetyl-L-cysteine, EAE: Enzyme-assisted extraction, UAE: Ultrasound-assisted extraction, HHPE: High hydrostatic pressure extraction, PEF: Pulse-electric field, PBS: Sodium phosphate buffer, PVP: polyvinyl propylene, DTT: dithiothretol, IEC: Ionic exchange chromatography, HPSEC: High performance size exclusion chromatography, IP: Isoelectric precipitation. n.s.: Not stated.

Besides glucanases, proteases are also used in EAE of SP, to achieve the release of proteins, peptides, and amino acids present in the supernatant of extracted samples [28].

2.3. Pulse-Electric Field Assisted Extraction

The use of electric pulses to break cell membranes and walls down has been growingly investigated to aid biomolecules' extraction. The application of PEFs can help in protein extraction from macroalgae by generating high voltage (kV) electric pulses of different length, ranging between micro and milliseconds, which result in reversible or irreversible electroporation of cell wall and membrane [43]. PEF is considered as a rapid and effective green technology that should cope with the own limitations, since conductivity and electrode gap may limit the widespread application of PEF at a larger scale [44]. PEF has been extensively applied to improve protein extraction from green seaweed species. For example, protein extraction from *Ulva* sp. was optimized using OS combined with PEF followed by hydraulic press treatment, increased protein extraction from 2.25% to 5.38% (w/v) [45]. Similar protein yields were reported in the same genus when using PEF combined with hydraulic pressure. Another study reported the application of PEF with a custom-made insulated gate bipolar transistor-pulsed generator coupled with a gravitation press-electrode to aid protein extraction from *U. ohnoi*, improving protein yield from 3.16% to 14.94% [23]. PEF coupled with mechanical pressing was employed for protein extraction from *Ulva* sp. An optimized protocol resulted in a seven-fold increase in total protein yield (~20% protein in the extract) when compared to an extract obtained using an OS [23]. Moreover, PEF has been regarded as a workable method for SP extraction and simultaneous hydrolyzation, as extracted proteins by this method display higher antioxidant activity than non-PFE extracted ones.

2.4. High Hydrostatyc Pressure Extraction

High hydrostatic pressure (HHP) improves extraction efficiency because of the application of pressurized conditions (up to 1000 bar) to induce cellular disruption [43]. Factors affecting HHPE efficiency include the choice of solvent along with the operating pressure, temperature, and duration. HHPE is considered as an effective green extraction technology due to its short processing time, mild operating temperature, and high recovery yields. Therefore, this technique may be suitable for heat sensitive compounds, although pressure-induced conformation changes/denaturation of proteins may need to be taken into consideration. The application of HHP (600 MPa for 4 min) to aid protein extraction from two brown seaweeds, *F. vesiculosus* and *Alaria esculenta*, and two red seaweeds, *P. palmata* and *C. crispus* was investigated [24]. HHP treatment appeared to be the most effective for protein extraction from *F. vesiculosus* (23.70% of total protein). On the contrary, autoclave treatment yielded higher protein content (21.50%) than the HHP treatment (14.90%) in the case of *P. palmata* [24]. However, in the case of *S. chordalis*, HPP treatment (400 MPa for 20 min) only resulted in a 2.60% increase in protein yield [24]. The use of HHPE in combination with other extraction techniques has also been investigated, particularly HHP-assisted enzyme extraction. Interestingly, it has been reported that lower temperatures and higher pressures could yield lower proportion of undesirable artifacts, such as polyphenols, and higher protein yields [36]. HHP treatment (400 MPa for 20 min) alone did not increase protein yield from dried ground *P. palmata*, while HHP-assisted hydrolysis with cellulase and hemicellulase resulted in a 17% increase in protein yield compared to the control. Managing extraction parameters to lower polyphenol extraction would contribute to the optimization and enhancement of SP yield, although further research is still needed to assess HHPE as a workable, specific SP extraction method.

2.5. Ultrasound-Assisted Extraction

The use of UAE whether as sonication pretreatment or central component of the extraction process has gained significant interest in maximizing algal protein extraction. This technique cause cell wall breakdown by the acoustic cavitation phenomenon, in which the implosion of air bubbles results in the generation of a potent mechanical energy that disrupts the cell wall [46]. The main advantages of this extraction method are its short processing time, the independence of temperature and the use of water as the solvent of choice, which also plays a meaningful factor in the case of algal samples, thanks to their susceptibility to OS [39]. However, the application of high ultrasound power for extended periods of time can lead to an excessive heat production that may significantly alter protein structure. UAE can be used simultaneously with other techniques, such as OS and EAE. These integrated approaches have led to increasing protein extraction yields. Combination of UAE and EAE with a cellulase cocktail promoted a significantly higher phycobiliprotein yield from the red seaweed *Grateloupia turuturu*, compared to treatment with EAE alone [32] (Table 2). UAE using NaOH as solvent allowed for obtaining a 3.4% protein yield (w/w) from the red seaweed *N. haitanensis* in just 20 min of sonication at room temperature [38]. In addition, O' Connor et al. proved that sonication combined with ammonium sulfate precipitation resulted in the highest protein recovery from *F. vesiculosus* and *Chondrus crispus*, with yields of 35.1% and 35.5% of total protein, respectively [24] (Table 2). This was compared to other approaches, like HHPE or laboratory autoclave treatment that yielded protein recoveries ranging from 16.1% to 24.3% out of total protein. Application of UAE as a food-grade extraction protocol at a larger scale has been previously proved in the protein extraction from *Ulva* sp. and *Gracilaria* sp., allowing to recover 70% and 86% of total proteins, respectively [39] (Table 2).

2.6. Microwave-Assisted Extraction

During the application of MAE, microwave energy is converted into heat by ion conduction and dipole rotation, and non-polar compounds are not heated [43]. Therefore, MAE may not be suitable for the extraction of heat-sensitive bioactive compounds. Although it has been recognized as an efficient low-energy extraction approach, MAE has to date been more widely used to extract carbohydrate or phenolic compounds rather than bioactive proteins/peptides from seaweed samples [40]. Microwave-derived heating and ionization can promote the release of intracellular components from the matrix into the extracting solution, partly because of the damage effect of microwave on cell wall and cell membrane. Because of the high ash content of edible seaweeds contributing to ionic conduction, MAE constitutes a powerful technique to be applied to macroalgae protein extraction. Compared with conventional extraction, MAE shortens extraction time and reduces solvent consumption, as reported for the application of acid/alkali SLE and MAE to *U. ohnoi*, where MAE achieved higher SP yield (23% dw) after 20 min, while SLE extraction required at least 24 h to yield a significant amount of protein from seaweeds [22] (Table 2). Most importantly, although SLE reached higher yields, in this study MAE was conducted in just 5 min and only with the aqueous SP fraction [40]. In summary, although MAE efficiency was reported to be lower than SLE in terms of SP yield, processing times can be reduced saving energy consumption and thus improving the efficiency of this technique [47].

3. Protein Purification

After extraction, SP should be purified to drop other co-extracted components, represented by polysaccharides, minerals, and phenolic compounds. Protein purification methods are based on molecular charge and size differences, and the most extensively used methods are ultrafiltration (UF), ionic-exchange chromatography (IEC), and dialysis.

3.1. Ultrafiltration

UF is an important and widespread purification technique developed by membrane filtration and based on the separation of biological molecules according to their molecular mass [48,49]. The method is suitable for purifying proteins from low-mass contaminating molecules and can be used to concentrate protein solutions at the same time (Figure 1). UF membranes must supply great separation ability, high flux value, and good mechanical and chemical properties. The membrane carrier must be chemically inert with excellent mechanical properties. The device should provide an easy way to remove the deposited layer as well as easy washing and sanitation of the membrane [50]. By the action of pressure force, solvents and molecules of low molecular weight pass through the membrane, while larger molecules stay trapped. If finer separation is needed, the UF method needs to be coupled to more selective methods, such as chromatography or electrophoresis [48,51].

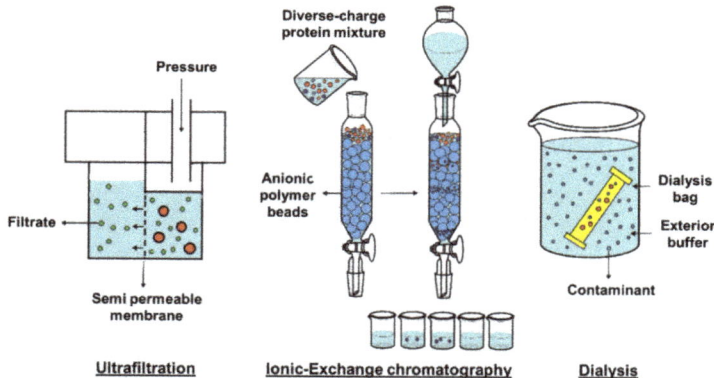

Figure 1. Depiction of ultrafiltration, ionic exchange chromatography and dialysis in protein purification.

3.2. Ionic-Exchange Chromatography

Regarding its use on SP purification, this method is more extensively used in SP hydrolysates fractionation. Therefore, use of UF allows separating very low-molecular weight compounds from the extracted matrix and is especially useful for purifying BAPs after enzymatic hydrolysis of SP. Indeed, different studies used UF membranes of <1 kDa molecular weight for purifying an enzymatic hydrolysate of *Ulva* sp. and yielded fractions with greater anti-inflammatory potential and inhibitory capacity against the angiotensin I-converting enzyme (ACE) [52]. Use of UF to separate low-molecular weight peptides from *Ulva rigida* hydrolysates doubled the ACE inhibitory activity of the sample in comparison to non-filtered hydrolysate [53]. Therefore, this technique may prove useful for concentrating BAPs and SP hydrolysates.

IEC is widely used for purification of charged biomolecules such as proteins, peptides, or amino acids [54,55]. IEC presents a high performance, because it can be applied to a large number of different proteins using high-affinity and cost-effective buffers. The basis of IEC is the interaction of charged molecules flowing in the mobile phase with charged groups of the stationary phase (column packing matrix). Amino acids present charges of different polarity, for example lysine and arginine have a positive charge, while aspartic acid and glutamic acid are negatively charged at physiological pH [56]. Thus, each protein has variable net charges based on its aminoacidic composition but also depending on the pH of the solution they are dissolved in. Thus, the proteins' IP is key to purify these by IEC, since it will find the best initial conditions for protein purification. Ion exchangers are divided into two classes: strong and weak. Strong ion exchange ligands keep their charge characteristics and ion exchange capacity in a wide range of pH, while weak ion exchange ligands show a more pronounced change in their exchange capacity with pH modifications [57]. If purification is conducted at a pH above 9 for anion exchange or below 6 for cation exchange, then a strong ion exchanger must be used. However, if purification is performed at less extreme pH values, then both strong and weak ion exchangers should be used, and the obtained results should be compared to optimize the purification process. Protein binding and elution is based on the competition between the charged amino acid groups on the protein surface and the charged conditions in the binding buffer for the oppositely charged groups in the stationary phase (Figure 1).

The protein sample is applied to an ion exchange column in a low salt solution [55–58]. The charged groups on the protein have a high binding affinity for the charged counterions on the ion exchange resin. Different affinity columns may be used to keep proteins and peptides, depending on their functional group. For example, sulfopropyl functional groups, as strong cation exchangers may keep molecules on a range of pH 4 to 13. Conversely, diethylaminoethyl is a weak anionic exchanger and may retain molecules in pH from 2 to 9 [59]. Regarding the use of this technique in SP, the most commonly used columns are anionic exchangers [60]. For example, IEC allowed for accurate fractionation of anticoagulant peptides from a *Neopyropia yezoensis* hydrolysate [61].

3.3. Dyalisis

Dialysis is a common method for removing contaminants by selective and passive diffusion through a semipermeable membrane, such as a dialysis tube. Dialysis is most used to remove small molecules in solution, such as salts, reducing agents, or preservatives, among others. This technique is a simple but time-demanding method since separation depends on diffusion rate. The dialysis system consists of a tube, which holds a semipermeable membrane, e.g., porous cellulose, closed on both sides to contain a protein solution [62]. The tube is immersed in a much larger vessel filled with buffer (Figure 1). Low-molecular weight particles will diffuse through the semipermeable membrane, while protein molecules, due to their larger size, will remain inside the tube. On the other hand, the buffers inside and outside the dialysis tube will change during diffusion until equilibrium is reached. This equilibrium obeys the Donnan effect, which keeps electrical neutrality on both sides of the membrane [63]. The process of diffusion of small molecules through the membrane is accompanied by the increased movement of protein molecules inside the dialysis tube. As they cannot diffuse due to their size, proteins remain inside the membrane. It should be noted that polyvalent proteins do not allow charged particles to move away from the membrane surface, thus preventing them from setting up an equilibrium potential [64]. On the other hand, the Donnan effect has a significant effect on the colligative properties of ions in the case of high concentrations of proteins or buffers with low ionic strength. Finally, during the dialysis process, the buffer inside the dialysis tube is gradually replaced with the solution in the outer vessel. In this way, efficient removal of small contaminants from the tube is achieved [48]. In summary, dialysis is indeed one of the most used techniques for separating peptides and proteins from natural matrixes. Hence, pairing high-yield extraction techniques with dialysis allows obtaining SP isolates with greater protein content compared to other purification methods [24,65].

4. Hydrolysis and Peptide Production

Protein hydrolysis allows producing protein hydrolysates and BAPs from seaweed. Figure 2 schematically depicts the steps involved in seaweed BAPs production. As mentioned above, pre-treatment strategies may be used to both simplify the extraction process and enhance hydrolyzed SP yield. While some SP hydrolysates have been reported to be biologically active, SP-derived BAPs have gained much attention due to their higher bioactive potential. Hence, once extracted and isolated, SP need to be hydrolyzed into smaller peptide sequences to become biologically active [66]. Hydrolysis can be done either chemically or using proteases. Chemical hydrolysis is typically performed using acids and/or alkali at temperatures over 40 °C. While the procedure is simple and inexpensive, the composition of the hydrolysate is difficult to control, also yielding products with modified amino acids in their peptide sequence [67]. For example, strong organic acids can efficiently hydrolyze hydrophobic peptide bonds, as a mixture of HCl and trichloroacetic acid was found to destroy tryptophan [68]. Conversely, alkaline hydrolysis with NaOH can reduce cystine, arginine, threonine, serine, and isoleucine; form unusual amino acid residues such as lysinoalanine or lanthionine; as well as induce isomerization of L-lysine residues into D-lysine ones [69]. Similarly, high temperatures may be used to induce hydrolyzation, without need of aiding chemicals [42].

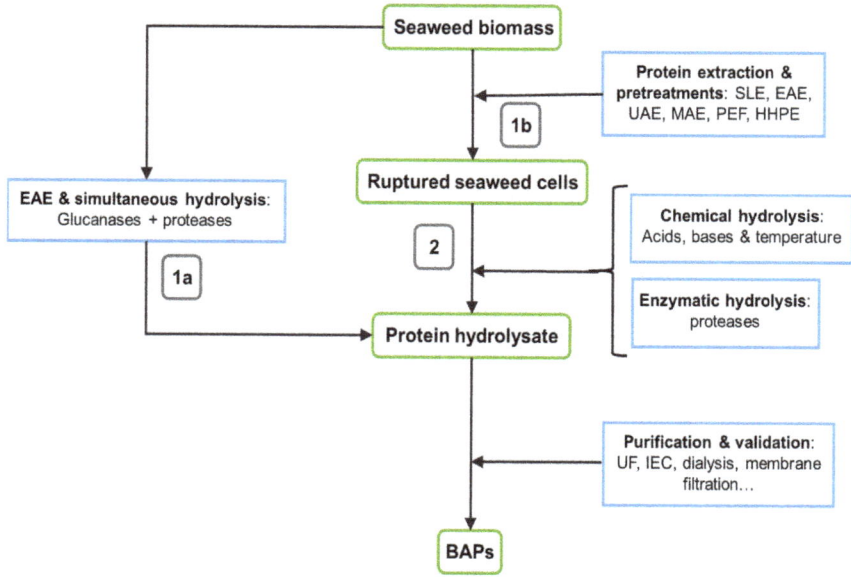

Figure 2. Schematic depiction of production of SP hydrolysates and bioactive peptides (BAPs) from seaweed. Proteins are extracted from seaweed cells and subsequently hydrolyzed in a single (1a) or multiple steps (1b and 2) to produce a protein hydrolysate. The protein hydrolysate is further separated into peptide fractions using diverse purification methods.

In contrast, enzymatic hydrolysis is performed at lower temperature in order to preserve the native structure of the used protease conducting the hydrolysis process. In addition, enzymatic hydrolysis is more specific to the desired peptides and results in higher peptide yield. Due to the lack of organic solvents, the purification steps are less labor-intensive and side reactions are less pronounced [70,71]. The experimental conditions of enzymatic hydrolysis are typically governed by the needs of the enzyme. The process can be done in a single or, at times, in multiple steps [72]. Substrate-to-enzyme ratio as well as the duration of the hydrolysis have a significant effect on the nature and yield of the final products [70]. Table 3 illustrates a range of bioactive peptides obtained by enzymatic hydrolysis from seaweed with the aid of a number of proteases. The most extensively used proteases to perform protein hydrolysis are trypsin, pepsin, papain, and α-chymotrypsin. They are used both individually and in combination with other proteases. More recently, commercially available enzyme cocktails including proteases and carbohydrases are used (Table 3).

Table 3. Bioactive SP-derived hydrolysates, peptides, aminoacidic sequence of bioactive peptides, and proteolytic methods used.

Seaweed	Hydrolysis Method	Peptide Sequence	Bioactivity Reported	Reference
		Rhodophyta		
Palmaria palmata	Papain, (E:S 20.7), pH 6, 24 h, 60 °C	IRLIIVLMPILMA, NIGK, IR	Renin, DPP IV, PAF-AH inhibition	[65,73,74]
	Corolase PP (E:S 1), pH 7, 2 h, 50 °C	ILAP, LLAP, MAGVDHI, FITDGNK., NAATIIK, ANAATIIK, SDITRPGGQM, DNIQGITKPA., LITGA., LITGAA., LITGAAQA., LGLSGK., LTLAPK, LTIAPK, ITLAPK ITIAPK, VVPT, QARGAAQA	Antioxidant, DPP IV inhibition	[75,76]

Table 3. Cont.

Seaweed	Hydrolysis Method	Peptide Sequence	Bioactivity Reported	Reference
Pyropia columbina	Fungal protease concentrate (E:S 5) pH 4.3, 3 h, 55 // Flavourzyme (E:S 2), pH 7, 4 h, 55 °C	N.A.	Antitumor, anti-inflammatory, antioxidant	[77]
Neopyropia yezoensis	Pepsin (E:S 0.025), 5 h, 45 °C	NMEKGSSSVVSSRM	Anticoagulant	[61]
Porphyra dioica	Alcalase + Flavourzyme (E:S 1), pH 7, 4 h, 50 °C	DYYLR, AGFY, YLVA, AFIT, SFLPDLTDQ, MKTPITE, TYIA, LDLW	ACE, DPP IV inhibition	[34]
	Prolyve 1000 (E:S 1), 2 h, 50 °C	N.A. (higher < 1 kDa peptides proportion)	Antioxidant	[78]
Porphyra sp.	Pepsin (E:S 5), pH 2, 4 h, 37 °C	GGSK, ELS	α-amylase inhibition	[79]
Mazzaella japonica	Thermolysin (E:S 1), pH 7, 5 h, 37 °C	YRD, VSEGLD, TIMPHPR, GGPAT, SSNDYPI, SRIYNVKSNG, VDAHY, YGDPDHY, NLGNDFGVPGHEP	ACE inhibition	[80]
Grateulopia lemaneiformis	α-chymotrypsin (E:S 4), pH 8, 2 h, 37 °C	ELWKTF	Antioxidant	[81]
	Trypsin (E:S 4) pH 8, 8 h, 37 °C	QVEY	ACE inhibition	[82]
Chlorophyta				
Ulva C lathrata	Alcalase (E:S 5), pH 7.6, 90 min, 25 °C // 10 min, 100 °C	PAFG	ACE inhibition	[83]
Ulva. intestinalis	Trypsin + Pepsin + Papain (E:S 4), pH 8.42, 5 h, 28.5 °C	FGMPLDR, MELVLR	ACE inhibition	[84]
Ulva rigida	Pepsin (E:S 1), pH 2, 20 h, 37 °C // Bromelain (E:S 1), pH 7, 20 h, 37 °C	IP, AFL	ACE, Renin inhibition	[53]
Ulva lactuca	Papain (E:S 1), pH 6, 24 h, 60 °C	Total of 58 non-allergenic, ACE inhibitory peptides identified	ACE inhibition	[85]
Ulva spp	Purazyme + Flavourzyme // Alkaline protease-Protex 6L + Flavourzyme	N.A.	Anti-inflammatory (IL10 expression & TNF-α inhibition)	[52]
Ochrophyta				
Sargassum maclurei	Pepsin (80 U/g S), pH 2, 2 h, 37 °C // Papain (60 U/g S), pH 7, 3 h, 50 °C	RVLSAAFNTR, IMNLEK, GGVQAIR, KAALMEK, GVFDGPCGT, SGVFDGPCGL QNIGDPR, AYSSGVSFK, RWDISQPY, LVYIVQGR, KPGGSGR, LGLSAKNYGR KEAWLIEK, REVADDK, ENFFFAGIDK, QEMVDK, EEEEEEQQQ	Antyhypertensive (ACE & ET-1 inhibition)	[86]

Table 3. Cont.

Seaweed	Hydrolysis Method	Peptide Sequence	Bioactivity Reported	Reference
Undaria pinnatifida	Protease S "Amano" (E:S 0.01), pH 8, 18 h, 70 °C	VY, IY, AW, FY, VW, IW, LW	Antihypertensive (ACE inhibition & in vivo)	[87]
	$_d$W (3:20), 20 min, 93 °C	YH, KY, FY, IY	Antihypertensive (ACE inhibition & in vivo)	[42]
Saccharina longicruris	Trypsin (E:S 0.05), pH 7, 24 h, 30 °C	TITLDVEPSDTIDGVK, ISGLIYEETR, MALSSLPR, ILVLQSNQIR, ISAILPSR, IGNGGELPR, LPDAALNR, EAESSLTGGNGCAK, QVHPDTGISK	Antimicrobial	[88]
Saccharina japonica	Alcalase + Papain + Trypsin (E:S n.s.), time n.s., pH 7.5, 55 °C	KY, GKY, STKY, AKY, AKYSY, KKFY, FY, KFKY	ACE inhibition	[89]

Abbreviations: //, Subsequent procedures; n.s., Not stated; N.A.: Not analyzed; DPP, Dipeptidyl peptidase; PAF-AH, Platelet activating factor acetylhydrolase; ACE, Angiotensin 1 converter enzyme; ET-I, Endothelin-1; $_d$W, Deionized Water.

A range of experimental conditions (temperature, pH, agitation speed, enzyme-to-substrate ratio, hydrolysis time) need to be optimized for best bioactivity. Typically, a mixture of peptides is obtained, of which only a few are biologically active. The active ones are typically isolated from the mixture using membrane filtration and reverse-phase chromatography techniques [90,91]. SP bioactive peptides range in sizes from 2 to 20 amino acids with the cut-off masses usually ranging from 5 kDa to 30 kDa [92]. Nonetheless, as the nature of SP varies for each seaweed, the resulting BAP profile will also be different depending on the hydrolysis conditions and protease of choice, as these account for different cut-off points [93]. The use of pepsin or trypsin may be also useful to obtain insight on in vivo SP degradation and potential bioavailability of BAPs. Indeed, a wide range of commercially available enzymes has been evaluated to screen out for the possible BAPs produced, such as Flavourzyme, Corolase, or fungal and bacterial proteases [75,76]. The type of the chosen proteolytic enzyme has been shown to have impact on the resulting bioactivity, as it defines the resulting BAP profile. In a recent study, *Gracilariopsis lemaneiformis* proteins were hydrolyzed by different proteases such as trypsin, pepsin, papain, α-chymotrypsin, or Alcalase and hydrolysates obtained by α-chymotrypsin hydrolysis displayed the highest antioxidant activity [81]. Studies performed by Fitzgerald et al. and Harnedy et al. proved that using papain or Corolase yielded highly different BAP in *P. palmata* protein isolates hydrolysis [73,75]. Hydrolysis is stopped by enzyme denaturation, often achieved with pH shifts or heating. One disadvantage of thermal deactivation is the fact that higher temperatures might speed up the kinetics of unwanted processes. An approach to overcome this problem is enzyme immobilization on solid substrates. The use of immobilized enzymes enables the enzymes to be separated from the hydrolysis mixture by filtration instead of increased temperature. An additional advantage is that immobilized enzymes are prevented from being aggregated with the peptides [94]. One challenge of enzymatic hydrolysis is the fact that the algal proteome needs to be known prior to hydrolysis so that enzymes with according cut sites are used. To improve the purity and yield of BAPs, enzymatic hydrolysis is often preceded by physical cell disruption methods, including PEF and bead milling [95,96]. Nonetheless, the hydrolytic activity of the chosen protease can be inhibited by co-extracted compounds such as polysaccharides or phenolic compounds, and optimization studies must be conducted [82,97]. Hydrolysates may be purified by the above-mentioned techniques to ensure concentration of lower molecular weight peptides or to obtain purified BAPs. In this sense, sequential purification processes seem to work best for obtaining high-purity peptides [39].

5. Bioactive Properties and Applications of Seaweed Proteins and Derived Products

As mentioned throughout this work, proteins and derived products obtained from seaweed show various biological activities, as reported by in vitro and a few in vivo tests, such as antioxidant, antimicrobial, anti-inflammatory, antihypertensive, or even antitumor [1]. Regarding SP, the extent of their displayed bioactivities varies upon protein composition, season, but also hydrolysis degree and purification methods applied. The three main bioactivities consistently reported for SP and BAPs from different species are antioxidant, anti-inflammatory and antihypertensive [97,98]. In vitro antioxidant activity is usually tested against oxidation-sensible molecules, such as 2,2-diphenyl-1-picrylhydrazyl (DPPH) or 2,2'-Azino-bis(3-ethylbenzothiazoline-6-sulfonic acid) (ABTS). It has been reported that SP derived peptides display higher antioxidant activity than SP hydrolysates [76]. These could be due to the concentration and better accessibility of released amino acids from folded proteins. Concentrated 1 < kDa BAPs from *P. dioica* hydrolysates showed significant antioxidant activity (20.88 µmol Trolox equivalents) in a wide range of assays, including DPPH and ABTS [78]. Comparing results with free aminoacidic composition of the isolated fractions, the authors suggested that higher presence of sulfated amino acids, like cysteine or methionine, could be related to these results, as proved by these in vitro assays. Different results were reported for *Macrocystis pyrifera* and *Chondracanthus chamissoi* BAPs, accounting for 193 and 167 µmol Trolox equivalents respectively, in a DPPH assay [37]. Antioxidant assays with *P. palmata* hydrolysates also suggested that a higher protein hydrolysis degree was related to higher antioxidant activity [93].

Anti-inflammatory assays are often conducted on cell culture tests, assessing production or inhibition of pro-inflammatory mediators, such as interleukins. SP hydrolysates produced using several proteases from *Ulva* sp. were found to exert significant anti-inflammatory activity by upregulating interleukin 10 and inhibiting tumor necrosis factor alpha (TNF-α) expression [52]. Hydrolysates obtained from *Pyropia columbina* also displayed anti-inflammatory properties in vitro with similar tested mechanisms, while also inhibiting expression of necrosis factor κB [77].

Yet, the most well studied bioactive property of SP, derived hydrolysates, and BAPs is their hypotensive activity [86]. These properties may be assessed in vitro by checking the inhibition capacity of these molecules against key cardiac tension enzymes such as ACE, being the most extensively used model, but also renin or endothelin I in a lesser extent [86]. Conversely, in vivo tests may be conducted monitoring blood pressure and cardiac rhythm in animal models. The previously mentioned study of Vasquez et al. showed that the *M. pyrifera* extract displayed an ACE inhibition of 38.8% compared to control and that the smaller the size of the purified peptides, the greater inhibition degree was [37]. However, *C. chamissoi* extracts did not show a detectable ACE-inhibitory activity. Authors proposed that this could be due to interactions between co-extracted compounds and ACE enzymatic reaction products [37]. Protein hydrolysates from *P. palmata*, showed that ACE inhibitory activity was independent from the time of harvesting, but was related to its hydrolysis degree [93]. Nine ACE-inhibitory peptides derived from phycobiliproteins were found, and the oligopeptide LRY demonstrated particularly high inhibitory activities, with an IC_{50} of 0.044 mM [99]. Similarly, the peptide PAFG, obtained from *U. clathrata* protein, showed an IC_{50} value of 35.9 mM on ACE-inhibitory activity [83] (Table 3). Moreover, since BAPs are obtained through different hydrolysis methods, these have shown to be stable towards gastrointestinal proteases like pepsin or trypsin, as well as the acidic pH of digestive reactions [37,83].

Other reported bioactivities include antidiabetic or antimicrobial, associated to phycobiliproteins and lectins, but also some SP hydrolysates [100]. Antidiabetic activity was characterized in *P. palmata* hydrolysates through in vitro inhibition of dipeptidyl peptidase IV (DPP-IV). Results showed that Corolase-hydrolyzed SP accounted for a much significant DPP-IV inhibition (IC_{50} = 1.65 mg/mL) [93]. BAPs from *Saccharina longicruris* displayed antimicrobial activity against several bacterial pathogens, such as *Escherichia coli*, *Staphy-*

lococcus aureus, or *Pseudomonas aeruginosa*, achieving a 40% growth inhibition at 2.5 mg peptides/mL [88].

Therefore, based on their reported bioactivities, these macroalgae molecules may be used for diverse industrial applications (Figure 3).

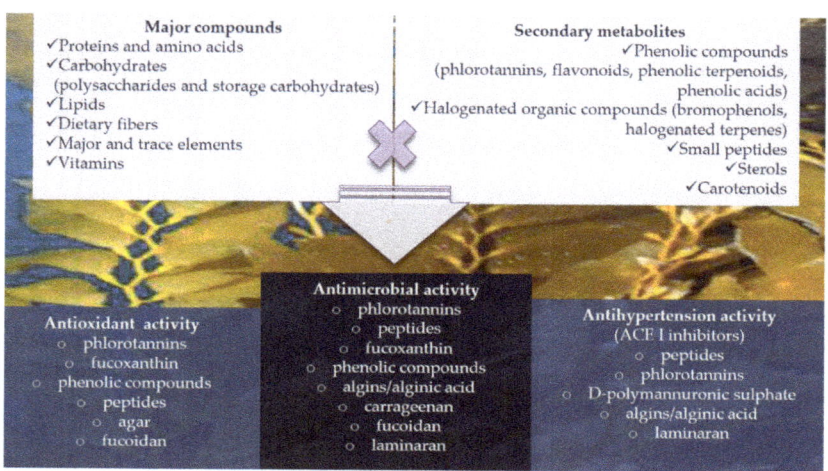

Figure 3. Reported bioactivities of different seaweed biomolecules with potential industrial application.

Both antioxidant and antimicrobial properties make SP hydrolysates a desirable choice for their use as food additives, preservatives, and protein fortifiers. Additionally, the ACE-inhibitory and anti-inflammatory activities widely apparent in several SP, could make them to be assessed as nutraceuticals, functional ingredients for food and feed, or cosmetic ingredients [101]. The fact that this effect has been assessed in vivo, with *Undaria pinnatifida* BAPs allowing for reduced blood pressure in rats, could be argued to also be the basis for developing new hypotensive pharmaceuticals [42,87]. Moreover, SP hydrolysates keep their bioactive properties when combined with other food matrices [17,102]. In the same way, the antioxidant properties attributed to BAPs make them excellent natural ingredients for cosmetic applications, as SP also hold significantly higher levels of taurine compared to other vegetal sources [91]. In summary, the full set of already reported bioactivities and the ongoing research to fully characterize the properties and production of SP and derived molecules will unveil the full extent of the potential applications of these natural molecules.

Development of such applications would thus confer an added value to this underexploited natural resource. Furthermore, these properties are also well accounted for co-extracted bioactive compounds in SP extractions, such as cell wall polysaccharides (e.g., carrageenan, fucoidan ...) or phenolic compounds, such as brown seaweeds phlorotannins [103]. Altogether, seaweed hold several different bioactive molecules with similar reported activities, that in the case of some extracts, could act in cooperation [104] Thus, SP could be considered as part of the whole composition of health-promoting compounds of seaweeds and their extracts be applied for a wide diversity of applications [105] (Figure 3).

6. Conclusions

SP and especially their hydrolysates and several identified BAPs, have been repeatedly reported to show significant bioactivities such as antioxidant or anti-inflammatory, but most importantly, antihypertensive. Their bioactivities raise potential applications in food and animal feed, whether as functional additives or colorants in the case of phycobiliproteins. On the other hand, BAPs may find use as cosmetic ingredients with antioxidant activity, while thanks to their antihypertensive activity, they can be used as nutraceuticals in the pharmaceutical industry. Nonetheless, these seaweed components need more extensive and in-depth research to fully characterize their bioactive properties, production methods, and potential in vivo effects.

Author Contributions: Conceptualization, J.E., M.F.-C., P.G.-P., J.X. and M.A.P.; Methodology, J.E., M.F.-C., J.X. and P.G.-P.; Software, J.E., M.F.-C. and P.G.-P.; Validation, M.F.-C. and P.G.-P.; Formal analysis, J.E., M.F.-C., J.P.-D., E.H.A. and M.R.; Investigation, J.E., M.F.-C., J.P.-D., E.H.A. and M.R.; Data curation, J.X.; Writing—original draft preparation, J.E. and M.A.P.; Writing—review and editing, J.E., M.F.-C., P.G.-P., J.P.-D., E.H.A. and M.R., Visualization, J.S.-G., J.X. and M.A.P.; Supervision, J.S.-G., J.X. and M.A.P. All authors have read and agreed to the published version of the manuscript.

Funding: The authors are grateful to the program Grupos de Referencia Competitiva (GRUPO AA1-GRC 2018) that supports the work of J. Echave, to the Bio Based Industries Joint Undertaking (JU) under grant agreement No. 888003 UP4HEALTH Project (H2020-BBI-JTI-2019) that supports the work of P. Garcia-Perez. The JU receives support from the European Union's Horizon 2020 research and innovation program and the Bio Based Industries Consortium. The project SYSTEMIC Knowledge Hub on Nutrition and Food Security has received funding from national research funding parties in Belgium (FWO), France (INRA), Germany (BLE), Italy (MIPAAF), Latvia (IZM), Norway (RCN), Portugal (FCT), and Spain (AEI) in a joint action of JPI HDHL, JPI-OCEANS, and FACCE-JPI, launched in 2019 under the ERA-NET ERA-HDHL (No. 696295).

Institutional Review Board Statement: Not applicable.

Data Availability Statement: Not applicable.

Acknowledgments: We would like to thank MICINN for supporting the Ramón y Cajal grant for M.A. Prieto (RYC-2017-22891), and Xunta de Galicia for supporting the program EXCELENCIA-ED431F 2020/12, the post-doctoral grant of M. Fraga-Corral (ED481B-2019/096). The authors acknowledge the Ministry of Education, Science and Technological Development of the Republic of Serbia for the support (grants nos. 451-03-9/2021-14/200026 and 451-03-09/2021-14/200378).

Conflicts of Interest: The authors declare no conflict of interest.

Abbreviations

SP	Seaweed proteins
dw	Dry weight
SLE	Solid–liquid extraction
HAE	Heat-assisted extraction
EAE	Enzyme-assisted extraction
UAE	Ultrasound-assisted extraction
MAE	Microwave-assisted extraction
PEF	Pulse-electric field
HHP	High-hydrostatic pressure
HHPE	High-hydrostatic pressure extraction
HAE	Heat-assisted extraction
EAE	Enzyme-assisted extraction
UAE	Ultrasound-assisted extraction
MAE	Microwave-assisted extraction
IP	Isoelectric point
Pr	Precipitation
Pu	Purification
DI	Dialysis
OS	Osmotic shock
Epr	Enzymatic pretreatment
Upr	Ultrasound pretreatment
$_d$W	Deionized water
AK	Alkaline
MAAs	Mycosporine-like amino acids
EAA	Essential amino acids
GRAS	Generally recognized as safe

RAAS	Renin–angiotensin–aldosterone system
IC$_{50}$	Half inhibitory concentration
DPP-IV	Dipeptidyl peptidase IV
MCF-7	Human breast cancer cell line
HepG2	Human liver cancer cell line
SGC-7901	Human gastric cancer cell line
A549	Human lung cancer cell line
HT-29	Human colon cancer cell line
UF	Ultrafiltration
IEC	Ionic-exchange chromatography
BAP	Bioactive peptide
DPPH	2,2-diphenyl-1-picrylhydrazyl
ABTS	2,2′-Azino-bis(3-ethylbenzothiazoline-6-sulfonic acid)
ACE	Angiotensin I converter enzyme

References

1. Carpena, M.; Caleja, C.; Pereira, E.; Pereira, C.; Ćirić, A.; Soković, M.; Soria-Lopez, A.; Fraga-Corral, M.; Simal-Gandara, J.; Ferreira, I.C.F.R.; et al. Red Seaweeds as a Source of Nutrients and Bioactive Compounds: Optimization of the Extraction. *Chemosensors* **2021**, *9*, 132. [CrossRef]
2. Garcia-Oliveira, P.; Fraga-Corral, M.; Pereira, A.G.; Prieto, M.A.; Simal-Gandara, J. Solutions for the sustainability of the food production and consumption system. *Crit. Rev. Food Sci. Nutr.* **2020**, 1–17. [CrossRef]
3. Bleakley, S.; Hayes, M. Algal proteins: Extraction, application, and challenges concerning production. *Foods* **2017**, *6*, 33. [CrossRef]
4. Pliego-Cortés, H.; Wijesekara, I.; Lang, M.; Bourgougnon, N.; Bedoux, G. Current knowledge and challenges in extraction, characterization and bioactivity of seaweed protein and seaweed-derived proteins. In *Advances in Botanical Research*; Elsevier Ltd.: Amsterdam, The Netherlands, 2020; Volume 95, pp. 289–326, ISBN 9780081027103.
5. Ohanenye, I.C.; Tsopmo, A.; Ejike, C.E.C.C.; Udenigwe, C.C. Germination as a bioprocess for enhancing the quality and nutritional prospects of legume proteins. *Trends Food Sci. Technol.* **2020**, *101*, 213–222. [CrossRef]
6. Lorenzo, J.M.; Agregán, R.; Munekata, P.E.S.; Franco, D.; Carballo, J.; Şahin, S.; Lacomba, R.; Barba, F.J. Proximate composition and nutritional value of three macroalgae: *Ascophyllum nodosum*, *Fucus vesiculosus* and *Bifurcaria bifurcata*. *Mar. Drugs* **2017**, *15*, 360. [CrossRef] [PubMed]
7. Denis, C.; Morançais, M.; Li, M.; Deniaud, E.; Gaudin, P.; Wielgosz-Collin, G.; Barnathan, G.; Jaouen, P.; Fleurence, J. Study of the chemical composition of edible red macroalgae *Grateloupia turuturu* from Brittany (France). *Food Chem.* **2010**, *119*, 913–917. [CrossRef]
8. Fleurence, J.; Morançais, M.; Dumay, J. *Seaweed Proteins*, 2nd ed.; Yada, R.Y.B.T.-P., Ed.; Elsevier Ltd.: Amsterdam, The Netherlands, 2018; ISBN 9780081007297.
9. Dumay, J.; Morançais, M.; Munier, M.; Le Guillard, C.; Fleurence, J. Phycoerythrins. In *Advances in Botanical Research*; Elsevier: Amsterdam, The Netherlands, 2014; Volume 71, pp. 321–343, ISBN 9780124080621.
10. Batista, S.; Pereira, R.; Oliveira, B.; Baião, L.F.; Jessen, F.; Tulli, F.; Messina, M.; Silva, J.L.; Abreu, H.; Valente, L.M.P. Exploring the potential of seaweed *Gracilaria gracilis* and microalga *Nannochloropsis oceanica*, single or blended, as natural dietary ingredients for European seabass *Dicentrarchus labrax*. *J. Appl. Phycol.* **2020**, *32*, 2041–2059. [CrossRef]
11. Bjarnadóttir, M.; Aðalbjörnsson, B.V.; Nilsson, A.; Slizyte, R.; Roleda, M.Y.; Hreggviðsson, G.Ó.; Friðjónsson, Ó.H.; Jónsdóttir, R. *Palmaria palmata* as an alternative protein source: Enzymatic protein extraction, amino acid composition, and nitrogen-to-protein conversion factor. *J. Appl. Phycol.* **2018**, *30*, 2061–2070. [CrossRef]
12. Dawczynski, C.; Schubert, R.; Jahreis, G. Amino acids, fatty acids, and dietary fibre in edible seaweed products. *Food Chem.* **2007**, *103*, 891–899. [CrossRef]
13. Biancarosa, I.; Espe, M.; Bruckner, C.G.; Heesch, S.; Liland, N.; Waagbø, R.; Torstensen, B.; Lock, E.J. Amino acid composition, protein content, and nitrogen-to-protein conversion factors of 21 seaweed species from Norwegian waters. *J. Appl. Phycol.* **2017**, *29*, 1001–1009. [CrossRef]
14. Ortiz, J.; Uquiche, E.; Robert, P.; Romero, N.; Quitral, V.; Llantén, C. Functional and nutritional value of the Chilean seaweeds *Codium fragile*, *Gracilaria chilensis* and *Macrocystis pyrifera*. *Eur. J. Lipid Sci. Technol.* **2009**, *111*, 320–327. [CrossRef]
15. Ortiz, J.; Romero, N.; Robert, P.; Araya, J.; Lopez-Hernández, J.; Bozzo, C.; Navarrete, E.; Osorio, A.; Rios, A. Dietary fiber, amino acid, fatty acid and tocopherol contents of the edible seaweeds *Ulva lactuca* and *Durvillaea antarctica*. *Food Chem.* **2006**, *99*, 98–104. [CrossRef]
16. Chen, X.; Wu, M.; Yang, Q.; Wang, S. Preparation, characterization of food grade phycobiliproteins from *Porphyra haitanensis* and the application in liposome-meat system. *LWT* **2017**, *77*, 468–474. [CrossRef]
17. Fitzgerald, C.; Gallagher, E.; Doran, L.; Auty, M.; Prieto, J.; Hayes, M. Increasing the health benefits of bread: Assessment of the physical and sensory qualities of bread formulated using a renin inhibitory *Palmaria palmata* protein hydrolysate. *LWT-Food Sci. Technol.* **2014**, *56*, 398–405. [CrossRef]

18. Deniaud, E.; Fleurence, J.; Lahaye, M. Preparation and chemical characterization of cell wall fractions enriched in structural proteins from *Palmaria palmata* (Rhodophyta). *Bot. Mar.* **2003**, *46*, 366–377. [CrossRef]
19. McLaughlin, C.M.; Harnedy-Rothwell, P.A.; Lafferty, R.A.; Sharkey, S.; Parthsarathy, V.; Allsopp, P.J.; McSorley, E.M.; FitzGerald, R.J.; O'Harte, F.P.M. Macroalgal protein hydrolysates from *Palmaria palmata* influence the 'incretin effect' in vitro via DPP-4 inhibition and upregulation of insulin, GLP-1 and GIP secretion. *Eur. J. Nutr.* **2021**. [CrossRef]
20. Fan, X.; Bai, L.; Mao, X.; Zhang, X. Novel peptides with anti-proliferation activity from the *Porphyra haitanesis* hydrolysate. *Process Biochem.* **2017**, *60*, 98–107. [CrossRef]
21. Lourenço-Lopes, C.; Fraga-Corral, M.; Jimenez-Lopez, C.; Pereira, A.G.; Garcia-Oliveira, P.; Carpena, M.; Prieto, M.A.; Simal-Gandara, J. Metabolites from macroalgae and its applications in the cosmetic industry: A circular economy approach. *Resources* **2020**, *9*, 101. [CrossRef]
22. Harnedy, P.A.; FitzGerald, R.J. Extraction of protein from the macroalga *Palmaria palmata*. *LWT-Food Sci. Technol.* **2013**, *51*, 375–382. [CrossRef]
23. Robin, A.; Kazir, M.; Sack, M.; Israel, A.; Frey, W.; Mueller, G.; Livney, Y.D.; Golberg, A. Functional Protein Concentrates Extracted from the Green Marine Macroalga *Ulva* sp., by High Voltage Pulsed Electric Fields and Mechanical Press. *ACS Sustain. Chem. Eng.* **2018**, *6*, 13696–13705. [CrossRef]
24. O' Connor, J.; Meaney, S.; Williams, G.A.; Hayes, M. Extraction of Protein from Four Different Seaweeds Using Three Different Physical Pre-Treatment Strategies. *Molecules* **2020**, *25*, 2005. [CrossRef]
25. Mendez, R.L.; Kwon, J.Y. Effect of extraction condition on protein recovery and phenolic interference in Pacific dulse (*Devaleraea mollis*). *J. Appl. Phycol.* **2021**, *33*, 2497–2509. [CrossRef]
26. Wong, K.; Chikeung Cheung, P. Influence of drying treatment on three *Sargassum* species 2. Protein extractability, in vitro protein digestibility and amino acid profile of protein concentrates. *J. Appl. Phycol.* **2001**, *13*, 51–58. [CrossRef]
27. Angell, A.R.; Paul, N.A.; de Nys, R. A comparison of protocols for isolating and concentrating protein from the green seaweed *Ulva ohnoi*. *J. Appl. Phycol.* **2017**, *29*, 1011–1026. [CrossRef]
28. Naseri, A.; Marinho, G.S.; Holdt, S.L.; Bartela, J.M.; Jacobsen, C. Enzyme-assisted extraction and characterization of protein from red seaweed *Palmaria palmata*. *Algal Res.* **2020**, *47*, 101849. [CrossRef]
29. Veide Vilg, J.; Undeland, I. pH-driven solubilization and isoelectric precipitation of proteins from the brown seaweed Saccharina latissima—effects of osmotic shock, water volume and temperature. *J. Appl. Phycol.* **2017**, *29*, 585–593. [CrossRef] [PubMed]
30. Garcia-Vaquero, M.; Lopez-Alonso, M.; Hayes, M. Assessment of the functional properties of protein extracted from the brown seaweed *Himanthalia elongata* (Linnaeus) S. F. Gray. *Food Res. Int.* **2017**, *99*, 971–978. [CrossRef]
31. Wijesekara, I.; Lang, M.; Marty, C.; Gemin, M.P.; Boulho, R.; Douzenel, P.; Wickramasinghe, I.; Bedoux, G.; Bourgougnon, N. Different extraction procedures and analysis of protein from *Ulva* sp. in Brittany, France. *J. Appl. Phycol.* **2017**, *29*, 2503–2511. [CrossRef]
32. Le Guillard, C.; Dumay, J.; Donnay-Moreno, C.; Bruzac, S.; Ragon, J.Y.; Fleurence, J.; Bergé, J.P. Ultrasound-assisted extraction of R-phycoerythrin from *Grateloupia turuturu* with and without enzyme addition. *Algal Res.* **2015**, *12*, 522–528. [CrossRef]
33. Kadam, S.U.; Álvarez, C.; Tiwari, B.K.; O'Donnell, C.P. Extraction and characterization of protein from Irish brown seaweed *Ascophyllum nodosum*. *Food Res. Int.* **2017**, *99*, 1021–1027. [CrossRef]
34. Cermeño, M.; Stack, J.; Tobin, P.R.; O'Keeffe, M.B.; Harnedy, P.A; Stengel, D.B.; FitzGerald, R.J. Peptide identification from a *Porphyra dioica* protein hydrolysate with antioxidant, angiotensin converting enzyme and dipeptidyl peptidase IV inhibitory activities. *Food Funct.* **2019**, *10*, 3421–3429. [CrossRef] [PubMed]
35. Hardouin, K.; Burlot, A.S.; Umami, A.; Tanniou, A.; Stiger-Pouvreau, V.; Widowati, I.; Bedoux, G.; Bourgougnon, N. Biochemical and antiviral activities of enzymatic hydrolysates from different invasive French seaweeds. *J. Appl. Phycol.* **2014**, *26*, 1029–1042. [CrossRef]
36. Suwal, S.; Perreault, V.; Marciniak, A.; Tamigneaux, É.; Deslandes, É.; Bazinet, L.; Jacques, H.; Beaulieu, L.; Doyen, A. Effects of high hydrostatic pressure and polysaccharidases on the extraction of antioxidant compounds from red macroalgae, *Palmaria palmata* and *Solieria chordalis*. *J. Food Eng.* **2019**, *252*, 53–59. [CrossRef]
37. Vásquez, V.; Martínez, R.; Bernal, C. Enzyme-assisted extraction of proteins from the seaweeds *Macrocystis pyrifera* and *Chondracanthus chamissoi*: Characterization of the extracts and their bioactive potential. *J. Appl. Phycol.* **2019**, *31*, 1999–2010. [CrossRef]
38. Wen, L.; Tan, S.; Zeng, L.; Wang, Z.; Ke, X.; Zhang, Z.; Tang, H.; Guo, H.; Xia, E. Ultrasound-assisted extraction and in vitro simulated digestion of *Porphyra haitanensis* proteins exhibiting antioxidative and α-glucosidase inhibitory activity. *J. Food Meas. Charact.* **2020**, *14*, 3291–3298. [CrossRef]
39. Kazir, M.; Abuhassira, Y.; Robin, A.; Nahor, O.; Luo, J.; Israel, A.; Golberg, A.; Livney, Y.D. Extraction of proteins from two marine macroalgae, *Ulva* sp. and *Gracilaria* sp., for food application, and evaluating digestibility, amino acid composition and antioxidant properties of the protein concentrates. *Food Hydrocoll.* **2019**, *87*, 194–203. [CrossRef]
40. Magnusson, M.; Glasson, C.R.K.; Vucko, M.J.; Angell, A.; Neoh, T.L.; de Nys, R. Enrichment processes for the production of high-protein feed from the green seaweed *Ulva ohnoi*. *Algal Res.* **2019**, *41*, 101555. [CrossRef]
41. Kandasamy, G.; Karuppiah, S.K.; Rao, P.V.S. Salt- and pH-induced functional changes in protein concentrate of edible green seaweed *Enteromorpha* species. *Fish. Sci.* **2012**, *78*, 169–176. [CrossRef]
42. Suetsuna, K.; Maekawa, K.; Chen, J.R. Antihypertensive effects of *Undaria pinnatifida* (wakame) peptide on blood pressure in spontaneously hypertensive rats. *J. Nutr. Biochem.* **2004**, *15*, 267–272. [CrossRef] [PubMed]

43. Silva, A.; Silva, S.A.; Lourenço-Lopes, C.; Jimenez-Lopez, C.; Carpena, M.; Gullón, P.; Fraga-Corral, M.; Domingues, V.F.; Fátima Barroso, M.; Simal-Gandara, J.; et al. Antibacterial use of macroalgae compounds against foodborne pathogens. *Antibiotics* **2020**, *9*, 712. [CrossRef]
44. Ade-Omowaye, B.I.O.; Rastogi, N.K.; Angersbach, A.; Knorr, D. Combined effects of pulsed electric field pre-treatment and partial osmotic dehydration on air drying behaviour of red bell pepper. *J. Food Eng.* **2003**, *60*, 89–98. [CrossRef]
45. Polikovsky, M.; Fernand, F.; Sack, M.; Frey, W.; Müller, G.; Golberg, A. Towards marine biorefineries: Selective proteins extractions from marine macroalgae *Ulva* with pulsed electric fields. *Innov. Food Sci. Emerg. Technol.* **2016**, *37*, 194–200. [CrossRef]
46. Silva, A.; Silva, S.A.; Carpena, M.; Garcia-Oliveira, P.; Gullón, P.; Barroso, M.F.; Prieto, M.A.; Simal-Gandara, J. Macroalgae as a source of valuable antimicrobial compounds: Extraction and applications. *Antibiotics* **2020**, *9*, 642. [CrossRef]
47. Singh, S.; Gaikwad, K.K.; Park, S.I.; Lee, Y.S. Microwave-assisted step reduced extraction of seaweed (*Gelidiella acerosa*) cellulose nanocrystals. *Int. J. Biol. Macromol.* **2017**, *99*, 506–510. [CrossRef]
48. Janson, J.-C. *Protein Purification: Principles, High Resolution Methods, and Applications*, 3rd ed.; John Wiley & Sons: Hoboken, NJ, USA, 2012; Volume 54, ISBN 9780471746614.
49. Baldasso, C.; Barros, T.C.; Tessaro, I.C. Concentration and purification of whey proteins by ultrafiltration. *Desalination* **2011**, *278*, 381–386. [CrossRef]
50. Chaturvedi, B.K.; Ghosh, A.K.; Ramachandran, V.; Trivedi, M.K.; Hanra, M.S.; Misra, B.M. Preparation, characterization and performance of polyethersulfone ultrafiltration membranes. *Desalination* **2001**, *133*, 31–40. [CrossRef]
51. Nordin, J.Z.; Lee, Y.; Vader, P.; Mäger, I.; Johansson, H.J.; Heusermann, W.; Wiklander, O.P.B.; Hällbrink, M.; Seow, Y.; Bultema, J.J.; et al. Ultrafiltration with size-exclusion liquid chromatography for high yield isolation of extracellular vesicles preserving intact biophysical and functional properties. *Nanomed. Nanotechnolo. Biol. Med.* **2015**, *11*, 879–883. [CrossRef] [PubMed]
52. Cian, R.; Hernández-Chirlaque, C.; Gámez-Belmonte, R.; Drago, S.; Sánchez de Medina, F.; Martínez-Augustin, O. Green Alga Ulva spp. Hydrolysates and Their Peptide Fractions Regulate Cytokine Production in Splenic Macrophages and Lymphocytes Involving the TLR4-NFκB/MAPK Pathways. *Mar. Drugs* **2018**, *16*, 235. [CrossRef]
53. Paiva, L.; Lima, E.; Neto, A.I.; Baptista, J. Isolation and characterization of angiotensin I-converting enzyme (ACE) inhibitory peptides from *Ulva rigida* C. Agardh protein hydrolysate. *J. Funct. Foods* **2016**, *26*, 65–76. [CrossRef]
54. Levison, P.R. Large-scale ion-exchange column chromatography of proteins. *J. Chromatogr. B* **2003**, *790*, 17–33. [CrossRef]
55. Cutler, P. *Protein Purification Protocols*, 2nd ed.; Humana Press Inc.: Totowa, NJ, USA, 2003; Volume 244, ISBN 1-59259-655-X.
56. Rathore, A.S.; Kumar, D.; Kateja, N. Recent developments in chromatographic purification of biopharmaceuticals. *Biotechnol. Lett.* **2018**, *40*, 895–905. [CrossRef]
57. Singh, C.; Sharma, C.S.; Kamble, P.R. Amino acid analysis using ion-exchange chromatography: A review. *Int. J. Pharmacogn.* **2014**, *3*, 3559–3567. [CrossRef]
58. Lenhoff, A.M. Ion-exchange chromatography of proteins: The inside story. *Mater. Today Proc.* **2016**, *3*, 3559–3567. [CrossRef]
59. Ljunglöf, A.; Lacki, K.M.; Mueller, J.; Harinarayan, C.; van Reis, R.; Fahrner, R.; Van Alstine, J.M. Ion exchange chromatography of antibody fragments. *Biotechnol. Bioeng.* **2007**, *96*, 515–524. [CrossRef]
60. Kim, E.Y.; Choi, Y.H.; Lee, J.I.; Kim, I.H.; Nam, T.J. Antioxidant Activity of Oxygen Evolving Enhancer Protein 1 Purified from Capsosiphon fulvescens. *J. Food Sci.* **2015**, *80*, H1412–H1417. [CrossRef]
61. Indumathi, P.; Mehta, A. A novel anticoagulant peptide from the Nori hydrolysate. *J. Funct. Foods* **2016**, *20*, 606–617. [CrossRef]
62. Tan, Z.; Li, F.; Xu, X.; Xing, J. Simultaneous extraction and purification of aloe polysaccharides and proteins using ionic liquid based aqueous two-phase system coupled with dialysis membrane. *Desalination* **2012**, *286*, 389–393. [CrossRef]
63. Whitford, D. *Proteins: Structure and Function*; John Wiley & Sons: Chichester, UK, 2005; ISBN 1118685725.
64. Filoti, D.I.; Shire, S.J.; Yadav, S.; Laue, T.M. Comparative Study of Analytical Techniques for Determining Protein Charge. *J. Pharm. Sci.* **2015**, *104*, 2123–2131. [CrossRef] [PubMed]
65. Fitzgerald, C.; Mora-Soler, L.; Gallagher, E.; O'Connor, P.; Prieto, J.; Soler-Vila, A.; Hayes, M. Isolation and Characterization of Bioactive Pro-Peptides with in Vitro Renin Inhibitory Activities from the Macroalga *Palmaria palmata*. *J. Agric. Food Chem.* **2012**, *60*, 7421–7427. [CrossRef] [PubMed]
66. Kim, S.-K.; Wijesekara, I. Development and biological activities of marine-derived bioactive peptides: A review. *J. Funct. Foods* **2010**, *2*, 1–9. [CrossRef]
67. Tavano, O.L. Protein hydrolysis using proteases: An important tool for food biotechnology. *J. Mol. Catal. B Enzym.* **2013**, *90*, 1–11. [CrossRef]
68. Tsugita, A.; Scheffler, J.-J. A Rapid Method for Acid Hydrolysis of Protein with a Mixture of Trifluoroacetic Acid and Hydrochloric Acid. *Eur. J. Biochem.* **2005**, *124*, 585–588. [CrossRef]
69. Provansal, M.M.P.; Cuq, J.L.A.; Cheftel, J.C. Chemical and nutritional modifications of sunflower proteins due to alkaline processing. Formation of amino acid crosslinks and isomerization of lysine residues. *J. Agric. Food Chem.* **1975**, *23*, 938–943. [CrossRef]
70. Hammed, A.M.; Jaswir, I.; Amid, A.; Alam, Z.; Asiyanbi-H, T.T.; Ramli, N. Enzymatic Hydrolysis of Plants and Algae for Extraction of Bioactive Compounds. *Food Rev. Int.* **2013**, *29*, 352–370. [CrossRef]
71. Castro, H.C.; Abreu, P.A.; Geraldo, R.B.; Martins, R.C.A.; dos Santos, R.; Loureiro, N.I.V.; Cabral, L.M.; Rodrigues, C.R. Looking at the proteases from a simple perspective. *J. Mol. Recognit.* **2011**, *24*, 165–181. [CrossRef]

72. Cian, R.E.; Martínez-Augustin, O.; Drago, S.R. Bioactive properties of peptides obtained by enzymatic hydrolysis from protein byproducts of *Porphyra columbina*. *Food Res. Int.* **2012**, *49*, 364–372. [CrossRef]
73. Fitzgerald, C.; Aluko, R.E.; Hossain, M.; Rai, D.K.; Hayes, M. Potential of a Renin Inhibitory Peptide from the Red Seaweed *Palmaria palmata* as a Functional Food Ingredient Following Confirmation and Characterization of a Hypotensive Effect in Spontaneously Hypertensive Rats. *J. Agric. Food Chem.* **2014**, *62*, 8352–8356. [CrossRef] [PubMed]
74. Fitzgerald, C.; Gallagher, E.; O'Connor, P.; Prieto, J.; Mora-Soler, L.; Grealy, M.; Hayes, M. Development of a seaweed derived platelet activating factor acetylhydrolase (PAF-AH) inhibitory hydrolysate, synthesis of inhibitory peptides and assessment of their toxicity using the Zebrafish larvae assay. *Peptides* **2013**, *50*, 119–124. [CrossRef] [PubMed]
75. Harnedy, P.A.; O'Keeffe, M.B.; Fitzgerald, R.J. Purification and identification of dipeptidyl peptidase (DPP) IV inhibitory peptides from the macroalga *Palmaria palmata*. *Food Chem.* **2015**, *172*, 400–406. [CrossRef]
76. Harnedy, P.A.; O'Keeffe, M.B.; FitzGerald, R.J. Fractionation and identification of antioxidant peptides from an enzymatically hydrolysed Palmaria palmata protein isolate. *Food Res. Int.* **2017**, *100*, 416–422. [CrossRef]
77. Cian, R.E.; López-Posadas, R.; Drago, S.R.; Sánchez De Medina, F.; Martínez-Augustin, O. A *Porphyra columbina* hydrolysate upregulates IL-10 production in rat macrophages and lymphocytes through an NF-κB, and p38 and JNK dependent mechanism. *Food Chem.* **2012**, *134*, 1982–1990. [CrossRef]
78. Pimentel, F.B.; Cermeño, M.; Kleekayai, T.; Harnedy-Rothwell, P.A.; Fernandes, E.; Alves, R.C.; Oliveira, M.B.P.P.; FitzGerald, R.J. Enzymatic Modification of *Porphyra dioica*-Derived Proteins to Improve their Antioxidant Potential. *Molecules* **2020**, *25*, 2838. [CrossRef] [PubMed]
79. Admassu, H.; Gasmalla, M.A.A.; Yang, R.; Zhao, W. Identification of Bioactive Peptides with α-Amylase Inhibitory Potential from Enzymatic Protein Hydrolysates of Red Seaweed (*Porphyra* spp.). *J. Agric. Food Chem.* **2018**, *66*, 4872–4882. [CrossRef]
80. Kumagai, Y.; Kitade, Y.; Kobayashi, M.; Watanabe, K.; Kurita, H.; Takeda, H.; Yasui, H.; Kishimura, H. Identification of ACE inhibitory peptides from red alga *Mazzaella japonica*. *Eur. Food Res. Technol.* **2020**, *246*, 2225–2231. [CrossRef]
81. Zhang, X.; Cao, D.; Sun, X.; Sun, S.; Xu, N. Preparation and identification of antioxidant peptides from protein hydrolysate of marine alga *Gracilariopsis lemaneiformis*. *J. Appl. Phycol.* **2019**, *31*, 2585–2596. [CrossRef]
82. Cao, D.; Lv, X.; Xu, X.; Yu, H.; Sun, X.; Xu, N. Purification and identification of a novel ACE inhibitory peptide from marine alga *Gracilariopsis lemaneiformis* protein hydrolysate. *Eur. Food Res. Technol.* **2017**, *243*, 1829–1837. [CrossRef]
83. Pan, S.; Wang, S.; Jing, L.; Yao, D. Purification and characterisation of a novel angiotensin-I converting enzyme (ACE)-inhibitory peptide derived from the enzymatic hydrolysate of *Enteromorpha clathrata* protein. *Food Chem.* **2016**, *211*, 423–430. [CrossRef]
84. Sun, S.; Xu, X.; Sun, X.; Zhang, X.; Chen, X.; Xu, N. Preparation and identification of ACE inhibitory peptides from the marine macroalga *Ulva intestinalis*. *Mar. Drugs* **2019**, *17*, 179. [CrossRef]
85. Garcia-Vaquero, M.; Mora, L.; Hayes, M. In Vitro and In Silico Approaches to Generating and Identifying Angiotensin-Converting Enzyme I Inhibitory Peptides from Green Macroalga *Ulva lactuca*. *Mar. Drugs* **2019**, *17*, 204. [CrossRef] [PubMed]
86. Zheng, Y.; Zhang, Y.; San, S. Efficacy of a novel ACE-inhibitory peptide from *Sargassum maclurei* in hypertension and reduction of intracellular endothelin-1. *Nutrients* **2020**, *12*, 653. [CrossRef]
87. Sato, M.; Hosokawa, T.; Yamaguchi, T.; Nakano, T.; Muramoto, K.; Kahara, T.; Funayama, K.; Kobayashi, A.; Nakano, T. Angiotensin I-Converting Enzyme Inhibitory Peptides Derived from Wakame (*Undaria pinnatifida*) and Their Antihypertensive Effect in Spontaneously Hypertensive Rats. *J. Agric. Food Chem.* **2002**, *50*, 6245–6252. [CrossRef] [PubMed]
88. Beaulieu, L.; Bondu, S.; Doiron, K.; Rioux, L.E.; Turgeon, S.L. Characterization of antibacterial activity from protein hydrolysates of the macroalga *Saccharina longicruris* and identification of peptides implied in bioactivity. *J. Funct. Foods* **2015**, *17*, 685–697. [CrossRef]
89. Chen, J.-C.; Wang, J.; Zheng, B.-D.; Pang, J.; Chen, L.-J.; Lin, H.; Guo, X. Simultaneous Determination of 8 Small Antihypertensive Peptides with Tyrosine at the C-Terminal in *Laminaria japonica* Hydrolysates by RP-HPLC Method. *J. Food Process. Preserv.* **2016**, *40*, 492–501. [CrossRef]
90. Chabeaud, A.; Vandanjon, L.; Bourseau, P.; Jaouen, P.; Chaplain-Derouiniot, M.; Guerard, F. Performances of ultrafiltration membranes for fractionating a fish protein hydrolysate: Application to the refining of bioactive peptidic fractions. *Sep. Purif. Technol.* **2009**, *66*, 463–471. [CrossRef]
91. Harnedy, P.A.; Fitzgerald, R.J. Bioactive proteins, peptides, and amino acids from macroalgae. *J. Phycol.* **2011**, *47*, 218–232. [CrossRef]
92. Jeon, Y.-J.; Samarakoon, K. *Recovery of Proteins and Their Biofunctionalities from Marine Algae*; John Wiley & Sons, Ltd.: Chichester, UK, 2013.
93. Harnedy, P.A.; FitzGerald, R.J. In vitro assessment of the cardioprotective, anti-diabetic and antioxidant potential of *Palmaria palmata* protein hydrolysates. *J. Appl. Phycol.* **2013**, *25*, 1793–1803. [CrossRef]
94. Homaei, A.A.; Sariri, R.; Vianello, F.; Stevanato, R. Enzyme immobilization: An update. *J. Chem. Biol.* **2013**, *6*, 185–205. [CrossRef]
95. Akaberi, S.; Gusbeth, C.; Silve, A.; Senthilnathan, D.S.; Navarro-López, E.; Molina-Grima, E.; Müller, G.; Frey, W. Effect of pulsed electric field treatment on enzymatic hydrolysis of proteins of *Scenedesmus almeriensis*. *Algal Res.* **2019**, *43*, 101656. [CrossRef]
96. Alavijeh, R.S.; Karimi, K.; Wijffels, R.H.; van den Berg, C.; Eppink, M. Combined bead milling and enzymatic hydrolysis for efficient fractionation of lipids, proteins, and carbohydrates of *Chlorella vulgaris* microalgae. *Bioresour. Technol.* **2020**, *309*, 123321. [CrossRef]

97. Admassu, H.; Gasmalla, M.A.A.; Yang, R.; Zhao, W. Bioactive Peptides Derived from Seaweed Protein and Their Health Benefits: Antihypertensive, Antioxidant, and Antidiabetic Properties. *J. Food Sci.* **2018**, *83*, 6–16. [CrossRef]
98. Lee, D.; Nishizawa, M.; Shimizu, Y.; Saeki, H. Anti-inflammatory effects of dulse (*Palmaria palmata*) resulting from the simultaneous water-extraction of phycobiliproteins and chlorophyll *a*. *Food Res. Int.* **2017**, *100*, 514–521. [CrossRef] [PubMed]
99. Nakamori, T.; Nagai, M.; Maebuchi, M.; Furuta, H.; Park, E.Y.; Nakamura, Y.; Sato, K. Identification of peptides in sediments derived from an acidic enzymatic soy protein hydrolysate solution. *Food Sci. Technol. Res.* **2014**, *20*, 301–307. [CrossRef]
100. Fontenelle, T.P.C.; Lima, G.C.; Mesquita, J.X.; de Souza Lopes, J.L.; de Brito, T.V.; das Chagas Vieira Júnior, F.; Sales, A.B.; Aragão, K.S.; Souza, M.H.L.P.; dos Reis Barbosa, A.L.; et al. Lectin obtained from the red seaweed *Bryothamnion triquetrum*: Secondary structure and anti-inflammatory activity in mice. *Int. J. Biol. Macromol.* **2018**, *112*, 1122–1130. [CrossRef]
101. Cermeño, M.; Kleekayai, T.; Amigo-Benavent, M.; Harnedy-Rothwell, P.; FitzGerald, R.J. Current knowledge on the extraction, purification, identification, and validation of bioactive peptides from seaweed. *Electrophoresis* **2020**, *41*, 1694–1717. [CrossRef]
102. Cian, R.E.; Caballero, M.S.; Sabbag, N.; González, R.J.; Drago, S.R. Bio-accessibility of bioactive compounds (ACE inhibitors and antioxidants) from extruded maize products added with a red seaweed Porphyra columbina. *LWT-Food Sci. Technol.* **2014**, *55*, 51–58. [CrossRef]
103. Popović-Djordjević, J.B.; Katanić Stanković, J.S.; Mihailović, V.; Pereira, A.G.; Garcia-Oliveira, P.; Prieto, M.A.; Simal-Gandara, J. Algae as a Source of Bioactive Compounds to Prevent the Development of Type 2 Diabetes Mellitus. *Curr. Med. Chem.* **2021**, *28*, 4592–4615. [CrossRef]
104. Charoensiddhi, S.; Conlon, M.A.; Franco, C.M.M.; Zhang, W. The development of seaweed-derived bioactive compounds for use as prebiotics and nutraceuticals using enzyme technologies. *Trends Food Sci. Technol.* **2017**, *70*, 20–33. [CrossRef]
105. Ibañez, E.; Cifuentes, A. Benefits of using algae as natural sources of functional ingredients. *J. Sci. Food Agric.* **2013**, *93*, 703–709. [CrossRef]

MDPI
St. Alban-Anlage 66
4052 Basel
Switzerland
Tel. +41 61 683 77 34
Fax +41 61 302 89 18
www.mdpi.com

Marine Drugs Editorial Office
E-mail: marinedrugs@mdpi.com
www.mdpi.com/journal/marinedrugs

www.ingramcontent.com/pod-product-compliance
Lightning Source LLC
LaVergne TN
LVHW070646100526
838202LV00013B/895